NCLEX-RN
SECRETS

Study Guide
Your Key to Exam Success

NCLEX Test Review for the
National Council Licensure Examination for Registered Nurses

Mometrix Test Preparation
NCLEX Exam Secrets Test Prep Team

Written and edited by the NCLEX Exam Secrets Test Prep Team

Printed in the United States of America

This paper meets the requirements of ANSI/NISO Z39.48-1992 (Permanence of Paper).

Mometrix offers volume discount pricing to institutions. For more information or a price quote, please contact our sales department at sales@mometrix.com or 888-248-1219.

NCLEX-RN was developed by the National Council of State Boards of Nursing (NCSBN), which was not involved in the production of, and does not endorse, this product.

ISBN 13: 978-1-61072-241-4
ISBN 10: 1-61072-241-8

Dear Future Exam Success Story:

Congratulations on your purchase of our study guide. Our goal in writing our study guide was to cover the content on the test, as well as provide insight into typical test taking mistakes and how to overcome them.

Standardized tests are a key component of being successful, which only increases the importance of doing well in the high-pressure high-stakes environment of test day. How well you do on this test will have a significant impact on your future, and we have the research and practical advice to help you execute on test day.

The product you're reading now is designed to exploit weaknesses in the test itself, and help you avoid the most common errors test takers frequently make.

How to use this study guide

We don't want to waste your time. Our study guide is fast-paced and fluff-free. We suggest going through it a number of times, as repetition is an important part of learning new information and concepts.

First, read through the study guide completely to get a feel for the content and organization. Read the general success strategies first, and then proceed to the content sections. Each tip has been carefully selected for its effectiveness.

Second, read through the study guide again, and take notes in the margins and highlight those sections where you may have a particular weakness.

Finally, bring the manual with you on test day and study it before the exam begins.

Your success is our success

We would be delighted to hear about your success. Send us an email and tell us your story. Thanks for your business and we wish you continued success.

Sincerely,

Mometrix Test Preparation Team

Need more help? Check out our flashcards at: http://MometrixFlashcards.com/NCLEX

TABLE OF CONTENTS

Top 20 Test Taking Tips

1. Carefully follow all the test registration procedures
2. Know the test directions, duration, topics, question types, how many questions
3. Setup a flexible study schedule at least 3-4 weeks before test day
4. Study during the time of day you are most alert, relaxed, and stress free
5. Maximize your learning style; visual learner use visual study aids, auditory learner use auditory study aids
6. Focus on your weakest knowledge base
7. Find a study partner to review with and help clarify questions
8. Practice, practice, practice
9. Get a good night's sleep; don't try to cram the night before the test
10. Eat a well balanced meal
11. Know the exact physical location of the testing site; drive the route to the site prior to test day
12. Bring a set of ear plugs; the testing center could be noisy
13. Wear comfortable, loose fitting, layered clothing to the testing center; prepare for it to be either cold or hot during the test
14. Bring at least 2 current forms of ID to the testing center
15. Arrive to the test early; be prepared to wait and be patient
16. Eliminate the obviously wrong answer choices, then guess the first remaining choice
17. Pace yourself; don't rush, but keep working and move on if you get stuck
18. Maintain a positive attitude even if the test is going poorly
19. Keep your first answer unless you are positive it is wrong
20. Check your work, don't make a careless mistake

Safe and Effective Care Environment

Management of Care

Nursing code of ethics

Since nursing involves providing for the care and well-being of the sick, injured, and those at risk, nurses must have a code of ethics to govern their behavior and practices. The American Nurses Association has developed a Code of Ethics to serve several purposes. First, the code describes the essential obligations to be upheld by every person who works as a nurse. These obligations set standards of practice that are universal to those throughout the nursing profession and include such concepts as patient autonomy and respect for human dignity. The ethics involved in the code are obligatory and are not optional practice. Finally, the code of ethics reflects the nurse's understanding of her role as a professional and the requirements of respect and compassion that she must give to her patients.

Ethics and morals

Although they may be used interchangeably, the terms "ethics" and "morals" have different meanings. Within nursing, ethics involves the personal choices the nurse makes about actions performed and care provided. The nurse may subscribe to certain ethical theories to guide these decisions, such as humanist or feminist theories. An example of an ethical issue might be when a nurse needs guidance about the quality of care to give to a client with a terminal illness. Morals are related to ethics and often guide a nurse's practice decisions; however, morals are also supported by the nurse's cultural or experiential background. An example of a moral issue is a nurse questioning the practices performed on a pregnant client because it interferes with the nurse's religious beliefs.

Ethical decision making

The steps in the ethical decision making process are:
1. Identify the health problem.
2. Define the ethical issue.
3. Gather additional information.
4. Delineate the decision maker.
5. Examine ethical and moral principles.
6. Explore alternative options.
7. Implement decisions.
8. Evaluate and modify actions.

Principles of ethical decision-making
The four principles are autonomy, nonmaleficence, beneficence, and justice. Autonomy is the patient's right to refuse treatment and to be his own person. A client also has the right to refuse case management, even if it would benefit him. Nonmaleficence is the theory that the nurse and the other health care providers will include nothing in a plan of care that is intended to harm a patient. Beneficence is the principle that obligates health professionals

to do as much good as possible. The final principle that helps a nurse deal with ethical issues is the principle of justice, meaning that the client should receive what he or she is owed. Problems arise when what the client wants or thinks he is owed is seen as excessive by health care providers and the nurse.

Ethical duties

Ethical duties of nurses are as follows:
1. Practice with compassion, forming professional relationships, offering respect and dignity to all patients, distinguishing and understanding the worth and uniqueness of every individual. The nurse should not be limited or make decisions based on economic or social status, personal attributes of the client or nature of the health problem.
2. Commitment to the patients they are caring for.
3. Promote, advocate for, and protect their patients.
4. Responsible for their individual actions, and the actions of individuals they supervise and delegate tasks to.
5. Provide optimal care.
6. Part of a team that establishes, maintains, and improves health care and health care environments.
7. Maintain integrity, promote optimal self and optimal care, maintain safety, and maintain competence while promoting growth and development.
8. Promote nursing practice by contributions of practice, education and administration, as well as increased knowledge development.
9. Promote community, self, national and international efforts when meeting health care needs.
10. Provide support to nurses, set standards and values and promote integrity and provide a scope of practice, and preservation of the profession with social policy.

Ethical issues

Nurses and other health care providers need to be aware that legal and ethical issues often go hand-in-hand. Often times legal and ethical issues may overlap, contradict, or interact with one-another. Nurses should be aware that the American Nurses Association sets standards of ethical practice that each nurse must follow, and that the nurse as well as the patient have ethical rights. Nurses should be aware of the decision making taking place with patient care. Often time's decisions that could be rendered ethical will not be legal, or decisions that might be considered legal might not be ethical. Issues most often found to cause conflict with legality and ethics include, but are not limited to privacy, right to share information, confidentiality and protection of the individual.

Bioethics

Bioethical principles used by the American Nurses Association include:
1. Autonomy: Autonomy is the individual's self-determination. Autonomy involves personal respect or others. Nurses have an obligation to respect the rights of patients to make uncoerced, voluntary decisions.
2. Beneficence: Beneficence involves doing well or doing what is best for the patient. Nurses have the responsibility to always do well by their patients. Acting in the best interest of the patient is at the core of beneficence.

3. Nonmaleficence: Nonmaleficence is the principle of doing no harm.

4. Justice: The principle of justice involves fair treatment and equal care for all.

5. Veracity: Veracity involves telling the truth. Health care providers are required and responsible to be truthful when providing care to patients.

6. Fidelity: Fidelity is the healthcare provider's obligation to keep the promises they make to their patients, maintain patient confidentiality, and patient information.

Bioethics is philosophy used to guide ethical decisions in health care and nursing. Theories of bioethics include:

1. Utilitarianism: Utilitarianism believes that ethical conflicts can be resolve by considering the individuals affected by the decision being made. Utilitarianism works under the premise of doing the most good for the greatest number of people. The theory of utilitarianism believes that maximization of good consequences automatically minimizes bad consequences.

2. Deontology: Deontology functions on the premise of duty or obligation. The deontological theory states that nurses are bound to always do what is right for their patients.

3. Virtue: Virtue is a theory that involves making ethical decisions or taking ethical stands related to health care. The intent is the driving force behind virtue. With virtue functioning under good intentions makes actions ethical.

4. Egoist: The egoist theory sites objectivism as the main focus. Egoist thought is centered on self-interest of the individual.

Patient rights

Patients have the right to appropriate care regardless of race, religion, ethnicity or economic status. Patients cannot be denied care based on age, sexual orientation, marital status, disability, or ability to pay. Patients have the right to be treated with respect. The patient's personal and individual needs should be respected. Patients have the right to privacy, pain management that is effective, psychosocial needs being met, spiritual needs being met, and recognition of cultural attributes as part of the health care to be provided. Patients have the right to make health care decisions. Patients have the right to be educated on procedures prior to making decisions related to health care. Patients are entitled to know who is making their health care decisions. Patients have the right to know the law regarding health care and procedures. Patients have the right to information regarding their health care, their illness, the course of treatment to be provided and prognosis of illness and treatment.

Patient bill of rights

The patient bill of rights clearly states that the patient has a right to health services and social services, and to have those services provided with dignity and respect. The patient has a right to privacy (as provided by HIPAA regulations) and a right to self-determination. The patient has a right to know the cost of health care services being provided and to receive notification if services are to be discharged or terminated. The patient has a right to withdraw from a case management program, to file a grievance if they feel they have been treated unfairly, and to choose a community service agency of their choice. The case manager has an obligation to protect the patient's rights when developing a plan of care and offering services.

Informed consent

Informed consent is the process of educating and obtaining consent from individual patients related to procedures and care. The client should be educated in a manner they will understand to make informed, reasonable decisions. Consent is the patient's voluntary, autonomous authorization to undergo a medical or surgical procedure. The nursing role in informed consent IS NOT to obtain conformed consent. The physician is responsible to obtain consent. The nurse may witness the consent and validate that the patient did indeed give informed consent. The nurse may educate the client on informed consent.

Informed consent must involve information on the disease process in terms the individual can understand. The informed consent must contain information on the prognosis. The informed consent must include benefits and burdens of the treatment being recommended. The informed consent must obtain information related to alternative treatments. Informed consent must explain the potential effects of no treatment. True informed consent must contain adequate information in terms of the individual, must include or account for the ability of the individual to make a reasonable and prudent decision, and must contain the consent of the individual who voluntarily provided the signature approving the treatment.

Informed consent is intended to facilitate appropriate, knowledgeable decision making among clients who are hospitalized, receiving specialty services and/or making any type of decision regarding health care. Informed consent should be directed toward the educational and cognitive level of the client. All possible outcomes and consequences of the procedure or treatment should be explained in as much detail as needed to ensure the client fully understands what is to be done and the potential outcomes. Informed consent must be signed and acknowledged by both the physician and the patient; nurses are no longer responsible for the information on and for obtaining informed consent, but do function as the witness to informed consent.

Nurse's role

Informed consent is the patient's agreement to participate in a procedure after having been fully advised of the process, the risks, the benefits and the alternatives. Informed consent involves informing the patient about the upcoming procedure as opposed to merely obtaining the patient's signature on a document. It is the physician's responsibility to talk with the patient to explain all of the necessary information so that he/she will make an informed decision. Nurses are responsible for assisting patients with signing forms once they have made decisions. However, a nurse may be held responsible if it is determined that a patient did not sign a consent form and the nurse failed to notify the physician before the procedure was started.

Patient's right to self-determination

A patient's right to self-determination is the right to make autonomous decisions regarding how to receive health care. In some cases, this may mean choosing not to accept treatment from the nurse, but this remains part of the right to autonomy. In cases where the patient is unable to make independent decisions, another person is appointed to make those decisions for him or her. Ideally, the second person has been selected ahead of time and chooses practices that are within the patient's best interests. As part of the Code of Ethics, the nurse must recognize the patient's right to self-determination and practice giving professional care that aligns with that respect. The nurse must continue to uphold the patient's decisions, even if he/she does not agree with them. Additionally, the nurse must

- 5 -

not coerce, convince, or bargain with the patient to change his/her mind. The nurse and the physician must provide enough information to ensure the patient is fully informed about all choices and their potential consequences.

<u>Self-determination and informed consent</u>
Each patient has the right to self-determination when making independent decisions about health care. The right to self-determination gives the patient the right to make an autonomous decision about what or what not to do with his/her body. Informed consent supports the patient's right to self-determination by giving the patient enough information to be able to make an independent choice. Without being informed prior to consent, the patient cannot be fully aware of the risks, benefits, or consequences of undergoing or declining a procedure. A patient can therefore not know or understand well enough to make an independent decision, which violates the inherent rights to care for oneself and to take responsibility for one's own welfare.

<u>Procedures when patient cannot give informed consent</u>
Since informed consent supports the patient's right to autonomy, the barriers to actual informed consent should be removed. If the barrier exists because the patient cannot make independent decisions, a person designated by the patient should be called upon to act on the patient's behalf. This person is responsible for weighing the information available to make an informed decision for the benefit of the patient. If the patient is unable to give informed consent due to other barriers, the nurse and physician must work to remove those barriers as completely as possible. For example, a patient may not understand the information due to a language barrier, so the nurse must make arrangements for an interpreter to explain the procedure as fully as possible. A patient is not informed when giving consent if he/she does not understand the language of the physician or nurse.

<u>Exceptions</u>
Informed consent may not be required in emergent situations where the client is unconscious, and where there is no legal representative of the client available to give consent for treatment. Informed consent may not be required where there are disclosures of therapeutic privilege; where these privileges would adverse effects on the client/patient. If the patient does not have the capacity to make decisions an informed consent may not have to be obtained. The patient may waive his/her right to informed consent. Informed consent may not have to be obtained if the physician does not believe the decisions being made are in the best interest of the individual; this will involve a court order to treat against patient/client will.

HIPAA

HIPAA stands for the Health Insurance Portability and Accountability Act. It protects a patient's privacy and prevents that patient from being denied insurance because of a pre-existing condition. It creates a standard for privacy protection among health care providers and institutions, and protects the patient's health record, which is currently an important issue because of electronic health records. It also allows the patient to know how and with whom their information will be shared. The regulations prevent information from being shared with everyone, and allow agencies and facilities to share what is needed for a specific purpose. Employers must train employees to practice confidentiality and ensure they understand the consequences of breaching that privacy.

Confidentiality

Confidentiality relates to maintaining privacy with client information, client status, client chart, and client condition. The nurse should be aware confidentiality is protecting the patients information that he or she may not want divulged to other individuals. Confidentiality respects the patients/clients autonomy and privacy, supports a trusting relationship between the nurse and the client, and assists in preventing harm to the patient. Confidentiality is based on the premise it will promote the greater good of society. Exceptions to patient confidentiality include testifying in court, reporting communicable diseases, reporting child abuse, spouse abuse and or elder abuse. The nurse is responsible for reporting suspicious or gunshot wounds if they are believed to have occurred as the result of a crime. Information relating to workers compensation issues is also an exception to the confidentiality of clients.

Nurses' rights and responsibilities

The primary responsibility of the nurse is to provide safety in healthcare for all individuals. Therefore nurses have the right to refuse assignments that jeopardize the client or the nurse, or place the client in immediate or serious danger. Nurses have the right to refuse to treat patients that are beyond their scope of practice. Nurses have the right to not be abused by clients, co-workers or employers. Nurses have the right to ask for clarity with assignments, assess his or her personal abilities as they relate to clients and client situations, and assist in identifying options that will fulfill the assignment. Nurses are responsible to know their scope of practice, the patient's rights, hospital policies and procedures, as well as standards of care and community norms.

Principles of statutory law

The nurse should know statutory laws are made by legislatures. The 10 principles include:
1. Nursing as a legal duty to always act in the best interest of the individuals they care for.
2. Informed consent is required for testing, procedures and treatment.
3. All patients should be informed of the consequences of refusing treatment. This should be documented as well in the permanent patient record.
4. All adult patients have the right to refuse treatment, including life saving treatment.
5. Patients have the right of advance directives to direct care when they are incapacitated.
6. The state may require documented evidence related to refusal of care.
7. Decisions that involve children should be made with the child's best interest in mind.
8. Adolescents are capable of making health care decisions.
9. Healthcare providers are legally bound to abide by privacy laws.
10. Privacy laws are only breeched when the client is endangering others with his or her decisions.

Negligence and malpractice

Negligence is an unintentional tort involving a breach of duty or failure (through an act or an omission) to meet a standard of care, causing patient harm. Malpractice is a type of professional liability based on negligence in which the health care professional is held accountable for breach of a duty of care involving special knowledge and skill.

Negligence is the concept of failing to provide care or thought in a way that any other reasonable, prudent person might provide in the same situation. This can become medical malpractice if a nurse is negligent while performing her professional duties. Negligence can impose risks and adverse outcomes on patients when nurses fail to communicate and update physicians about changes in patient status, perform interventions based on the plan of care, or document those interventions. The nurse can also impose risk by failing to follow facility policies, refusing to use equipment appropriately, or acting in a personal manner that is unsafe or unjustifiable.

Five rights of delegation

The five rights of delegation are as follows:
- Right task
- Right circumstances
- Right person
- Right directions and communication
- Right supervision and evaluation

Advocacy

Advocacy is the act or incidence of beseeching for, supporting, urging public argument, and recommending publicity, and espousing actively things that promote the health and well being of individuals. Nurses are responsible to advocate for their vulnerable clients who may not be able to advocate for themselves. Patient advocacy is done to ensure the highest level of care and treatment is maintained. Nurse advocates accept responsibility to safeguard patient rights, and ensure quality of care for the client or patients they care for. The role of nurse advocate involves three aspects; these include informing patient of rights in any particular situation, providing information in making informed decisions, and supporting patient decisions. All nurses are responsible to advocate for their patients. Things the nurse should know about advocacy include:
1. Understanding advocacy is ethical in concept.
2. Realizing the relationship of advocacy and practice.
3. Analyze and develop communication skills that are effective for advocation of clients and health care.
4. Identification of needed advocacy situations.
5. Action taking or becoming involved on behalf of the patient.

Standards of care

Standards of care are the current practice standards utilized to ensure capable and skillful health care delivery. Standards of care are used as a measurement tool for providing quality care. This type of established norm is a mechanism of providing safe and appropriate care to the public. Nursing standards discuss what would be done in and under the same circumstance by any other nurse with the same level of expertise and knowledge. By following standards of care or practice standards the nurse reduces his/her chances of being found negligent in a court of law.

Barriers to communication

Barriers to communication exist when the nurse is unable to effectively communicate the wants, needs, and desires of the patient, as well as to effectively discuss and explain the care and rational for the care needed and to be provided. Barriers to communication include, but are not limited to minimalization of concerns, offering false reassurance, or approval to the client, rejecting individuals, choosing sides.

Choosing sides can be associated with the client, the family, or the physician. Placing blame on external factors, having conflicting opinions from the client or family, placing blame on family or client, giving advice, belittling the client, family or other health care team member, and offering minimal feedback to questions (example: giving a one word response to a question) are all forms of ineffective communication and can cause barriers with communication. Other barriers to communication include shifting the focus of concern, using medical terminology the client, or family does not understand, and offering unrealistic ideation or ignoring what is important to the client.

Managed care and case management

Managed care is a broader term referring to an organized delivery of care or services. Managed care usually involves a select panel of care providers who give out their services based on a prepayment arrangement between the provider and the managed care organization. For instance, a hospital may be the managed care organization, and the physicians who are part of the hospital staff are prepaid for the services they render to patients who seek care from that institution. HMOs and PPOs are examples of those types of managed care services. Case management is an individual patient care delivery system specific to the patient, their diagnosis, and their individual needs. The main difference is that managed care is the function of the healthcare reimbursement system, while case management is the structure used to provide individual patient care to affect expected treatments and outcomes.

Case management plan

Case management has been in practice for 20 years. It began with the introduction of case management plans, or critical pathways. A good case management plan must include all of the disciplines that are relevant to the patient's care, and it must be clinically specific to the patient and their condition. The plan must be outcome based, with the best possible outcome for the patient as the goal. The plan must be flexible so that it can be adapted to each individual patient. It must also, however, be standardized for each disease process so that a healthcare team from any institution could easily implement the plan for a patient with the same condition. An example of this would be a case management plan with community-acquired pneumonia as the disease process. The standard treatments and expected outcomes would be listed in the plan, but the entire plan would be individualized for each patient with pneumonia based on factors such as age, response, health history, and compliance. The plan must also have a financial component emphasizing the most cost-effective way to care for the individual patient.

Plan of care

<u>Data management to develop plan of care</u>
The interdisciplinary team would meet to discuss the goals for the meeting, the expectations, and the process for developing the plan of care. They would discuss and determine who would collect the data and where the data should come from. The following couple of meetings would be held to analyze the data and begin evaluating the information. The fourth or fifth meeting would be held to report all of the data, the analysis, and the evaluation, and to begin documenting the care plan for any patient with the disease. They would discuss and develop expected outcomes and interventions needed to get those outcomes. They would also develop the treatment plan. The ultimate purpose of all meetings would be to put together a clinical pathway or plan of care for a specific disease. Subsequent meetings would be held to get input and approval for the document, make changes, and set a time for putting the document into practice. The entire process of developing a pathway for each disease entity takes several months, and requires evaluation after the initial application in the clinical setting.

<u>Elements in a patient care plan</u>
The items on a care plan may vary from patient to patient, but some routine items must always be documented by the nurse. Items which must appear on any care plan include the assessment of the patient and any monitoring which is mandatory for particular patients. Cardiac patients must have telemetry for most hospitalizations, for instance. All tests and procedures must be documented, as well as any consultations or referrals. Medications, intravenous therapy, activity, and nutrition, along with patient teaching and any nursing interventions should be recorded. Wound care interventions, physical therapy, and pain management should be documented. Outcome indicators and projected/desired responses should be documented as the standard for what the plan predicts. Finally, safety issues, a psychosocial assessment, and discharge planning should be documented.

<u>Inclusion of patient</u>
The nurse may include the patient in the plan of care by interviewing the patient personally, along with the family. The nurse should allow the patient to have input and to verbalize the needs they feel they have. Asking the patient what goals they have and what they expect the outcomes of their care to be help the nurse to be realistic about the plan of care. Including the family, the health care team members, and the physician add information, which can be important, but knowing where the patient stands in terms of knowledge, expectations, and needs will help the plan of care be successful.

Outcomes

<u>Expected outcome example</u>
The expected outcomes for a female or male patient who has suffered a myocardial infarction would first be that chest pain would be absent for 48 hours after the initial onset and treatment, and that the ischemia damage would be kept to a minimum. You would want ischemia changes on the EKG to be resolved, and for any signs of a further attack to be absent. You would expect the cardiac enzymes to be returning to normal after 48 hours, and you would expect the physician to have converted all intravenous medications to oral doses by 48 hours. You would want the patient to be able to return as quickly as possible to the activity level they were at pre-infarction, and for the patient to be pain free and not short of breath on exertion. Discharge planning would include teaching the signs and symptoms to

look for so early intervention could be started if another infarction occurs, and also teaching the steps to take if chest pain reoccurs. You would also teach about the risk factors for heart disease, and set up a plan to address those risk factors that the patient can control. This might include, for instance, a smoking cessation program. Finally, educate about medications, diet, and balancing rest with activity.

Expected outcome example

When it is documented that a patient or his or her family has a knowledge deficit regarding the patient's diagnosis, teaching must be done. The results must be documented in the patient record as an expected outcome for the case manager. The nurse would look for documentation to prove the patient can describe the signs and symptoms of diabetes. The chart should show that the patient can describe both hypoglycemia and hyperglycemia, and that the patient can describe injection sites for insulin. The patient should also be able to demonstrate injection and blood glucose monitoring skills. If the patient does not possess these skills, documentation regarding which family member will be taking over this job and their compliance should be present. The documentation should also include proof that the patient can describe preventive measures for foot care, can recognize signs and symptoms of infection, and knows when to call the physician.

If outcome is not met

If an outcome has not been met in the charting by exception system by assessing the patient, then additional documentation is needed to record the actual outcome. The actual outcome is called the variance. Additional documentation must include the actual outcome, or variance, along with the action plan to correct the issue. The case manager may have to develop an entirely new plan, or may need to make adjustments to the plan to change the variance or outcome. Subsequent charting must include the new outcomes and new expectations or a new plan of care with the new actual outcomes. Each time a case manager sees a variance or negative outcome, they must log it in the documentation and indicate the reason why it occurred. This helps to organize data and track trends, which can improve the case management system or process down the road, and also improves the care providers give.

Discharge planning

Discharge planning begins as soon as a patient is admitted to hospital. The health care team starts educating the patient right away about what to expect and what milestones need to be met before discharge. They also interview the patient about what they want to see happen upon discharge. A patient may have had many admissions, and will know from the beginning that they can no longer handle self care at home. The case manager would take this information into account when developing a plan of care for this hospitalization and start making contacts with facilities that may be able to handle the patient upon discharge. Discharge planning must be started early to shorten the length of the hospital stay and plan appropriate post-hospital care. These issues are interconnected, and the nurse assists with coordination of and communication between all providers and payers.

End of life care and advanced directives

The nurse helps the patient discuss personal wishes for end of life care with family and friends. The nurse helps the patient obtain copies of Advanced Directives and/or a living will and a medical power of attorney. The nurse helps the patient choose a trusted family member or friend willing to be an advocate for the patient's health and welfare. The nurse helps to make sure forms are filled out correctly. The nurse educates the patient and their family about keeping papers in a safe place and submitting copies to the physician, attorney, and others who may need them. The nurse ensures that copies of all documents are in the chart, and that they are copied and sent if the patient is transferred.

<u>Advance directive</u>
An advance directive is a legal list of the wishes a patient may have regarding the level and type of health care they want provided in a specific situation. The document is witnessed, and clearly states the wishes of the client regarding healthcare-related situations. The list or directive is drawn up when the patient is of sound mind and mentally and emotionally capable of making these types of decisions. The directives most often state the client's wishes regarding end-of-life issues, including feeding decisions, life support, and resuscitation wishes if the client should stop breathing or have a sudden cardiac arrest.

Documentation

Documentation is an essential component of nursing to support communication between caregivers, to prevent errors and adverse outcomes, and to maintain a record of work in case care or judgment comes into question. Documentation should be fair and exact, avoiding opinion or blaming others or the patient. The nurse should document all actions that were performed for the patient's plan of care, communication with and instructions from physicians, and any educational information given to the patient and family. If mistakes are made with documentation, the nurse should draw a single line through the error and mark the document with his/her initials. Charting that is performed late should be noted within documentation that it is a late entry, to avoid questions about time lapses.

<u>Electronic documentation</u>
Electronic documentation, while being implemented in many health care facilities throughout the country, speeds the charting process and maintains patient medical records while cutting back on paper charts. However, because of access and advanced capabilities of electronic documentation, there are some potential risks associated with this practice. Computerized records may allow many people to access files on patients from different locations, and measures should be taken to prevent unauthorized users from accessing patient information and violating confidentiality. Nursing documentation may differ when charting electronically as well, since computerized records may automatically record dates and times that differ from that of the nurse's documented actions. Nurses should make changes to the medical record carefully, as they would with a written record, to avoid potential liability or questionable charting that needs to be justified.

Safety and Infection Control

Nosocomial infections (HOSPital-acQUIRED)

The different types of nosocomial infections are:
- Exogenous infections: Caused by microorganisms that are not found in normal flora.
  Ex: Aspergillus, Salmonella
- Endogenous infections: Microorganism overgrowth causes a different area of the body to become infected.
  Ex: Enterococci (GI) to wound site or E. Coli (GI) to urinary tract via foley catheter.
- Iatrogenic infections: Infections that are caused by procedures.
  Ex: UTI after foley insertion or bacteremia after IV insertion.

Nosocomial infections among children

Primary bloodstream infections (28%), pneumonia (21%), and urinary tract infections (15%) are the most frequent nosocomial infections among children found in ICUs and high-risk nurseries. An invasive device, such as a catheter, almost invariably has a role in the infection. Infection sites and pathogens involved are not uniform but are of several types of infections distributed over various sites in patterns related to age. The illnesses also are not, in general, the same as those reported for the occupants of adult ICUs. In addition to an association with intrinsic risk factors such as low birth weight and gestational age, outbreaks of *Klebsiella pneumoniae* BSIs in high-risk nurseries have been associated with extrinsic factors. These include procedures necessary to intravenous therapy, use of antimicrobials, and cross-transmission. Bloodstream hospital-acquired infections (BSIs) are a leading cause of morbidity and mortality for neonates in high-risk nurseries.

Surgical asepsis

The following are the principles of surgical asepsis:
- A sterile object remains sterile only when touched by another sterile object.
- Only sterile objects may be placed on a sterile field.
- A sterile object or field out of the range of vision or an object held below a person's waist is contaminated. ✳
- A sterile object or field becomes contaminated by prolonged exposure to air.
- When a sterile surface comes in contact with a wet, contaminated surface, the sterile object or field becomes contaminated by capillary action.
- Fluid flows in the direction of gravity.
- The edges of a sterile field or container are considered to be contaminated about 1-inch from the outer edge.
- When opening sterile supplies, avoid crossing over the sterile object or sterile field.

CDC Standard Precautions

Before CDC issued its Standard Precautions, Blood and Body Fluid Precautions designed to reduce the risk of transmission of bloodborne pathogens and Body Substance Isolation had been in effect. Their intent was to cut the risk of transferring pathogens from moist body substances to people and surfaces. Promulgated to further reduce the risk of transmission of microorganisms from both recognized and unrecognized sources of infection in hospitals, Standard Precautions combines and synthesizes the major features of those two earlier sets of precautions, applying them to all patients receiving care in hospitals, regardless of their diagnosis or presumed infection status. Standard Precautions apply to blood; all body fluids, secretions, and excretions (except sweat), regardless of whether or not they contain visible blood; nonintact skin; and mucous membranes.

Handwashing and use of gloves

Gloves, not necessarily sterile but clean, are to be worn when touching blood, body fluids, secretions, excretions, and contaminated items. They should be donned before touching mucous membranes and non-intact skin. After contact with material that may contain a high concentration of microorganisms on one part of a patient's body, health care personnel should change gloves before performing any task or procedure on another part of the same patient's body. This ensures against the possibility of cross-contamination between infection sites. Remove gloves promptly after use, before touching non-contaminated items and environmental surfaces, and before going to another patient. Plain soap is acceptable for routine hand washing; an antimicrobial agent or a waterless antiseptic agent should be used during outbreaks.

Occupational health and bloodborne pathogens and patient placement

The Standard Precautions regarding bloodborne pathogens basically boil down to avoiding cuts from sharp, contaminated instruments. Used, disposable hypodermic syringes, for instance, are never to be recapped but immediately placed in the closest puncture-resistant container for transport to a reprocessing area. Health care workers are directed to never point a needle toward any part of their body or manipulate them using both hands. Should mouth-to-mouth resuscitation become necessary, it must be performed only with the use of mouthpieces, resuscitation bags, or other ventilation devices. A patient who contaminates the environment and will not (or cannot) follow rules of proper hygiene and environmental control, must be placed in a private room. If none is available, the problem must be taken up with infection control professionals.

Handwashing

All patients are considered potentially infectious, so handwashing must be done before and after every direct contact with a patient or when removing gloves. Contamination of the hands is one of the most common causes of person-to-person transmission of infection and all medical personnel must be trained in handwashing techniques and observed regularly for compliance:

- Handwashing is done under running water with plain soap rather than antimicrobial soap because of issues related to resistance.
- Hands must be lathered thoroughly, covering all areas of the hands and wrists with soap, and then rinsed.
- After handwashing, care should be taken to avoid contact with surfaces that might serve as vectors, such as faucet handles and doorknobs.
- The faucet should be turned off by using the elbow or upper forearm or holding a piece of paper towel as a barrier.
- Hands should be dried using disposable towels.

<u>Washing hands within a risk-laden environment</u>
Remove all rings and bracelets. Adjust the water to comfortably warm temperature and rinse hands from the wrist downward. (If hand washing is done frequently, as it is in hospital situations, using cold water will avoid the dermatitis that can come from frequent washing in warm water.) Apply soap and lather thoroughly, beginning at the wrist and working downward. Scrub vigorously with friction for 15-30 seconds. Interlace the fingers and continue scrubbing by sliding the fingers back and forth. After hand washing with soap and water, apply a hand rub with an alcoholic base formulation (70%) if possible to enhance resident skin flora destruction or inhibition. Use dry toweling to turn off the water and use a clean paper towel to open the door when leaving a public restroom. When bar soap is in use, it should not be allowed to stay wet between washings, for microorganisms grow in moist conditions, even on soap.

<u>Surgical hand disinfection and hygienic washing</u>
Surgical hand washing aims to remove and kill transient flora and decrease resident flora toward reducing the risk of wound contamination should surgical gloves undergo damage. Agents are the same as those used for hygienic hand washes, the primary difference between the surgical scrub and the hygienic hand wash being that, for the former, more time is spent in scrubbing – an extra 2-3 minutes – and it includes both wrists and forearms. Sterile disposable or autoclave-able nailbrushes may be used to clean the fingernails only, but not to scrub the hands. A brush should only be used for the first scrub of the day. After hand washing with soap and water, a hand rub with an alcohol base formulation (70%) should be used if possible. This enhances the destruction or inhibition of resident skin flora. If an alcohol preparation is used, two applications of 5ml each is suggested, both rubbed to dryness. Sterile towels should be used to dry the hands thoroughly after washing and before alcohol is applied.

Triclosan

In the United States, 79 percent of liquid soaps and 29 percent of bar soaps contain the antibacterial agent triclosan, an antibiotic designed to kill a wide variety of germs. The germicide has been put into soaps and toothpastes for the last 30 years, a prominent brand containing it being Procter & Gamble's Dial. It may be contributing to the rise of drug-resistant microorganisms, says a recent study. The triclosan used by hospital personnel in soaps to prevent the spread of infection comes in much higher doses, about 10 times as much as is found in soap used in the home. The irony is that the doses found in supermarket soaps are too small to prevent infection but large enough to make microorganisms resistant to the ingredient over time. Germs that can resist triclosan have already been observed in laboratories. Right now, *Escherichia coli*, a major offender in cases of food poisoning, has the ability to fight off triclosan if it mutates only a single gene.

Alcohol-based rub

While soap and water handwashing has been the standard for many years, in fact studies have proven that alcohol-based rubs kill twice as much bacteria in the same amount of time. They are waterless and act quickly to kill bacteria and are less irritating to the hands than repeated washing. *Hand disinfection* is done for at least 15 seconds by using an alcohol-based rub, such as Purell®, and should be done before and after contact with a patient or after removal of gloves. All hand surfaces should be thoroughly coated with the alcohol-rub, including between the fingers, the wrists, and under the nails, and then the hands rubbed together until the solution evaporates. Hands should not be rinsed. Alcohol-based rubs disinfect but do not mechanically clean hands, so hands that are dirty or contaminated should be washed first with soap and water.

Antiseptic solutions and occlusive adhesive drapes

Lister, in 1865, introduced the practice of using carbolic acid for antisepsis in the operating theater. Today, skin may be washed with a variety of solutions such as those listed below to sterilize hands and instruments and produce a sterile field for surgery; it also maintains microorganism-free environments for laboratory work and on hospital wards. No evidence indicates any one of these solutions being superior to another:

- Alcohols: Most commonly used is ethanol (60-90%), 1-propanol (60-70%) and 2-propanol/isopropanol (70-80%) or mixtures of the two. Short-acting bactericidals effective against gram-positive and gram-negative organisms, they are also a fungicidal and virucidal.
- 0.5% Chlorhexidine: Used to treat gingivitis, as a bactericidal it's persistent and has a long duration of action. It's effective against gram-positive organisms but does not kill spore forming organisms, instead disrupting the bacterial cell wall.
- Mercurichrome: Because of concerns about its mercury content, this organomercury antiseptic is now obsolete, no longer being recognized as safe and effective by the FDA.

Occlusive adhesive drapes are sometimes used during surgery, but there is no evidence that they reduce infection rate and they may actually increase skin bacterial count during surgery.

Iodine

Used as a pre- and post-operative antiseptic, usually in an alcohol solution called tincture of iodine or as Lugol's iodine solution, iodine is no longer recommended as a disinfectant for minor wounds because it induces scar tissue formation and increases healing time. Gentle washing with mild soap and water or rinsing a scrape with sterile saline is a better practice. Novel iodine antiseptics (such as Betadine) containing iodopovidone/PVP-I are far better tolerated, don't adversely affect wound healing, and have a persistent effect. They have the widest scope of antimicrobial activity, are lethal to all principal pathogens and, given enough time, kill even spores, considered the most difficult form of microorganism to destroy with disinfectants and antiseptics. One bactericidal active against spore forming organisms, both gram-positive and gram-negative, 70% Povidone – iodine, has drawbacks in that some people have skin reactions to it and it is rapidly inactivated by organic material such as blood.

Ideal disinfectant

The properties of the ideal disinfectant are as follows:
- Inexpensive
- Non-caustic, non-corrosive
- Environmentally safe, won't harm other forms of life (except for pathogens)
- Effective

Ideal disinfectants don't exist. Even if they could meet the other conditions, all disinfectants, without exception, are potentially harmful and even toxic to humans or animals. A "sure kill" rate on bacteria, molds, funguses, and viruses cannot be obtained without using a compound also harmful to higher forms of life. Besides, bacteria reproduce rapidly and evolve over relatively short periods, so any bacteria that survive a chemical attack will go on to give rise to the next generation. Over a period of a few years, a new "super race" of the bugs emerges that develop, over many generations, resistance to hostile chemicals. Creating and maintaining conditions not conducive to bacterial survival and multiplication is, as an alternative to killing them with chemicals, an idea now getting a great deal of attention.

Barrier precautions

Barrier precautions are used to prevent infection in accordance with mode of transmission and likelihood of contamination with blood or other body fluids or wastes.

Gloves
Gloves are worn when hands may make contact with body fluids, including mucous membranes, or instruments that have made contact with body fluids, or any skin that is not intact, such as cuts, scrapes, or chapped. Gloves should be worn to protect the patient from any cuts or other breaks in the skin of the caregiver. Sterile gloves are used for sterile procedures. Gloves are used not only to prevent the spread of pathogenic agents from one patient to another but also to protect the healthcare worker. There are limitations to the degree to which gloves can control infections because transmission is complex. For example, gloves offer no protection to infections caused by endogenous flora.

Goggles and face shields
The face is particularly vulnerable to splashing and splattering of blood and body fluids because staff are often leaning over the patients during procedures. The mucous membranes of the eyes, nose, and mouth can become contaminated, so protective eyewear and face shields should be worn when contamination of the face is possible:
- Goggles should be non-vented or indirectly vented with an anti-fog coating and should allow for direct and peripheral vision. They should be large enough to cover eyeglasses if necessary and still fit snugly to provide protection.
- Face shields provide protection to the eyes and face. The shields should have both crown and chin protection and should extend around the face to the ears. Small, thin disposable shields that attach to surgical masks provide more limited protection.

Both goggles and face shields should be washed with soap and water after each use and disinfected with 70% alcohol if contaminated.

Gowns
The CDC guidelines for barrier precautions call for the use of a clean non-sterile gown. Sterile gowns are reserved primarily for surgical procedures. There are a variety of different types of aprons and gowns that are available, primarily for the protection of the healthcare worker, but gowns also reduce contamination of uniforms and thus protect patients. Gowns should be moisture-resistant and easily cover clothing. They are worn to prevent contamination from blood or body fluids during activities or procedures that may result in splashing or splattering. They should be changed after caring for the patient or procedures that may have resulted in contamination. Gowns should be handled as little as

possible, sliding down raised arms and fastening at the neck, with gloves pulled over sleeves. Gown should be removed before gloves to reduce hand contamination, and the hands should be washed immediately after gloves are removed.

<u>Masks and respirators</u>

Masks can provide protection from droplets, but they do not provide protection from smaller airborne microorganisms. Respirators that contain filters must be used for airborne precautions. Masks are used primarily to protect patients from droplets during sterile procedures, but are used when working within 3 feet of a patient on droplet precautions. They provide protection of the mucous membranes of the nose and mouth from spraying or splattering of blood or body fluids. Respirators must be used for protection against airborne transmission. The National Institute for Occupational Safety and Health (NIOSH) establishes requirements for respirators, which must filter 95% of 0.3um-sized particles in order to protect against *Mycobacterium tuberculosis*. These are referred to as N95 respirators. The disposable N95 can be reused if not visibly damaged or dirty with TB patients but must be disposed of after use if patients are also on contact precautions (smallpox, SARS).

Special ventilation systems

Special hospital ventilation systems are designed to prevent the acquisition and/or spread of nosocomial infections in operating theatres and patient care areas such as isolation areas for severely immunocompromised patients. Rooms intended to house patients with suspected or known airborne infectious diseases – pulmonary tuberculosis, chickenpox, or measles, for instance – should be designed with special ventilation and seals permitting them to be maintained at negative air pressure. This minimizes opportunities for infectious pathogens to escape from the room. The opposite should be true for operating theatres as well as rooms that will house immunocompromised patients, where positive air pressure and seals should be used to impede infectious pathogens in the surrounding atmosphere from coming inside the area. Certain aerosolized medications such as pentamidine, given for conditions like pneumonia associated with AIDS, must be administered in rooms with increased ventilation, as must certain chemotherapy drugs, because they could otherwise contaminate the immediate environment.

[handwritten margin note: Airborne infectious diseases = neg. air pressure room.]

Patient placement

The use of standard precautions obviates most patient placement in private rooms, but private room placement is necessary under some conditions:
- Airborne transmission: Airborne precautions must be used. Room should have negative pressure if possible.
- Droplet transmission: Droplet precautions must be used. Patient may share a room with another patient infected with the same microorganism if there are no other contraindications.
- Microorganism transmitted by contact: Contact precautions must be used. Patient may share a room with a patient colonized or infected by the same microorganism.
- Contaminated environment: Patients producing large amounts of body fluids or waste, such as blood or stool, that cannot be contained should be placed in a private room.
- Poor hygiene: Patients not willing or are too confused or unable to properly maintain hygiene should be placed in private rooms.

Private rooms should be assigned when possible by Admissions utilizing a list of specific diagnoses.

Positive pressure and laminar air flow rooms

A positive pressure room creates a protective environment for patients who are immunocompromised. In these rooms, the pressure is positive within the room so that clean air flows out of the room to the "dirty" area of the hallways, protecting the patient from pathogens. Air exchanges are >12 per hour, and filtration is by 99.97% HEPA filters. Windows should be sealed for protection and the room outfitted with self-closing doors. Positive pressure rooms are used for those who are immunocompromised:

(handwritten margin note: positive pressure room = allows clean air to flow out, to dirty.)

- HIV/AIDs patients with reduced immunity.
- Oncology patients with bone marrow suppression.
- Solid organ transplant patients.

Laminar air flow (LAF) rooms provide more protection than a positive pressure room because one entire wall is composed of HEPA filters and fans blow air at high velocity through the filters with >100 air exchanges per hour, creating drafts and noise. Staff should work "down wind" of patients, who are severely immunocompromised: Bone marrow transplant patients.

Protective positive pressure environment in the operating room

In an operating room, a positive pressure environment must be maintained with the area of the operating table and the patient considered "clean." Filtered air in large volumes washes over the table from the ceiling and then is drawn to the air returns around the margin of the room. Air displacement must assure that any pathogens shed by the operating room personnel are moved away from the patient by the force of air. Windows should remain sealed and doors closed to maintain the proper pressure and air flow. Air exchanges are 15-25 per hour and 90% filters are used. It is also very important that barriers, such as masks and gowns, be used by all staff to prevent the shedding of bacteria into the operative area and that all surfaces be clean. Local exhaust and filtration systems to capture odors or aerosols generated during operative procedures may be used in addition to the room filtration system.

Isolation guidelines and Universal Precautions

By 1980, the primary need for isolation precautions was becoming nosocomial in nature rather than the previous concern with the spread of infectious diseases brought into the hospital from the community. The CDC's 1983 guideline changed the categories of isolation to Strict Isolation, Contact Isolation, Respiratory Isolation, Tuberculosis Isolation, Enteric Precautions, Drainage/Secretion Precautions, and Blood and Body Fluid Precautions. As with its previous categorical approach, the CDC tended to over-isolate some patients. But an alternative approach, attacking each disease individually, was also recommended to correct for this. A CDC-issued chart listed all diseases posing the threat of in-hospital transmission; the epidemiology of each infectious disease was considered individually by advocating only those precautions (e.g., private room, mask, gown, and gloves) needed to interrupt transmission of the infection.

In 1985, driven largely by the growing HIV epidemic, the CDC altered isolation practices dramatically by introducing a new strategy which became known as Universal Precautions (UP). For the first time, emphasis was put on applying to everyone universally the already existing Blood and Body Fluid Precautions regardless of presumed infection status. UP expanded precautions to using masks and eye coverings to prevent exposure of mucous membrane exposures and taking greater precautions against needle-stick infections. Reports in 1987 and 1988 emphasized blood as the single most important source of HIV and that infection control must focus on preventing exposures to it. A new system, Body Substance Isolation (BSI), focused on isolating all moist and therefore potentially infectious body substances (blood, sputum, feces, urine, wound drainage, saliva, etc.) from all patients, regardless of their presumed infection status, primarily through the use of gloves. Recommendations for Tuberculosis (AFB) Isolation were updated in 1990 after heightened concern about nosocomial transmission of drug-resistant TB, particularly around persons with human immunodeficiency virus (HIV).

1996 revision to the Centers for Disease Control's isolation guidelines

By the early 1990s, there was considerable confusion about which body fluids or substances required precautions under UP and BSI. The CDC released a 1996 guideline containing three important changes to eliminate confusion. It:
- Melded into a single set of precautions the major features of UP and BSI, calling them Standard Precautions, to cover all patients regardless of their presumed infection status.
- Collapsed the old categories of isolation precautions (Strict Isolation, Contact Isolation, Respiratory Isolation, Tuberculosis Isolation, Enteric Precautions, and Drainage/Secretion Precautions) along with the old disease-specific precautions into three sets of precautions based on routes of transmission and called Transmission-Based Precautions; these were intended to be used additional to Standard Precautions.
- Listed specific syndromes highly suspicious for infection and identified appropriate Transmission-Based Precautions to be used on an empirical, temporary basis until a diagnosis could be made.

Isolation precautions noted in the 1996 CDC guidelines:
- Standard Precautions – applies to the care of all patients
- Airborne Precautions -- for patients known or suspected to have serious illnesses such as measles or tuberculosis that are transmitted by airborne droplets
- Droplet Precautions –deal with larger particle droplets than are true for Airborne Precautions; they are applied to patients known or suspected of having serious illnesses such as meningitis, pneumonia, diphtheria (pharyngeal), mycoplasma pneumonia, or serious viral infections (influenza, mumps, rubella)
- Contact Precautions -- patients known or suspected to have serious illnesses (GI, wound infections, diphtheria, colonization with multi-drug-resistant bacteria) easily transmitted by direct patient contact or by contact with objects.

Isolation of patients with communicable diseases

In 1996, the CDC revised its *Guideline for Isolation Precautions in Hospitals* that identifies appropriate precautions to use on an empiric, temporary basis until a diagnosis can be made. It also lists specific clinical syndromes or conditions that should be regarded as highly suspicious for infection. The first tier of precautions are the Standard Precautions, to be practiced with all patients regardless of their diagnosis or presumed infection status – including patients with whom transmission-based precautions should also be followed. In the second tier of the *Guideline* are listed precautions intended only for the care of specified patients known to be or suspected of being infected or colonized with pathogens transmittable through any or all of three routes: airborne, droplets, or contact that is either direct with another person or indirect through the medium of contaminated surfaces.

Protection against acquiring communicable diseases
Devices and wearable items such as surgical gowns, gloves, masks and respirators act as barriers between infectious materials and the skin, mouth, nose, eyes and other mucous membranes. FDA evaluates the performance of personal protective equipment (PPE) such as this before it is cleared for marketing. Proper use of PPE by workers involved in patient care helps prevent the spread of infection because:

- It helps protect wearers from infection or contamination from blood, body fluids, or respiratory secretions
- It reduces the chance that healthcare workers will infect or contaminate others
- It reduces the chance of transmitting infections from one person to another.

The use of PPE alone does not fully protect against acquiring an infection, however. Hand-washing, isolation of patients, and care in coughing or sneezing are also important to minimize risk of infection, and protective clothing should be changed whenever torn or ripped.

Handling permanent medical equipment
Medical equipment may be cleaned to remove contaminants -- dust, soil, large numbers of micro -organisms and organic matter (e.g. blood, vomit); as a necessary prelude to disinfecting and sterilizing it. Whilst disinfecting reduces the number of smaller micro-organisms so that they are not immediately harmful to health, bacterial spores will still remain. Sterilization removes them. Each medical instrument that has come into contact with a patient is a potential source of infection. It should be considered a high risk item when it has made close contact with broken skin or mucous membranes or has been introduced into a body; it requires sterilizing. Intermediate risk items – mainly respiratory equipment -- need only to be disinfected. Stethoscopes, blood pressure cuffs, and such make only slight skin contact and therefore need only cleaning and drying. Boiling equipment in water for 10 minutes disinfects, killing all organisms except for a few bacterial spores. Autoclaving sterilizes by using steam under pressure at a temperature of 134°C for 3 minutes or 121°C for 15 minutes.

Airborne precautions
Precautions are to be taken with infected patients against transmitting disease through airborne droplets containing suspended microorganisms that can be dispersed by air currents.

- Place infected patients in a private, closed-off room equipped with a monitored, high-efficiency air filtration system and negative air pressure system.
- If no private room is available, the patient may be cohorted – placed in a room with another patient with the same infection.

- There should be no hospital personnel susceptible to measles or chickenpox, as, if they have not had the diseases, they should be inoculated against them. So there should be no worry concerning their entering the room of patients known to have (or suspected of having) either of those diseases. If there is any question, they should wear respiratory protection.
- All personnel must wear respiratory protection when entering the room of a patient with known or suspected infectious pulmonary tuberculosis.
- Limit movement and transport of patients outside the room to essential purposes only, at which time the patient must wear a surgical mask to minimize dispersal of droplet nuclei.

Contact precautions

Contact precautions reduce the risk of transmitting microorganisms by skin-to-skin contact, whether direct, as occurs when health care personnel perform activities requiring physical contact with a patient, or indirect via contaminated intermediate objects in the patient's environment. Standard contact precautions cover:

- Patient placement -- a private room when possible
- Gloves and hand washing -- wear gloves, dispose of them and wash hands before leaving a patient's room
- Gowns -- wear when there's any chance of clothing touching a contaminated person or surface),
- Patient transport -- limit movement and use barriers to prevent spread of infection
- Patient-care equipment – avoid, if possible, using a piece of durable equipment with more than one patient.

Additional precautions deal with preventing the spread of vancomycin resistance.

Droplet precautions

Unlike the pathogens transmitted by airborne mechanisms, microorganisms transmitted through droplets consist of particles larger than 5 µm in size. They infect by making contact with the mucous membranes of the nose or mouth of a target. They are contained in droplets generated from a carrier's cough or sneeze, or even talking. They may also be producing in the performance of suctioning or bronchoscopy. Precautions in isolating a patient are exactly the same as for the patient whose disease is transported through means other than large droplets – except for one thing: Because large droplets do not remain suspended in the air and generally travel only short distances, usually 3 ft or less, special air handling and ventilation is not necessary, and the room's door may remain open. While some hospitals may prefer staff to wear a mask upon entering the room, at the very least, a mask should be worn when working within 3 ft of the patient. Transport advisories are exactly the same as those for patients with airborne pathogens. SPIDERMAN can help you to remember common microorganisms that require droplet precautions.

S- sepsis/scarlet fever/ streptococcal pharyngitis
P- parovirus B19/pneumonia/pertussis
I- influenza
D- diptheria (pharyngeal)
E- epiglottitis
R- rubella
M- mumps/meningitis/mycoplasma/meningeal pneumonia
An- Adenovirus

Isolation of tuberculosis patients

Barrier protection and decontamination
It is estimated that *Mycobacterium tuberculosis* causes the greatest number of deaths of any infectious pathogen – three million deaths annually worldwide. Hospital staff should therefore use extra precaution against infection when treating tubercular patients by wearing gowns and gloves and using HEPA filtration masks. Should a staff member suspect he or she has had any possible exposure, it has got to be reported immediately to a supervisor for referral to a screening exam. While a Mantoux skin test helps identify those infected with *M tuberculosis* but not yet showing symptoms, sputum or other bodily secretions can be cultured for growth of mycobacteria to confirm the diagnosis. It may take 1-3 weeks to detect growth and 8-12 weeks to be certain. With a positive test result, a daily dose of isoniazid (also called INH) may be prescribed. It will be taken for up to a year, with periodic checkups.

Respiratory protection and duration of isolation
Admit patients into negative pressure isolation rooms when:
- Coughing and chest X-ray suggest there may be tuberculosis
- There is a positive acid-fast smear
- Multi-drug resistant tuberculosis is known when admitted or re-admitted
- There is a known HIV infection
- There is an undiagnosed cough or pulmonary condition.
- Medical conditions, with cough and an undiagnosed pulmonary infiltrate, predispose to tuberculosis.

Isolation should be maintained until there is evidence of response to therapy. Such evidence consists of:
- Three consecutive negative AFB smears with no organisms on smear
- Decreased cough
- Decrease in maximum daily temperature
- Resolution of night sweats
- Improved appetite.

Ventilation and patient management
Crowded living conditions and poor ventilation are conducive to the transmission of *M. tuberculosis*. Epidemics of tuberculosis were quite common in American big city slums of the early 20th Century, and there are still troubling incidences of the disease in such overcrowded conditions as those found in many prisons.

Improvements in housing conditions help prevent outbreaks. In hospitals, ventilation systems may be supplemented with high- efficiency particulate air (HEPA) filtration (which will also remove droplet nuclei from the air) and ultraviolet germicidal irradiation (UVGI) in high-risk areas. UVGI lamps can be used in ceiling or wall fixtures or within air ducts of ventilation systems. Such systems may be used along with negative pressure systems in rooms used for isolation of TB patients.

Communicable diseases associated with respiratory infections

RSV
Respiratory syncytial virus (RSV), though first observed in chimpanzees having colds, was soon found to cause colds in man as well. (In fact, the chimps probably got infected by some human handlers carrying the disease to begin with.) Soon thereafter, it was also found to be associated with severe pulmonary infections in infants – especially bronchiolitis, for which RSV is the prime cause; in Great Britain, it accounts for 78% of URI infections among children. Inflammation of terminal bronchioles marks acute bronchiolitis in small children, leading to hyperinflation of air sacs distal to bronchiole. Complete plugging of bronchiole with air resorption leads to collapse that can be life-threatening. Bronchiolitis appears in seasonal epidemics but can also be seen year round in poorer communities throughout the world. It is usually preceded by coryzal symptoms which later develop into a major pulmonary illness. Clinically there is fever, rapid respiration, exhausting cough, and wheezing.

Adenoviruses
The 49 distinct types of adenoviruses can cause a number of illnesses such as gastroenteritis, conjunctivitis, and cystitis. Epidemics of febrile disease with conjunctivitis are associated with waterborne transmission of some adenovirus types, often centering on inadequately chlorinated swimming pools and small lakes. But most commonly, adenoviruses cause respiratory illnesses ranging from the common cold to pneumonia. Unusually resistant to chemical or physical agents and adverse pH conditions, they can sustain prolonged survival outside the body. First encountered by World War 2 GI's, acute respiratory disease (ARD) may be related to a combination of adenovirus infections and conditions of crowding and stress. ARD, an epidemic form of acute pneumonic disease, can be prevented by enteric capsulation of a live vaccine strain activated in the gut.

Rhinoviruses
With more than 100 serotypes of one virus family of rhinoviruses, *Picorna,* causing half of all URI inhalational infections – the common cold, goes far to explain why colds are so readily spread by droplets from the nose and mouth. It also explains why colds are acquired simply by taking breaths in a poorly ventilated room in which there are cold carriers, who are in the first two days of infectious coryza. Though an infection resolves in about a week, it may temporarily upset the mucosal cilia and predispose to secondary invaders, especially bacterial infections, anything from sinusitis to pneumonia, which may require antibiotic treatment. A short period of immunity to all colds follows a rhinovirus cold, but a prolonged immunity forms against the specific serotype that caused the most recent infection.

Transmission of HIV/AIDS

HIV can be transmitted from an infected person to another through:
- Unprotected sexual contact. Direct blood contact, including injection drug needles, blood transfusions, accidents in health care settings or certain blood products. Mother to baby (before or during birth, or through breast milk)
- Sexual intercourse (vaginal and anal): In the genitals and the rectum, HIV may infect the mucous membranes directly or enter through cuts and sores caused during intercourse (many of which would be unnoticed).
- Oral sex (mouth-penis, mouth-vagina): The mouth is an inhospitable environment for HIV (in semen, vaginal fluid or blood), meaning the risk of HIV transmission

through the throat, gums, and oral membranes is lower than through vaginal or anal membranes. There are however, documented cases where HIV was transmitted orally.

- Sharing injection needles: An injection needle can pass blood directly from one person's bloodstream to another. It is a very efficient way to transmit a blood-borne virus.
- Mother to Child: It is possible for an HIV-infected mother to pass the virus directly before or during birth, or through breast milk.

The following "bodily fluids" are NOT infectious: Saliva, Tears, Sweat, Feces, Urine.

Multidrug-resistant microorganisms in respiratory infections

Antimicrobial resistance is found in such organisms as multidrug-resistant *Mycobacterium tuberculosis*, methicillin-resistant *Staphylococcus aureus* (MRSA), vancomycin-intermediate-resistant *S. aureus* (VISA), vancomycin-resistant enterococci (VRE), and penicillin-resistant pneumococci. Few new antibiotics to replace them are in development. Concern has been increasing over nosocomial transmission of multidrug-resistant disease, particularly in settings where persons with human immunodeficiency virus (HIV) infection are receiving care. This has led in the early 1990's to new guidelines on the isolation of patients with multidrug-resistant tuberculosis. Hospital patients with confirmed or suspected tuberculosis began to be placed in private rooms that had been reengineered to have lower, or negative, air pressure compared with surrounding areas. Ventilating systems which reduced through dilution and filtration mycobacterial contamination of air were installed; and hospital personnel replaced standard surgical masks with particulate respirators when put in contact with infectious tubercular patients.

Neisseria gonorrhoeae

Sexually transmitted neisseria gonorrhoeae, unable to survive dehydration or cool conditions, causes urethritis with dysuria and purulent discharge in the male and, in the female, most commonly infects the endocervix, from whence it produces purulent vaginal discharge and bleeding and, if not treated, can ascend to cause salpingitis (PID). This can lead to sterility, ectopic pregnancy, or Fitz-Hugh-Curtis syndrome. However, it is often asymptomatic during early infection. One outcome, ophthalmia neonatorum (a purulent conjunctivitis), in the past was passed from mother to infant but is now rare, thanks to the initiation of treatment by prophylactic erythromycin eye ointment (formerly AgNO3 solution) applied at birth. Though disseminated gonorrhoeae infections can sometimes lead to endocarditis and meningitis, more often they cause septic arthritis. As the disease is penicillin resistant, it must be countered with ceftriaxone/ spectinomycin or ciprofloxacin (though it is developing new resistance to Cipro). Chlamydia should be treated concurrently with gonorrhea using tetracycline or erythromycin.

Escherichia coli

Escherichia coli, more commonly known as *E. coli,* is a group containing four classes that cause gastroenteritis in humans, the most familiar being *Escherichia coli* serotype 0157:H7. It's a normal inhabitant of the intestines, suppressing the growth of harmful bacterial species and synthesizing vitamins. However, some varieties that have "gone bad" produce large quantities of one or more toxins causing severe damage to the lining of the intestine.

This produces hemorrhagic colitis with its severe cramping and bloody diarrhea. The illness, usually self-limited, lasts for an average of 8 days. Undercooked or raw ground beef has been behind many of the documented outbreaks, but also cited have been alfalfa sprouts, dry-cured salami, lettuce, unpasteurized fruit juices, game meat, and cheese curds. Young victims may develop hemolytic uremic syndrome (HUS); this can produce permanent loss of kidney function. HUS is combined with two other symptoms, fever and neurologic distress, to make up the condition, thrombotic thrombocytopenic purpura (TTP) having a mortality rate in the elderly as high as 50%.

Escherichia coli, the coliform bacteria most abundant in the colon and normally innocuous can, upon acquiring a virulence factor, cause enteric infections such as traveler's diarrhea. This can then lead to osmotic diarrhea by inhibiting uptake of salt. It can also cause Hemolytic uremic syndrome (HUS), making possible acute renal failure as well as urinary tract infections like cystitis and pyelonephritis, neonatal meningitis, respiratory infection, and bacteremia. *Escherichia* comes in several species:

- *Enteropathogenic escherichia coli*, a problem in developing nations, especially among children.
- *Enteroinvasive escherichia coli* has the same virulence factor as shigella, with plasmid mediated invasion and destruction of the colon.
- *Enterohemorrhagic Escherichia coli* inhabit undercooked meat and causes blood-heavy diarrhea without fever or inflammation but with severe abdominal cramps (a syndrome called hemorrhagic colitis).

Treatment of the GI symptoms brought on by *eschericina* begins with rehydration. Antibiotics are discouraged, due to the germ's resistance; urinary tract infections can be treated with Bactrim or ampicillin, and meningitis with 3rd generation cephalosporin (ceftriaxone).

Enterobacter

Important nosocomial pathogens responsible for various infections, *Enterobacter cloacae* and *Enterobacter aerogenes* rarely cause disease in a healthy individual and are seldom seen in community outbreaks. Particularly lethal among very young and very old hospitalized patients and those already suffering from serious underlying conditions, the average mortality rate is estimated at 20 to 46%, and possibly higher.
Risk factors for nosocomial *Enterobacter* species infections include:
- Extended hospitalization
- An invasive procedure within the last three days
- Treatment with antibiotics in the past month
- A central venous catheter.

For infection with nosocomial multidrug-resistant strains, specific risk factors are the recent use of broad-spectrum cephalosporins or aminoglycosides and ICU care. Certain antibiotics, particularly third-generation cephalosporins, should be avoided because resistant mutants can appear quickly, and multiple antibiotic resistances complicate management of the infection.
The source of infection may be exogenous or via colonization of the skin, gastrointestinal tract, or urinary tract.

Campylobacter jejuni

While seldom deadly, campylobacter, being the most common cause of diarrhea in the United States, is the cause of considerable misery. Of some 100,000 who contract it yearly in the USA, only about 100 die. It can sometimes occur in outbreaks, and there may be long-term consequences of infection. Some people may have arthritis following campylobacteriosis; others may develop Guillain-Barré syndrome.
This is a rare autoimmune disease that affects nerves throughout the body beginning several weeks after the diarrheal illness. Paralysis that may last several weeks usually requires intensive care. As many as 40% of Guillain-Barré syndrome cases in this country may be triggered by campylobacteriosis, usually as a result of eating or handling raw or undercooked poultry meat. An outbreak in 1988 was caused by milk that had been improperly pasteurized.

Clostridium botulinum

Foodborne botulism is a toxin that's destroyed if heated at 80°C for 10 minutes or longer. The heat-resistant spores of *Clostridium botulinum* can produce, however, a deadly neurotoxin in poorly processed foods, with most of the outbreaks reported annually in the United States (from 10 to 30) associated with home-canned foods. Occasionally, though, commercially produced foods are at fault -- canned meat products, canned vegetables, and canned seafood products being the most frequent sources. A victim must be treated immediately upon ingestion with an antitoxin; otherwise, there is an elevated chance of death. The organism and its spores occurs widely in soils as well as stream, lake, and ocean sediments, intestinal tracts of fish and mammals, and in the gills and viscera of crabs and other shellfish. It also appears in honey, which is definitively linked to infant botulism but not in any cases involving adults. Foods are not involved in the botulism sometimes found in wounds; it results when *C. botulinum* infects a wound, producing toxins which travel via the blood stream to infect other parts of the body.

Vibrio cholerae Serogroup 01

Unsanitary conditions pollute waters providing the breeding grounds for Vibrio cholerae Serogroup 01, the bacterium responsible for epidemic cholera. Cholera reported in 1991 in Peru grew to epidemic proportions, spreading north to Mexico, infecting 1,099,882 and killing 10,453. It was the only cholera epidemic in the Western Hemisphere in the 20th Century. The last major outbreak in the United States was 1911, but sporadic cases reported between 1973 and 1991 suggest that strains of the organism may now be found in the temperate coastal waters surrounding the USA. Ingested viable bacteria attach to the small intestine and produce cholera toxin. Dehydration and loss of essential electrolytes bring death. Individuals infected with cholera require rehydration, either intravenously or orally, with a solution containing sodium chloride, sodium bicarbonate, potassium chloride, and dextrose (glucose). The illness is generally self-limiting. Antibiotics such as tetracycline have been demonstrated to shorten the course of the illness.

Listeria monocytogenes

Listeriosis, caused by *Listeria monocytogenes* finds expression in encephalitis, meningitis (or meningoencephalitis), and septicemia. It is also a factor in intrauterine or cervical infections in pregnant women. (It can result in stillbirth or spontaneous abortion.) It has been associated with consuming raw or badly pasteurized milk, raw meats of all types, ice cream, and uncooked vegetables. Cheeses, raw and cooked poultry, fermented raw-meat sausages, and raw and smoked fish are thought to be other sources. It can grow in refrigerated foods. Listeriosis is effectively treated with penicillin, ampicillin, or Trimethoprim-sulfamethoxazole. Onset to GI symptoms may take more than 12 hours, whereas the time to serious forms of listeriosis may range from a few days to three weeks. At least 1,600 cases of listeriosis end in 415 deaths per year in the U.S. Overall mortality attributed to the bacillus ranges from 50% in septicemia to as high as 70% in listeric meningitis; it may go beyond 80% in perinatal/neonatal infections. For infections during pregnancy, the mother usually survives.

Giardia lamblia

Giardia lamblia is the causative agent of giardiasis, the most frequent source of non-bacterial diarrhea in North America. Ingestion of one or more protozoan cysts may bring on diarrhea within a week, though, for most bacterial illnesses, at least thousands of organisms may have to be consumed to produce illness. Illness normally lasts for 7-14 days, but there are cases of chronic infections lasting months to years. Chronic cases, both those with defined immune deficiencies and those without, are difficult to treat. Giardiasis most frequently results from drinking contaminated water, though outbreaks have been traced to food contamination, and it's impossible to rule out contaminated vegetables eaten raw as sources of infection. It is more prevalent in children, possibly because many adults seem to have a lasting immunity after infection. This organism is implicated in 25% of the cases of gastrointestinal disease and may be present asymptomatically.

Shigella

The illness caused by *Shigella* (shigellosis) accounts for less than 10% of the reported outbreaks of foodborne illness in this country, at an estimated 300,000 cases. Infants, the elderly, and the infirm are susceptible to the severest symptoms of the disease, but all humans are susceptible to some degree. Fatalities may be as high as 10-15% with some strains. Shigellosis is a very common malady suffered by individuals with acquired immune deficiency syndrome (AIDS). The organism is frequently found in water polluted with human feces. Infection, which requires as few as 10 cells, depending on age and condition of the host, is characterized by abdominal pain, cramps, diarrhea, fever, vomiting, blood, pus, or mucus in stools. The usual medium is food contamination, usually through the fecal-oral route as a result of unsanitary food handling.

Cryptosporidium parvum

Severe watery diarrhea marks intestinal cryptosporidiosis, while tracheal cryptosporidiosis has as its symptoms coughing, mild fever; and sometimes severe intestinal distress. They are both caused by a single-celled obligate intracellular parasite. Herd animals (cows, goats, sheep) and humans may be infected with the *Cryptosporidium parvum* sporocysts, which are resistant to most chemical disinfectants. Drying and the ultraviolet portion of sunlight are deadly to them. Presumably, one organism in infected food touched by a contaminated food handler can initiate an infection. Incidence is high in child day care centers where food is served. Another possible source of human infection is raw manure that has been spread over garden vegetables, but large outbreaks invariably have contaminated water supplies as their source. Up to 80% of the population has been infected with cryptosporidiosis. There is no effective treatment, and the severe watery diarrhea is often a contributor in the death of AIDS victims; invasion of the pulmonary system may also be fatal.

Entamoeba histolytica

Amebiasis (or amoebiasis), the infection caused by *E. histolytica*, can last for up to four years with no symptoms, some gastrointestinal distress, or dysentery, complete with blood and mucus. Potential complications include pain from ulcers or abscesses and, rarely, intestinal blockage. The amoeba's cysts survive, especially under moist conditions, in water and soils and on foods. They result in infections when they are swallowed; they excyst to the trophozoite stage in the digestive tract, with the possibility of other tissues being invaded. Ingestion of one viable cyst, it is thought, is enough to cause an infection. Amebiasis is transmitted primarily by fecal contamination of drinking water and foods and also through direct contact with dirty hands or objects. Because sexual contact may also transmit the disease, AIDS / ARC patients are very vulnerable. Fatalities are infrequent.

Hepatitis A Virus

Primarily transmitted person-to-person through contact through fecal contamination, hepatitis A virus (HAV) is most often found in areas of poor sanitation and overcrowding, though epidemics from contaminated food and water also occur. In the latter, water, shellfish, and salads are the most frequent sources. When contaminated foods are the source, infected workers in food processing plants and restaurants are commonly behind it. Hepatitis A has a worldwide distribution. Outbreaks are common in crowded housing projects, institutions, prisons, and military installations. Major epidemics in foreign countries occurred in 1954, 1961, and 1971. Sudden onset of fever, malaise, nausea, anorexia, abdominal discomfort, and jaundice are indicative of infection. The period of communicability extends from early in the incubation period to about a week after the development of jaundice. Most cases resolve within three weeks and there are seldom fatalities. (Hepatitis E, which has symptoms similar to Hepatitis A, has a fatality rate of 20% among pregnant women.)

Anisakis simplex and related worms

Anisakid nematodes (roundworms) are a hazard for those who consume raw or undercooked seafood, as are *Anisakis simplex* (herring worm), and *Pseudoterranova (Phocanema, Terranova) decipiens* (cod or seal worm). Reported encounters are rare in North America, typically less than 20 per year. However, it's suspected that many cases may be suffered after eating sushi or sashimi and go undetected. Symptoms appear anywhere between an hour and two weeks. Anisakids rarely reach full maturity in humans because they are generally expelled from the GI tract spontaneously within three weeks. Severe cases, while rare, are extremely painful and require surgical intervention. Should an individual cough up or manually extract a nematode after feeling a tingling or tickling sensation in the throat, he can be certain it is a definite indication of anisakiasis. In severe cases there is acute abdominal pain, much like acute appendicitis, accompanied by nausea. The larvae of *Ascaris lumbricoides*, a large roundworm and a terrestrial relative of anisakines, may sometimes also crawl up into the throat and nasal passages.

Copyright © Mometrix Media. You have been licensed one copy of this document for personal use only. Any other reproduction or redistribution is strictly prohibited. All rights reserved.

Rotaviruses

Rotaviruses, transmitted by the fecal-oral route, are spread most commonly by dirty hands. Commonly found in day care centers, pediatric and geriatric wards, and family homes, they may also be found in uncooked food contaminated by infected food handlers. Sanitary measures adequate for bacteria and parasites seem to be ineffective in controlling rotavirus; a similar incidence of infection is observed in countries with both high and low health standards. Sufferers from severe diarrhea who don't get quick access to fluid and electrolyte replacement may die; otherwise, recovery from infections is usually complete. Childhood mortality due to rotavirus is relatively low in the U.S., with an estimated 100 cases/year, but approaches nearly a million cases per year worldwide. Of childhood cases of severe diarrhea that require hospitalization, about half can be attributed to Group A rotavirus. Group B rotavirus is endemic primarily to China.

Shellfish associated toxins

Though good statistical data on the occurrence and severity of cases stemming from eating shellfish which feed upon algae that can produce a variety of toxins are largely unavailable, we know that mollusks can pass on four types of poison:
- Paralytic Shellfish Poisoning (PSP): attacks the nervous system, causing tingling, burning, numbness, drowsiness, incoherent speech, and respiratory paralysis; it comes from cockles, mussels, scallops, or clams and is the most serious.
- Diarrheic Shellfish Poisoning (DSP): derived from mussels, oysters, and scallops, leads to no more than a mild gastrointestinal disorder.
- Neurotoxic Shellfish Poisoning (NSP): from shellfish harvested along the Florida coast and the Gulf of Mexico causes dizziness, tingling, and numbness of lips, tongue, and throat, muscular pain, reversal of the sensations of hot and cold, diarrhea, and vomiting.
- Amnesic Shellfish Poisoning (ASP): from mussels, produces GI disorders and neurological problems (confusion, memory loss, disorientation, seizure, and coma). All fatalities to date have involved elderly patients.

Norwalk family of viruses

Viral gastroenteritis, more commonly known as food poisoning, has at its root a member of the Norwalk family of viruses. It is a preeminent cause of illness in the U.S. It is estimated that Norwalk viruses are behind about a third of all viral gastroenteritis cases, and the only viral illness reported to a greater extent is the common cold. Though not permanent (people can become reinfected), half the population over 18 develops immunity because it gradually increases with age. Norwalk gastroenteritis is transmitted through drinking water or foods that have been contaminated with human feces, water being the most common source of outbreaks. Eating raw or insufficiently steamed clams and oysters that come from polluted beds makes for a high risk for Norwalk virus infection. But other foods, not just shellfish, may be contaminated by food handlers. Illness usually comes on about 24 to 48 hours after eating or drinking. The disease is self-limiting, lasting between one day and 60 hours, and is mild. It's characterized by diarrhea, nausea, vomiting, and abdominal pain.

Legionnaire's Disease

At an American Legion convention in 1976, one Legionnaire after another became ill with an acute pneumonia-like illness; 34 of the 221 who were stricken died. A CDC investigation ensued to track down the cause, a bacterium they named *Legionella.* It thrived in the convention hotel's cooling tower from which the bacteria were actively pumped into the hotel through the air conditioning system. (This led to new worldwide restrictions requiring more stringent cleaning for cooling towers and large scale air conditioning systems.) Since 1977, 41 species of *Legionella* species containing 62 serogroups have been characterized; one of them, *Legionella pneumophila,* is responsible for more than 80% of Legionnaires' disease cases, and among its 13 serogroups, Serogroup 1 is responsible for 95% of these cases. The *Legionella* bacteria are widely distributed at a low concentration, flourishing in both warm and cold water, from lakes to shower heads. They cause disease only if inhaled.

Pseudomonas aeruginosa

Pseudomonas aeruginosa is an opportunistic pathogen, exploiting breaks in host defenses to initiate urinary tract infections, respiratory system infections, dermatitis, soft tissue infections, bacteremia, bone and joint infections, gastrointestinal infections, and just a whole big variety of nosocomial infections. Particularly active in patients with cancer, cystic fibrosis, severe burns, or immunosuppressed AIDS, this disease has a fatality rate of 50 percent in these patients. Accounting for 10% of all hospital-acquired infections, *Pseudomonas aeruginosa* is the fourth most commonly-isolated nosocomial pathogen. Only the antibiotics, fluoroquinolones, gentamicin, and imipenem are effective against it, and even these drugs are not effective against all strains. The futility of treating *Pseudomonas* infections with antibiotics is most dramatically illustrated in cystic fibrosis patients, virtually all of whom eventually become infected with a strain so resistant that it cannot be treated, and death is the general outcome.

Proteus mirabilis

As a cause of non-nosocomial acquired urinary tract infections, the *proteus Enterobacter* is second only to *E. coli,* but also causes wound infections, septicemia, and pneumonia, mostly in hospitalized patients by emitting *urease,* an enzyme which catalyzes the splitting of urea into ammonia and carbon dioxide. This causes the pH of urine to rise, allowing unchecked growth of the bacteria. The higher pH is also toxic to renal cells, making possible urinary stones that can make *proteus* infections chronic. Over time the stones may grow large enough to cause obstruction and renal failure. In addition, they block the free flow of urine, inhibiting one of the body's natural cleansing mechanisms. Bacteria permeating the stones reinitiate infections even after antibiotic treatment. *P. mirabilis* is generally susceptible to most antibiotics apart from tetracycline. However, some strains are resistant to first generation cephalosporins and ampicillins.

Meningitis

Neisseria bacterium causes *Neisseria meningitides,* which is transmitted by airborne droplets that bring on nasopharyngeal colonization and spread to other organs via the circulatory system. Epidemic meningitis, seen most frequently in college dormitories and military barracks, can underlie an even more serious condition, Waterhouse-Friderichsen

Syndrome. This can quickly be fatal if glucocorticoid and mineralocorticoid replacement of salts, glucose, and steroids is not begun immediately. Military recruits and college students are inoculated as a defense with capsular polysaccharides during outbreaks, while G. Rifampin is used for prophylaxis of suspected contacts. Meningitis is successfully treated with penicillin.

RCV

Infecting nearly all infants by the age of two years, respiratory syncytial virus (RSV) is the most common respiratory pathogen found in young children. Easily spread by physical contact with contaminated secretions, it can live for half an hour or more on hands, five hours on countertops, and several hours on used wipes. RSV is usually a mild respiratory illness for adults because healthy people can and do produce antibodies against the virus. But in infants and young children, RSV can cause pneumonia, inflammation of the small airways of the lungs, and croup, incidence of which is about 125,000 infants yearly with cases serious enough to be hospitalized, of whom 1-2% die. It is imperative, then, that infants with RSV in a high risk nursery be isolated from others and that special care be taken that any physical contact does not result in cross-contamination. Premature infants, immuno-compromised infants, and infants with either chronic lung disease or certain forms of heart disease are at increased risk for severe RSV disease.

Prions

Prions, though disease-producing, are not cellular organisms or viruses, being normal proteins of animal tissues that can misfold and become infectious. They are associated with a group of diseases called Transmissible Spongiform Encephalopathies (TSEs). Both the cattle disease, bovine spongiform encephalopathy (BSE), and the human disease vCJD (a variant of Creutzfeldt-Jakob disease) that results from eating infected beef, are known as "mad cow" disease and appear to be caused by the same agent. Significant numbers of vCJD cases have occurred only in the United Kingdom; isolated cases have been reported in other countries. The United Kingdom epidemic that began in 1986 and affected nearly 200,000 cattle has been waning. There is a possibility, however, that large numbers of apparently healthy persons might be incubating the disease. Though government agencies in many countries continue to implement new measures to minimize this and other associated risks, the possibility of "phantom carriers" raises concerns about iatrogenic transmission of the disease through insufficient sterilization of instruments used in surgery and medical diagnostic procedures and through blood and organ donations from unsuspected carriers.

Acinetobacter and Brucella

Acinetobacter baumannii is frequently found in the hospital environment, commonly colonizing irrigating solutions and intravenous solutions. Though capable of causing infection, it is an organism of low virulence, and most found in respiratory secretions and urine represent colonization rather than infection. *Acinetobacter* pneumonias occur in outbreaks and are usually associated with colonized respiratory support equipment or fluids. Nosocomial meningitis may occur in colonized neurosurgical patients with external ventricular drainage tubes. It has always been an organism inherently resistant to multiple antibiotics. *Brucella* is a strictly aerobic, Gram-negative coccobacillus which causes Brucellosis, a disease similar in its symptoms to influenza, though there can be chronic recurrent fever, joint pain, and fatigue. Carried by animals, it causes only incidental infections in humans. Rare in the USA (about 200 cases per year), afflicted individuals are usually treated with streptomycin or erythromycin. The disease is more common in countries that do not have good, standardized, and effective public health and domestic animal health programs.

Infection control strategies

<u>Obstetrics</u>
Infection control strategies for obstetrics comprise efforts to identify and prevent infections:
- Temperature monitoring will identify most infections for inpatients.
- Post-discharge questionnaires or telephone surveys of patients and physicians can identify potential problems.
- Preoperative shaving should be replaced with clipping and depilatories or done immediately prior to procedures.
- Glucose/blood sugar control increases resistance to infection.
- Antibiotic prophylaxis should be with 60 minutes of incision and discontinued within 24 hours to provide protection and prevent resistance.
- Central venous lines using internal jugular of femoral sites should be avoided if possible or used for short periods of time. PICCs have lower infection rates. Coated catheters and use of heparin flushes may also lower chances of infection.
- Alcohol-based hand sanitizers should be used properly before and after all patient contact.
- Nursing/breast care instruction should be provided to all maternal patients.

<u>Neurology/ spinal cord injuries</u>
Infection control strategies for neurology/ spinal cord injuries target the most common types of infection:
- Urinary tract infection: Patients should be monitored for fever and/or changes in spasms or voiding habits that may indicate infection. When possible, intermittent catheterization (sterile rather than clean in the hospital) should be used rather than continuous. Antibiotic prophylaxis has not proven to be effective but bacterial interference, colonizing of the urinary tract with nonpathogenic E. coli 83972, has shown promising results.
- Decubitus: Procedures for regular monitoring of skin condition, turning patients, and avoiding friction to prevent pressure from developing are critical. Both staff and patients must be educated about prevention and skin care and cleanliness. Nutrition and hydration must be adequate to maintain integrity of the skin.
- Respiratory infections: Proper use of ventilation equipment must be monitored. Assisted coughing, such as through respiratory therapy and postural drainage, can reduce infections. Prophylactic antibiotics are not recommended, but patients should receive immunizations for pneumonia.

<u>Oncology</u>
Infection control strategies for oncology are aimed first at preventing infections:
- Transmission-based precautions are appropriate for some patients, especially those immunocompromised.
- Handwashing and aseptic techniques are especially important for person-to-person transmission.

- Central venous line precautions include using antimicrobial/antiseptic-coated catheters, using clear dressings that do not obscure site, and observing carefully for signs of infection.
- Protective isolation with use of glove and gown barriers has proven to be effective in reducing the spread of infection but is costly and not recommended for all patients.
- Total protected environments can be difficult to provide and expensive but may be used in selected case.
- Air filtration using HEPA-filtered air can be used to maintain ultra-clean air in a patient's room. The use of particulate respirators, such as the HEPA and N95 mask, by either the patient or the staff, can help to reduce inhaled pathogens.

Cystic fibrosis

Cystic fibrosis (mucoviscidosis) is a progressive congenital disease that particularly affects the pancreas and lungs causing digestive and respiratory problems. It is caused by a genetic defect that affects sodium chloride movement in cells, including mucosal cells that line the lungs, causing the production of thick mucus that clogs the lungs and provides a rich medium for bacteria. Cystic fibrosis patients usually suffer from recurrent respiratory infections of the lower respiratory tract. The most common infective agents are *Pseudomonas aeruginosa* and *Burkholderia cepacia* complex. Patients with chronic infections serve as reservoirs for patient-to-patient transmission of infection, with proximity and duration of contact as precipitating factors. Cystic fibrosis patients should be maintained on universal and droplet precautions and placed in private rooms or cohorted with someone with the same pathogen.

Operating rooms

Strategies for preventing and controlling transmission of infection in operating rooms include:
- Preoperative surgical scrubs for 3-5 minutes and aseptic techniques at all times.
- Positive-pressure ventilation with respect to corridors and adjacent areas.
- ≥15 air exchanges per hour (ACH) with at least 3 fresh air.
- Filtering of all recirculated and fresh air though filters with 90% efficiency.
- Horizontal laminar airflow or introduction of air at ceiling and exhaust near the floor level.
- Operating room closed except to allow passage of essential equipment and staff.
- Clean visible soiling with approved disinfectants between patients.
- Wet-vacuum operating room at end of each day.
- Sterilize surgical equipment and avoid use of flash sterilization.
- Perform environmental sampling of surfaces or air as part of epidemiological investigation.
- Establish protocols for patients with airborne precautions, such as tuberculosis.

Urinary catheters

Strategies for reducing infection risks associated with urinary catheters include:
- Using aseptic technique for both straight and indwelling catheter insertion.
- Limiting catheter use by establishing protocols for use, duration, and removal, training staff, issuing reminders to physicians, using straight catheterizations rather than indwelling, using ultrasound to scan the bladder, and using condom catheters.
- Utilizing closed-drainage systems for indwelling catheters.

- Avoiding irrigation unless required for diagnosis or treatment.
- Using sampling port for specimens rather than disconnecting catheter nd tubing.
- Maintaining proper urinary flow by proper positioning, securing of tubing and drainage bag, and keeping drainage bag below the level of the bladder.
- Changing catheters only when medically-needed.
- Cleansing external meatal area gently each day, manipulating the catheter as little as possible.
- Avoid placing catheterized patients adjacent to those infected or colonized with antibiotic-resistant bacteria to reduce cross-contamination.

Short-term intravascular devices
Strategies for reducing infection risks associated with intravascular devices include:
- Site selection away from the internal jugular or femoral veins, using PICC if possible.
- Tunneled catheter or ports used if possible because of lower infection rates than non-tunneled catheters.
- TPN catheters used only for TPN and not other procedures.
- Experienced trained staff to insert intravascular devices.
- Dressings may be transparent or gauze, but insertion site should be examined frequently by palpation and dressing removed for inspection on any tenderness. Change dressings at least 1 time weekly.
- Using maximum aseptic technique for insertion.
- Catheter material of Teflon® or polyurethane, which demonstrates lower rates of infection than polyvinyl chloride or polyethylene; catheters impregnated with antimicrobials have demonstrated reduction in infections.
- Rotation of catheter sites every 72-96 hours (for adults) for short peripheral venous catheters but only as needed for others.
- Avoid antibiotic ointments at insertion site because of danger of fungal infections or resistance.

Infection in transplant patients

Infections pose a serious threat to transplant patients, especially during the first year. While opportunistic infections have decreased, nosocomial infections have increased, most related to bacterial infections. Transplant patients consistently show higher rates of infection than other patients. There are numerous potential sources:
- Donor-infected organs can transmit HBV, HBC, Herpesvirus, HIV, Human-T-cell leukemia virus, type I. Additionally, donors who are immunocompromised prior to harvesting of the organs may have nosocomial bacterial or fungal infections that can be transmitted. Organs can also become infected during harvesting.
- Healthcare workers may transmit pathogens through droplets, airborne particles, or contact, frequently transmitting pathogens on their hands or clothing.
- Blood and blood products can transmit CMV, but transmission is rare. HCV transmission has been reduced to <1%.
- Environmental reservoirs/sources can include the water system, demolition activities, equipment, and surfaces. Some pathogens, such as MRSA and VRE, may be endemic to the hospital environment.

CMV
Cytomegalovirus (CMV) is the most common pathogen related to transplant infections affecting 40-90% of recipients. There are 3 types:
- Primary infection: seropositive organ is transplanted into a seronegative recipient, posing the most risk of rejection and other complications.
- Reactivation infection: latent viral infection reactivates in response to immunosuppression.
- Superinfection: new strain of the virus infects a seropositive recipient.

Infection control strategies may vary:
- Serologic matching of donor and recipients can prevent transmission; however, the limited number of seronegative transplant organs may preclude transplant surgery for many patients.
- Early diagnosis with the CMV antigenemia assay can yield information about the degree of infection and likelihood of CMV disease.
- Targeting patients at the highest risk for disease through surveillance methods, such as monitoring with CVM antigenemia assay and instituting prophylaxis to prevent asymptomatic disease from activating, is the most practical infection control.

Time of onset for infection
Time of onset for infections is significant as an indicator of nosocomial infection in transplant patients:
- Days 1-30: Infections that arise in the early postoperative period are often surgical site infections or other nosocomial infections.
    o Bacterial infections are most common.
    o Fungal infections, especially *Candidiasis* and *Aspergillus* usually occur early.
    o Viral infections are less common but usually involve HSV or the herpesvirus, HHV-6.
- Days 31-180: Most infections during this time period are opportunistic infections rather than nosocomial because of continued immunosuppression that increases susceptibility.
    o CMV is the most common pathogen for all types of transplants.
    o HBV and HCV may reactivate about 90 days after surgery.
    o Various pathogens may cause infections, including *Mycobacterium tuberculosis and Nocardia.*
- Days 181 and onward: Infections acquired after 6 months are usually community-acquired rather than hospital-acquired although the risk of opportunistic infections remains as well. Varicella zoster virus and dematiaceous fungi infections are late infections, usually after 6 months.

HHV-6
Human herpesvirus-6 is the newest identified viral pathogen of transplant patients, infecting 31-55% of solid organ transplants with the usual onset of symptoms (bone marrow suppression, encephalopathy, fever, and pneumonia) about 2-4 weeks after transplant. HHV-6 is a DNA virus distinct from other herpesvirus but most like CMV. There are 2 variants of the disease HHV-6A and HHV-6B. HHV-6A is more virulent than HHV-6B, but at the current time HHV-6B is the most common infection. HHV-7 is a closely related virus that often co-infects, but its significance is not yet established. Most infection with

HHV-6 is endogenous from reactivation of latent virus acquired in early childhood, but primary donor transmission can also occur.
Infection control strategies include:

- Early diagnosis with culture assay.
- Antiviral medications ganciclovir and foscarnet are effective against HHV-6 infection.
- Antiviral prophylaxis with ganciclovir has been given BID for a week prior pre-stem cell transplant and 120 posts. Studies demonstrated a significant reduction in infection for those receiving prophylaxis.

HSV and VZV
Herpes simplex virus infection may occur from reactivation or primary transmission from the donor. Infection may become disseminated, most frequently affecting the liver with a high mortality rate. Infection control strategies include:

- Serologic matching can prevent primary transmission but the limited supply of organs may make this impractical.
- Antiviral prophylaxis with low dose Acyclovir (200-400 mg TID) for 1-3 months has proven very effective in preventing HSV infections.

Varicella-zoster virus infection may result in primary infection over 2 years from the time of transplant, resulting in visceral dissemination and sometimes death. This delay time may cause the symptoms to be misdiagnosed.
Infection control strategies include:

- Immunization has proven to be safe and highly effective, reducing the incidence of infection and the severity.
- VZ immunoglobulin is given to susceptible transplant patients exposed to VZV, but is not completely protective.
- High dose acyclovir during the 2-3 week incubation period may reduce incidence and severity of infection.

HCV
Hepatitis C virus causes end-stage liver disease in about half of the liver transplant patients, and 95% remain viremia after transplant, resulting in recurrence in 30-70% of patients within a year. HCV is also common in hemodialysis patients as it is a bloodborne pathogen, and 10-60% of rental transplant patients develop chronic liver disease. Co-infection with HGV occurs in about 25% without clinical impact. Most infections are reactivation, but primary transmission can occur. Infection control strategies include:

- Standard precautions prevent bloodborne transmission. Up to 10% of those with needlestick injuries develop HCV.
- Antiviral prophylaxis using HBIG developed for hepatitis B has been shown to reduce incidence of HVC viremia because it also contains some antibodies to HCV. A new investigational Hepatitis C Immune Globulin, Civacir, is currently in trials to evaluate its prevention of recurrence of HCV infection in liver transplant patients. Civacir is made from pooled blood and serum of individuals with antibodies to HCV.

HBV
Hepatitis B virus is a concern for both liver and kidney transplant patients because infection markedly increases mortality rates. HBV is transmitted in blood, semen, and vaginal fluids. Recurrence of HBV is most common in those already seropositive (about 83%) compared to

those seronegative (about 58%) at the time of transplant, but both figures are high. Mutant varieties of HBV (precore mutants) pose an even greater threat of graft loss. HBV progresses more slowly in kidney transplant patients than in liver transplant patients, with cirrhosis and death occurring in 6-8 years compared to 2-2.5 years for liver transplant patients.

Infection control strategies include:
- Standard precautions should prevent bloodborne transmission.
- Antiviral prophylaxis with Hepatitis B Immune Globulin (HBIG) has markedly reduced recurrence rates.
- Combination therapy with HBIG and lamivudine prevents recurrence disease in >90% of liver transplant patients infected with HBV.
- Hepatitis B vaccine should be provided to adults at risk, especially staff working with patients with HBV. Children are now routinely immunized.

AdV
Adenoviruses (AdV) comprise at least 49 serotypes and cause infections in up to 10% of pediatric transplant pediatric patients and 15% of adult, especially affecting those receiving bone marrow transplants. AdV can cause disseminated disease resulting in hemorrhagic cystitis (kidney transplants), hepatitis (liver transplants), conjunctivitis, and pneumonitis (lung transplants). AdV 11, 34, 35 are implicated in hemorrhagic cystitis while 2, 5, 7, and 9 are implicated in pulmonary infection, especially in children. Infection may be from seropositive donors or reactivation. Nosocomial outbreaks have occurred. A recent military study demonstrated serotypes 4 and 7 were transmitted through asymptomatic shedders via the respiratory tract. Infection control strategies include:
- Ribavirin, ganciclovir, and IgG have been tried with varying reports as to effectiveness.
- Vaccine (serotypes 4 and 7) was available to the military from the 1970s to 1990s and was successful, but the vaccine was lost. Phase I trials for a new vaccine are underway and show good results.
- Droplet precautions should be considered, especially with respiratory infection.

BKV
BK virus (BKV) has recently emerged as a cause of renal dysfunction after transplant, resulting in loss of graft. BKV is a DNA polyomavirus, and is ubiquitous, with about 80% of the population seropositive. The transmission mode is not yet established. JC virus (JCV) often co-infects and may be a cause of nephropathy as well. About 5% of kidney transplant patients develop BKV infection (hemorrhagic and non-hemorrhagic urinary infection, nephritis, increase in creatinine, and replication of decoy cells of the urinary epithelium), usually reactivation, within 3 –24 months after surgery. Diagnosis is by PCR assay. Infection control strategies include:
- Reduction in immunosuppressive medications with the addition of cidofovir (10-20% of the recommended dose of cidofovir) has been the treatment of choice with varying degrees of effectiveness.
- Leflunomide at immunosuppressive doses was shown in one study to eradicate BK virus. Other studies are ongoing or in progress.

Mycobacterium tuberculosis

Mycobacterium tuberculosis in transplant patients occurs in 0.35-5% of patients, a relatively low number, but the mortality rate for those infected is 30%. About a third of those infected develop disseminated disease involving extrapulmonary sites that include the gastrointestinal tract, the urinary tract, and the central nervous system. While most M. tuberculosis infection is reactivation of latent disease, nosocomial transmission of infection has occurred, especially if patients are undiagnosed so that airborne precautions are not used. Transmission has also occurred from living and cadaveric donor organs.

Infection control strategies include:

- Airborne precautions for diagnosed or suspected infections.
- Identifying infected patients/staff includes tuberculin skin testing followed by confirming radiography.
- Prophylaxis with Isoniazid:
    - Tuberculin reactivity $\geq$ 5mm
    - Newly-converted positive tuberculin.
    - Chest-x-ray showing old active TB with no prior treatment or inadequate treatment.
    - Close contact with infected individual.
    - Seropositive TB donor organ.

Staphylococcus aureus (MRSA) and Enterococci (VREF)

Staphylococcus aureus is the most common cause of bacterial infection in liver, heart, kidney, and pancreas transplant patients with >50% of infections occurring in the ICU. Intravascular cannulas cause about 54% of MRSA infections, but nosocomial transmission occurs. While nasal colonization has been implicated in infection in liver transplant patients, using mupirocin to eradicate nasal colonization has not affected infection rates, probably because of nosocomial transmission with exogenous colonization. Isolate studies have demonstrated nosocomial cross-transmission. Enterococci are a primary concern for liver transplant patients. Vancomycin-resistant *Enterococcus faecium* (VREF) cause 10-15% of liver failures, according to recent studies. Nosocomial transmission occurs frequently, especially with prolonged hospitalization and ICU stay. Intra-abdominal infections occur about 40 days after surgery with mortality rates of 23-50%. VREF colonization puts patients at continued risk for infection and poses a reservoir for nosocomial infections. Antibiotics have been ineffective in reducing mortality rates.

Nocardia

Nocardia infections occur in about 2-4% of organ transplant recipients with onset from 2-8 months after surgery with pulmonary infection common but 17-38% of those infected have central nervous system involvement which often includes brain abscesses. Lung, heart, and intestinal transplants have the highest rates of infection. Mortality rates are high for those who are infected. *Nocardia* is found in the soil and decaying vegetation, and transmission is through inhalation. Some species are more virulent than others. Nosocomial infections have occurred in clusters in transplant units related to environmental dust. Risk factors include high dose cortisone, high levels of calcineurin inhibitors (cyclosporine and tacrolimus), and CMV infection within 6 months. Calcineurin inhibitors are commonly used for immunosuppression for kidney transplants.

Infection control strategies include:
- Environmental monitoring
- Antibiotic prophylaxis with trimethoprim-sulfa-methoxazole is effective.
- Airborne precautions of those infected have been recommended by some.

Legionella

Legionella pneumonia occurs in 2-9% of solid organ recipients with *Legionella pneumophila* and *Legionella micdadei* the most common forms. Some studies have reported incidence as high as 17% in heart transplant patients. Inhalation of aerosols may transmit the disease but aspiration of the bacteria occurs more frequently. *Legionella* has been traced to potable water systems providing hospital drinking water, ice machines, and ultrasonic nebulizers. Patients may develop pneumonia with or without characteristic dense nodular areas and cavitation, pericarditis, necrotizing cellulitis, and graft rejection.

Infection control strategies include:
- Routine annual culturing of water supply to check for *Legionella,* especially important if there are large numbers of transplant patients.
- Positive water culture should result in the laboratory having diagnostic tests, such as urinary antigen, available.
- Early diagnosis of high-risk patients should be done by routine urinary antigen testing up to 2 times weekly.
- Water disinfecting methods:
  - Superheating water to 70° C and flushing distal outlets.
  - Installing copper-silver ionization units.

Candidiasis

Candidiasis is the most common fungal infection in transplant patients, with the exception of heart transplants. While some infections are mild, thrush and cystitis, others are invasive and life threatening, especially with the immunocompromised patient. Infection of all organs is about 5%, but liver and pancreas transplant patients have infection rates of 15-30%. Infection may occur in the surgical site or be disseminated, posing a serious threat to the site of anastomosis. Almost all transmission of Candida is nosocomial. Endogenous transmission is common in liver transplants, but heart and lung transplants are often infected from the donor organs. Some cases have been traced to contaminated medical equipment. Infection control strategies include:
- Antiviral prophylaxis with 1-2 months of fluconazole post-transplant is used at some centers, but azole-resistant strains are appearing, and there is an associated increase in *aspergillus*, so prophylaxis may be considered for only high-risk patients.
- Monitoring of invasive devices to ensure that they are not contaminated with *candida*.

Aspergillus

Aspergillus infections primarily involve pneumonia and sinusitis, but 25-35% disseminate systemically, and *Aspergillus* pneumonia infections have mortality rates to 85%. *Aspergillus* is a serious fungal infection in immunocompromised transplant patients, especially lung transplant patients with 8% infection rates within 9 months of surgery. Liver transplant patients have infection rates of 1-4% but disease occurs earlier, within 2-4 weeks. Heart transplant infection rates are 1-6% with disease within 1-2 months. Aspergillus affects renal transplants the least with <1% infection rates. Prophylaxis with antifungals has not proven to be effective.

Infection control strategies include:

- Monitoring environment and improving air filtration with HEPA filtration or use of laminar air flow rooms for patients at high risk.
- Construction precautions to prevent dust and debris from circulating in patient care areas.
- Standard precautions
- High resolution CT scans should be used for early diagnosis rather than chest x-rays so treatment with voriconazole (drug of choice) can begin.

Pneumocystis jiroveci

Pneumocystis jiroveci (formerly *carinii*) was classified for many years as a Protozoan, but DNA analysis has caused it to be reclassified as a fungus, but it does not respond to antifungal treatment. The variety that causes *Pneumocystis* pneumonia, commonly referred to as PCP, has been renamed as *Pneumocystis jiroveci*. While most infection is thought to be endogenous, there is sufficient evidence that person-to-person transmission has occurred in nosocomial outbreaks affecting transplant patients in contact with PCP infected HIV patients. While renal, heart, and liver transplant patients are vulnerable to *Pneumocystis,* without prophylaxis 80% of lung transplants become infected, with infection usually occurring 4 months after surgery although the length of time varies depending upon the degree of immunosuppression.

Infection control strategies include:

- Transmission precautions to separate PCP-infected patients from contact with transplant patients.
- Prophylaxis with trimethoprim-sulfa-meth oxazole should be given to all transplant patients. There is not consensus on the length of prophylaxis with durations varying from 6-12 months to indefinite.

Burn infections

Burn wound cellulitis

Burn patients are at exceptional risk for infection because the barrier of protective skin is breached, eschar provides a medium for microorganisms, and immunosuppression occurs. Classifying burn infections can be done in different ways. NNIS/CDC proposed a classification system for unexcised burns, but with early excision this system often does not apply. A newer system classifies burn infections by 4 types: cellulitis, invasive infection in unexcised burns, impetigo, and open burn-related surgical wound infection.

Burn wound cellulitis is characterized by erythema of uninjured tissue around burns that is more than the usual irritation and includes one of the following:

- Pain, tenderness and edema.
- Systemic signs of infection.
- Progressive erythema and edema.
- Lymphangitis/lymphadenitis.

This type of infection usually suggests a need for different antimicrobial treatment. When the erythema spreads beyond 1-2 cm from the burn, it may be indicative of infection with β-hemolytic *Streptococcus.*

Burn wound impetigo

Burn wound impetigo is an infection of previously healing and re-epithelialized partial-thickness burns, skin grafts, or donor sites. One important criterion for burn wound impetigo is that the deterioration is not caused by mechanical disruption of the tissue or by a failure to completely excise the wound but by an invading organism. Burn wound impetigo can occur with or without indications of systemic infection, such as temperature >38.4°C, leukocytosis, and/or thrombocytopenia, may be present as well. The wound may develop multiple small superficial abscesses that infect and erode the tissue. The most common cause of burn wound impetigo is *Staphylococcus aureus.* Prompt debridement of the abscesses, cleansing of the area, and application of topical antimicrobials, such as Bactroban®, must be done in order to stop the spread of the infection. A change in antimicrobial treatment may be necessary as well.

Common reservoirs for organisms

There are a number of reservoirs for organisms that infect burns. Many of these reservoirs can serve as sources for transmission on the hands of healthcare workers:

- Burn wounds are colonized within the first few hours by Gram-positive organisms from sweat glands and hair follicles and within days by Gram-negative organisms, so collectively the burn wounds of all patients on the unit may harbor organisms that can spread from one patient to another.
- Gastrointestinal tract flora can contaminate burn wounds directly if wounds are in proximity to fecal material or indirectly through cross contamination.
- Normal flora, especially Gram-positive cocci, on the skin are the cause of early burn infections and an increasingly important reservoir, with nasal colonization often implicated in burn infections.
- Environment can harbor organisms on many inanimate surfaces. Hydrotherapy equipment has been a frequent cause of wound infection as contaminated equipment spreads the infection to subsequent patients being treated.

Preventing and controlling transmission of infection

Strategies for preventing and controlling transmission of infection in burn units include the following:

- Handwashing and sanitizing before and after every patient contact.
- Barriers such as gloves and water-impermeable aprons or gowns to reduce contact transmission.
- Environmental controls include providing patients with individual equipment, such as stethoscopes and blood pressure cuffs, and thorough cleaning and disinfecting of all surfaces. Mattress covers should be checked. Gloves should be worn to use computers and keyboard covers cleaned daily.
- Raw fruits and vegetables should not be fed to patients or allowed to contaminate kitchen utensils.
- Surveillance of all burn patients that might serve as reservoirs of infection, including convalescent patients no longer in acute care.
- Use of topical antimicrobials, such as silver sulfadiazine, to control infection, but with testing of outbreak strains for resistance.
- Protocol for systemic antimicrobial to treat active infection but avoid development of resistance.
- Early wound excision and closure to reduce wound infection.

Issues related to hydrotherapy

Hydrotherapy has been used in burn treatment but implicated in a number of nosocomial outbreaks, primarily of *Pseudomonas aeruginosa*. In some cases, rigorous cleaning protocols have reduced infection; in others, suspension of hydrotherapy treatments was needed. Because of problems with infection, there has been decrease in the use of hydrotherapy. Methods to control transmission of infection include:

- Protocol for draining tub after use and cleaning and disinfecting all parts of the hydrotherapy tub and agitators, with a chlorine germicidal agent circulated through agitators. Tank to be rinsed and dried thoroughly.
- Environmental cleaning and disinfecting of complete area and transportation equipment.
- Disinfectant may be added to filled tank.
- Disposable plastic liners, shown to reduce but not eliminate infection.
- Barriers such as long gloves and aprons or gowns impervious to fluid to prevent contact with water or patient.
- Faucets without stream diverters or aerators, which might harbor organisms, flushed with hot and cold water before use.

Initiating and discontinuing special protective environment isolation

While isolation is usually intended to protect others from an infected patient, protective environments (PE) are usually used to protect a severely immunocompromised patient. Most often, protective environments are provided in specialized hospital units, such as those for stem-cell transplant. Patients who are identified by diagnosis should be placed immediately in the protective environment and maintained in the environment until immune or clinical status improves. Protective environments include:

- Placing patient in a private room (or room shared by cohort) with positive airflow from the room to the outside so that contamination from the hallway or other rooms is avoided. ACH is ≥ 12 and HEPA filtration is used to prevent contamination.
- Gown and gloves are used to reduce transmission of pathogens, but mask is not needed unless the patient is also on droplet precautions.
- One to one nursing should be utilized.
- Patient should leave room only if medically necessary and in clean linens with face mask if necessary and 2-person transport.

Initiating and discontinuing isolation for airborne infection

Airborne infection isolation should be initiated with suspicion or confirmation of a diagnosis of disease that has airborne transmission, such as varicella-zoster virus (VZV), measles, variola (smallpox), and tuberculosis, with droplet size <5μm, or patients with multiple drug-resistant strains of organisms. Isolation should be continued until confirmation that patient is not infective. Isolation procedures include:

- Placing patient in a private room with ≥ 12 air exchanges per hour (ACH) under negative pressure with air from the outside in and exhaust, preferably, to the outdoors, or recirculation provided through high-efficiency particulate air (HEPA) filters.
- Door to the room should remain closed and sign or color/coding should be used at door to alert medical staff to isolation.

- Respirator use for personnel entering room when indicated because of disease transmission (TB and smallpox) or lack of immunity (measles, VZV).
- Patient transported in clean linens and wearing a facemask.
- Procedures done in the room whenever possible.

Infection control and transfer/discharge planning

Infection control and transfer/discharge planning must be a joint effort so that the transfer and discharge documents provide the information that the individual or staff at transfer facilities need. Information should include:
- Contact telephone numbers/email addresses/street addresses for IPC to contact patient for discharge surveillance and patient or transfer facility staff to contact IPC if problems arise.
- An outline of risk factors for infection incurred during hospital stay, including stay in ICU or specialized units and use of invasive devices, such as central venous lines, ventilators, and/or urinary catheters.
- Information sheets outlining signs of infection for all risk factors, especially if patient is discharged home without nursing care.
- Public Health notification if indicated by local or state regulations.
- Follow-up appointment dates, with physicians or infection control.
- Specific directions for medication or treatments, especially important for antibiotics or wound treatment.

Infection control for medical wastes

Medical waste management is mandated by Federal and state laws, which require that certain types of medical waste be separated from others. This regulated medical waste (RMW) is eventually packaged, transported, and disposed of according to specific regulations for the type of waste material. Separate trash containers, lined with red plastic bags or containers and labeled as "Biohazard," must be provided for RMW, which includes:
- Sharps include needles, syringes, small vials, pins, probes, and lancets.
- Blood and body fluid contaminated material that can drip fluid: sponges, specimen containers, drainage bags (such as Hemovacs), and contaminated tubing.
- CDC Bio-safety Class 4- associated waste, such as those related to Marburg hemorrhagic fever.
- Laboratory materials, including cultures, infectious agents, and contaminated materials.
- Animal waste related to medical research.
- Human tissue includes body parts removed during surgery or autopsy.
- Chemotherapy waste containing over 3% antineoplastic drugs.

Sharps disposal
Injuries, especially needle-sticks, related to medical instruments such as scalpels and needles (sharps), are very common but pose a serious risk of infection. Care should always be used when sharp instruments or needles, and assistance should be obtained when using sharps with people who are confused or uncooperative, increasing the chance of injury. The following guidelines should be used:
- A special sealed sharps container should be available in every room where treatment is done (patients rooms, clinics, operating rooms).

- Disposable needles should not be removed, recapped, or touched but deposited immediately into the sharps container. If recapping cannot be avoided, the scooping method of recapping using only one hand must be used.
- The sharps container must be checked daily and removed for disposal when about 3/4 full and a new container provided.
- Any non-disposable sharps must be placed in a covered container that is leak and puncture proof and returned to the central supply department for cleaning and sterilization.

Fit testing of respirators

Respirators that are not properly fitting will not provide adequate protection against airborne particles. Fitting must be done prior to use for anyone who will use a respirator. OSHA has established guidelines for fitting and use of respirators. The staff must be tested with the same make, model, and size of respirator they will use. Numerous factors can affect seal: facial hair, makeup, bone structure, scars, and dentures. Sensitivity testing involves placing the subject's head into a hood and then squeezing a test solution of saccharine or denatonium benzoate into the hood in increments to determine when the subject can taste the solution. The qualitative fit test involves wearing the respirator for 5 minutes; then, the hood is placed over it and the test solution is squeezed into the hood to determine if the respirator fits tightly enough to prevent the subject from tasting the solution. Exercise, such as talking, moving, bending, and jogging must be done to check security of seal.

Emerging infectious diseases

SARS
Severe Acute Respiratory Syndrome (SARS) is caused by a corona virus (Co-V) and presents as a respiratory illness with fever, cough, dyspnea, and general malaise is extremely virulent, spreading easily from person to person through close contact by way of contaminated droplets produced by coughing or sneezing. SARS has a high mortality rate. Some possibility exists that SARS may also have airborne transmission in some cases with aerosol-producing procedures. High rates of infection have occurred in healthcare workers and others in contact with infected patients, so prompt diagnosis and proper isolation are essential.
Precautions:
- Contact and droplet precautions, including eye protection and appropriate personal protection equipment.
- Airborne precautions (recommended by the CDC), especially with aerosol-producing procedures (ventilators, nebulizers, intubation).
- Immediate notification of public health authorities and institution of contact tracing.
- Activity restrictions of exposed health care workers planned in coordination with public health officials.

Pandemic influenza
Pandemic influenza is a worldwide epidemic of influenza that causes serious respiratory illness and/or death in large populations of people. Pandemics can occur when a virus mutates, creating a new subtype that infects humans and spreads easily from person to person. The influenza of most concern recently has been avian flu, which primarily affects birds, but has infected other animals, including humans, primarily those in contact with

infected flocks. There are a number of subtypes of avian flu and symptoms may range from typical influenza-like respiratory infections to severe pneumonia. Should a further mutation occur and a pandemic occur, the implications for health care are profound because of the potential number of infected patients overwhelming the medical system. Precautions:

- Standard precautions with careful hand hygiene.
- Contact precautions with gloves and gown for all patient contact and goggles when within 3 feet.
- Dedicated equipment.
- Airborne precautions in isolated negative pressure rooms and use of N-95 filter respirator.

Medical maggots

Medical use of maggots is slowly regaining acceptance since FDA approval in 2004 as a medical device for wound debridement. Used extensively before the introduction of antibiotics, they fell out of favor, but maggots eat infected or necrotic tissue, cleaning the wound effectively and stimulating new tissue. The eggs are sterilized so the maggots do not transmit infection unless they become contaminated so careful handling is critical. They arrive in a sterile container, which should be examined to be sure it's intact. The maggots should be used right away, following prescribed procedures. Maggots excrete enzymes that can be very irritating to healthy tissue if too many are applied or if they are left in place for too long. Maggots are left in the wound for 48 hours and then must be carefully collected and disposed of in a red plastic biohazard bag tied and placed inside another bag to ensure that none escape and exposed of as hazardous waste.

Medical leeches

In 2004, the FDA approved medical leeches as a medical "device" to relieve venous congestion, especially in skin grafts and reattachment/reimplantation. *Hirudo medicinalis* is about 1-2 inches long before feeding. It has 3 jaws and bites into the tissue with teeth, which are surrounded by an oral sucker that aids attachment along with the rear ventral sucker. The teeth leave a bite mark. Leeches must be maintained in non-chlorinated water before use. While feeding, they will swell with about 15 ml of blood and then drop off after feeding. The wound will continue to bleed slowly, forming new venules. The leech should be retrieved with tweezers and immediately placed in a container of 70% alcohol and disposed of as medical waste. *Aeromonas hydrophila* lives in the gut of the leech and is necessary for the leeching function, but approximately 20% of patients develop infection, so prophylactic antibiotics are often given with treatment, especially for the immunocompromised.

Infection implications of products and durable medical equipment

Oxygen equipment
Oxygen equipment can easily become contaminated and implicated in nosocomial infections. Control includes:

- Use standard precautions, including washing hands and wearing gloves when working with oxygen equipment to avoid spreading contamination.
- Avoid humidification when possible. Flow rates of 1-4 l/m per mask or nasal cannula allow for adequate humidification from the respiratory tract, but higher

flow rates or flow directly to a trachea requires humidification. In-line fine particle nebulizers have become contaminated when oxygen is mixed with ambient air from an oxygen wall outlet.
- Decondensate any tubing as needed.
- Use only sterile solutions for humidification or inhalation.
- Use disposable equipment (regulators, masks, tubing, humidifiers) and replace according to manufacturer's directions. Equipment should never be shared among patients. Nasal cannulas and facemasks should be cleaned regularly as replaced scheduled intervals.
- Store oxygen cylinders (green tanks) properly in upright position and only in areas that are designated as clean.

Wheelchairs and walkers
Wheelchairs are ubiquitous in the healthcare facility and often are used to transport many different patients between various units in the hospital without intervening cleaning or disinfection. However, they may become contaminated with urine, feces, and food. Organisms on the hands can be easily transmitted to the arms of the chairs or walkers and then to the next occupant. Walkers, while often dedicated to one patient, pose a similar danger if used for multiple patients. Control of transmission should include:
- Barriers for transportation, such as a clean sheet between the patient and the wheelchair with waterproof disposable pads if necessary to protect against urine, feces, blood, or other discharge.
- Inspection after use should be done each time and if soiled, it should be immediately removed from service, washed, and disinfected with an approved EPA disinfectant.
- Scheduled cleaning should be done on a regular basis for all wheelchairs and walkers in use, including either manual cleaning and disinfecting or use of automated cleaning and infection control systems.

Bioterrorism

The ICP and the infection control team should develop specific plans for dealing with different bioterrorism agents and training should be provided to staff. An organized approach should include the following:
- Be on the alert for possible bioterrorism-related infections, based on clusters of patients or symptoms.
- Use personal protection equipment, including respirators when indicated.
- Complete thorough assessment of patient, including medical history, physical examination, immunization record, and travel history.
- Provide a probable diagnosis based on symptoms and lab findings, including cultures.
- Provide treatment, including prophylaxis while waiting for laboratory findings.
- Use transmission precautions as well as isolation for suspected biologic agents.
- Notify local, state, and federal authorities as per established protocol.
- Conduct surveillance and epidemiological studies to identify at risk populations.
- Develop plans to accommodate large numbers of patients:
- Restricting elective admissions.
- Transferring patients to other facilities.

Biological weapons

Anthrax

There are a number of different infections that could be part of a bioterrorism attack. The type of barrier/isolation needed is dependent upon the symptoms and the mode of transmission. Knowledge of typical presenting symptoms and prompt precautions are essential to prevent spread of disease. Anthrax (*Bacillus anthracis*) usually occurs from contact with animals, but as a bioterrorism weapon, anthrax would most likely be aerosolized and inhaled. It is not transferred from person to person. There are 3 types:

- Inhalation: fever, cough, fever, shortness of breath, and general debility
- Cutaneous: small non-painful sores that blister and ulcerate with necrosis at the center.
- Gastrointestinal: nausea, vomiting, diarrhea, and abdominal pain.

The inhaled form of anthrax is the most severe with about a 50% mortality rate. The vaccine for anthrax is not yet available to the public.

Precautions:

- Prophylaxis with antibiotics after exposure.
- Standard precautions
- Contact precautions for wounds if there are cutaneous lesions.

Pneumonic plague

Yersinia pestis causes pneumonic plague, which is normally carried by fleas from infected rats but can be aerosolized to use as a biologic weapon. There are 3 forms of plague, but they sometimes occur together and bubonic and septicemic plague can develop into pneumonic, which is the primary concern related to bioterrorism:

- Bubonic occurs when a person is bitten by an infected flea.
- Pneumonic occurs with inhalation and results in pneumonia with fever, headache, cough, and progressive respiratory failure.
- Septicemic occurs when Y. pestis invades the bloodstream, often after initial bubonic or pneumonic plague.

Pneumonic plague can spread easily from person to person. There is no vaccine available.

Precautions:

- Immediate antibiotics within first 24 hours are necessary, so early diagnosis is critical.
- Prophylaxis with antibiotics may protect those exposed.
- Droplet precautions should be used with appropriate barriers, such as surgical mask.

Botulism

Clostridium botulinum produces an extremely poisonous toxin that causes botulism. The organism can be aerosolized or used to infect food. There are 3 primary forms of botulisms:

- Food borne botulism results from contamination of food. This type poses the greatest threat from bioterrorism. Symptoms usually appear 12-36 hours after ingestion but may be delayed for 2 weeks and include nausea, vomiting, dyspnea, dysphagia, slurred speech, progressive weakness and paralysis
- Infant botulism results from C. botulinum ingested into the intestinal tract. Constipation, poor feeding, and progressive weakness are presenting symptoms.

- Wound botulism results from contamination of open skin, but symptoms are similar to food borne botulism.

Botulism is not transmitted from person to person, but contaminated food has the potential to infect many people, especially if the contaminated food is manufactured and widely distributed.

Precautions:
- Antitoxin after exposure and as early in disease as possible.
- Standard precautions.

Tularemia

Francisella tularensis causes tularemia, which is usually transmitted from small mammals to humans through insect bites, ingestion of contaminated food or water, inhalation, or handling of infected animals. Although there is no evidence of person-to-person transmission, *F. tularensis* has the potential to be aerosolized for use as in bioterrorism because it is highly infective and requires only about 10 organisms to infect. Flu-like symptoms appear in 3-5 days after exposure and progress to severe respiratory infection and pneumonia. A vaccine for laboratory workers was available until recently, but the FDA is reviewing it at present, so there is no vaccine available now. Prophylaxis with antibiotics within 24 hours may prevent disease. Standard precautions are sufficient. Biologic safety measures should be used for laboratory specimens. Autopsy procedures that may cause tissue to be aerosolized should be avoided.

Smallpox

The variola virus causes smallpox, which has been eradicated worldwide since 1980, but has the potential for use as a biological weapon because people are no longer vaccinated. Smallpox is extremely contagious and has a high mortality rate (about 30%). Flu-like symptoms appear about 7-17 days after exposure with fever, weakness, vomiting and rash that begins on the face and arms and spreads. The rash becomes pustular, crusts, scabs over and then sloughs off, leaving scars. People remain infective from the first rash until all scabs are gone. The disease can spread through contact with infective fluid from lesions or from contact with clothes or bedding. Aerosol spread is theoretically possible. Precautions:
- Vaccination must be done before symptoms appear and as soon as possible after exposure as vaccination after rash appears will not affect the severity of the disease.
- Maximum precautions should be used, which includes the use of gowns and gloves to enter the room and keeping the patient in a patient or cohorted room.

Viral hemorrhagic fevers

Viral hemorrhagic fevers are zoonoses (spread from animals to humans) and comprise a number of different diseases: Ebola, Lassa, Marburg, yellow, Argentine and Crimean-Congo. Some hemorrhagic fevers can spread person to person, notably Ebola, Marburg, and Lassa through close contact with body fluids or items contaminated. Hemorrhagic fevers are extremely contagious multi-system diseases, and those in contact with infected patients are at risk of infection   Symptoms vary somewhat according to the disease but present with flu-like symptoms that progress to bleeding under the skin and internally, and some people develop kidney failure and central nervous system symptoms, such as coma and seizures. Treatment is supportive although ribavirin has been used to treat Crimean-Congo hemorrhagic fever. Mortality rates are high. Only yellow fever and Argentine have vaccines. Precautions: Maximum precautions must be used with full barrier precautions, with care used in any handling of blood and body fluids or wastes.

Risk factors of falls and restraints

Falls

The following are some risk factors along with prevention for falls:
- Orthostatic hypotension: Rise and move slowly; stand in place for several seconds; walk short distance
- Urinary frequency or incontinence: bedside commode; assist
- Weakness: disease process or therapy; call for help; monitor tolerance
- Current medications: sedatives, hypnotics, tranquilizers, narcotic analgesics, diuretics; bed in low position, side rail up on one side or half rails maintained. Monitoring devices: use if available

Restraints
- Must have a physician's order to apply restraints in acute care and long-term care.
- Must know correct application of restraints.
- Must follow policy and procedure of the health care facility.
- Can be delegated to non-licensed personnel; however, nurse is responsible for monitoring.
- Restraints are a major issue with JCAHO.

R.A.C.E.

The (NFPA/OSHA fire safety) R.A.C.E. acronym is as follows:
- Rescue
- Activate alarm
- Confine the fire
- Evacuate/Extinguish (NFPA/OSHA fire safety)

Pharmacological order taking

The nurse should check any orders that are written or given verbally for errors in dose, medication, and route as these errors can prove fatal to the client. The nurse should know the five rights: right patient, right dose, right medication, right route, and right time of administration. Nurses need to be aware of look-alike and sound-alike medications. Often time's abbreviations and symbols are misinterpreted. Facilities and institutions are now beginning to be required by accrediting bodies to have uniform abbreviations and symbols. It is the nurse's responsibility to be sure the orders are transcribed correctly; this is a criminal negligent act upon the part of the nurse if not done. The nurse is responsible to confirm the order with the practitioner prescribing by method of phone. The nurse should know the normal parameters of dose to be able to safely administer medications to clients.

Health Promotion and Maintenance

Freud, Erikson, and Piaget

<u>Freud</u>
All human behavior is energized by psychodynamic forces of
- Id: The unconscious mind—"Pleasure and gratification"
- Ego: Conscious mind—"The reality principle"
- Superego: Conscience/moral arbitrator—"The ideal"

<u>Erik Erikson's Stages of Psychosocial Development</u>
- Trust vs. Mistrust (birth to 1 yr)
- Autonomy vs. Shame and doubt (1 to 3 yrs)
- Initiative vs. Guilt (3 to 6 yrs)
- Industry vs. Inferiority (6 to 12 yrs)
- Identity vs. Role confusion (12 to 18 yrs)

<u>Jean Piaget's Stages of Cognitive Development</u>
- Intuitive (the stars have to go to bed just as they do)
- Concrete operational (conservation- realize that physical factors remain the same even if outside appearance changes)
- Formal operational (think in abstract terms such as; if A is larger than B, and B is larger than C, which is the largest?)

<u>Jean Piaget's Development of Logical Thinking</u>
- Sensorimotor (birth to 2 yrs)
- Pre-operational (2 to 7 yrs)
- Concrete operations (7 to 11 yrs)
- Formal operations (11 to 15 yrs)

Erikson's psychosocial theory

The 8 stages of Erik Erikson's psychosocial theory are as follows:
- Oral-Sensory, Birth to 12 to 18 months, Trust vs. Mistrust
- Muscular-Anal, 18 months to 3 years, Autonomy vs. Shame/Doubt
- Locomotor, 3 to 6 years, Initiative vs. Guilt
- Latency, 6 to 12 years, Industry vs. Inferiority
- Adolescence, 12 to 18 years, Identity vs. Role Confusion
- Young Adulthood, 19 to 40 years, Intimacy vs. Isolation
- Middle Adulthood, 40 to 65 years, Generativity vs. Stagnation
- Maturity, 65 to Death, Ego Integrity vs. Despair

Infancy

<u>Theorists and theories of development</u>
According to Freud and the Psychosocial Theory of Development the infant is in the oral stage of development. The infant in the oral stage of development gains pleasure from eating, sucking, rooting, and biting, and is impulse dominated.

Erikson: Erikson's Psychosocial Theory of Development states that the infant is developing trust v/s mistrust (meeting the needs of the infant is how this trust is developed). The infant is learning they are their own identity separate from the mother, and accepts that the mother will return upon absence.

Piaget: Piaget's theory of Cognitive Development places the infant in the sensorimotor stage of development, and determines the infant to have egocentric thought processes.

<u>Gross motor development</u>
Gross motor development is the development of large muscle coordination. At age two months the infant will be able to move from side to back, lift head and chest while lying in a prone position, follow objects both vertically and horizontally. At age 3 to 4 months the infant will be able to turn from back to side, balance head while in an erect position, and follow objects at 180 degree angles. At age 5 to 6 months the infant will be able to roll from abdomen to back and then back to abdomen. At seven to eight months the infant will begin to crawl, and begin to pull self into a sitting position. During months nine and ten the infant should be able to stand holding onto objects, stand alone for seconds, and pull self into an upright position. The infant will begin to ambulate around the eleventh and twelfth month, and can return to a sitting position.

<u>Language development</u>
At 2 months the infant will make noises in his/her throat, and have a variation of cries depending upon the situation. At age 3 or 4 months the infant will laugh out loud, respond with coos and gurgles when spoken to, vocalize with a familiar voice, and be able to pronounce consonants such as n, k, g, p, and b. During age five or six months the infant will begin to make vowel sounds such as ah, eh, and uh, and vocalize syllables that may be well defined. At seven to eight months the infant will begin to make sounds such as da, and ba, will imitate sounds, combine syllables, and make consonant sounds such as t, d, and w. An infant age nine and ten months will say mama or dada and realize who they are speaking of, will have a vocabulary of approximately 3 to 5 words, understand bye, and may begin to respond to simple one step commands. At age eleven and twelve months the infant will have a 5+ word vocabulary, and will begin to imitate animal sounds.

<u>Fine and gross motor development</u>
The basics of fine and gross motor development in the 0-12 months timeframe are as follows:
- Fine Motor Development:
  - Grasping object—age 2-3 months
  - Transfer object between hands—age 7 months
  - Pincer grasp age—10 months
  - Remove objects from container—age 11 months
  - Build tower of two blocks—age 12 months

- Gross Motor Development
    - Head control
    - Rolling over—5-6 months age
    - Sit alone—age 7 months
    - Move from prone to sitting position—age 10 months
- Locomotion
    - Cephalocaudal direction of development
    - Crawling age—6-7 months
    - Creeping age—9 months
    - Walk with assistance—11 months
    - Walk alone—12 months

Fine motor development

Fine motor development consists of skills that take precise direction and action of the muscles. At two months of age the hands of an infant are open often; this demonstrates a natural fading of the grasp reflex. At 3 or 4 months the infant will be able to hold onto objects that are placed into the hand (rattles/toys), grasp with both hands, begin to reach out for objects, plays with his/her own hands, and will begin to bring objects to his or her mouth. During months five or six the infant uses a palmer grasp, plays with his or her feet, can retrieve a dropped object, and can hold his or her own bottle. At seven and/or eight months the infant will begin to transfer objects from hand to hand, and use the pincer grasp. At age nine and ten months the infant will show a preference for a dominant hand, and begin showing signs of hand release. At age eleven or twelve months the infant will begin to hold and mark with a crayon, pencil or marker, and begin to eat finger foods.

Personal social development

At age 2 months the infant will have a social smile. The infant is able to recognize his/her mother at age 3 to 4 months, as well as anticipate feeding, and initiate social play activities. At age five and six months the infant will reach to be picked up, fuss to get attention, smile in the mirror at him/her self, and show definite likes and dislikes. At age seven and eight months the infant will experience and show stranger anxiety, play games such s peek-a-boo, and respond to his or her own name. At nine and ten months the infant will wave goodbye, and play games such as pat-a-cake. During month eleven and twelve the infant will demonstrate fear, anxiety, anger, affection, sympathy and jealousy, enjoy being the center of attention, and give kisses upon request, and shake his/her head for no.

Vision development

Vision development during the 0-12 months time frame is as follows:
- Birth to four months: When they're born, babies can see patterns of light and dark and shades of gray. Because newborns can only focus eight to twelve inches, much of their vision is blurred.
- Four to six months: As babies learn to push themselves up, roll over, sit, and scoot, eye/body coordination develops as they learn to control their own movements in space. Normal visual acuities, or a child's sharpness of vision, has usually developed to 20/20 by the time the child reaches six months.

- Six to eight months: Most babies start crawling during this time, further developing eye/body coordination. They learn to judge distances and set visual goals, seeing something and moving to get it.
- Eight to twelve months: Babies can now judge distances well. Eye/hand/body coordination allows them to grasp and throw objects fairly accurately.

Toddler years

Theorists and theories of development
Freud's Psychosexual Theory of Development. Freud believed a child age 12 to 36 is in the anal stage of development, will display principles of reality, and have a distinct id and ego. Freud also discusses the ability of the toddler to be in control of his or her own situation and environment by controlling his or her impulses. Pleasure comes from letting go and holding on.

Erikson's Psychosocial Theory of Development discusses the toddler's sense of autonomy vs. shame and doubt. The child at this age is able to handle demands the parent places on them such as toileting, nap time, and limits to behavior. At this stage the child is undecided about his/her parent. As demands are placed on the child they may exhibit increased temper tantrums, episodes of undesirable behavior, experience negative thoughts, and express ritualistic behavior as coping mechanisms.

Piaget's theory of Cognitive Development describes a child who is capable of solving more complex problems, understanding complex issues, utilize methods of trial and error to determine outcome of actions, and recognize relationships as causal, temporal, or spatial. Piaget's thought process discusses the child who begins to utilize mental images, realizes objects are consistent, and can organize thoughts.

Attributes of the child
During years 1 and 3 of a child's life they will gain 4 to 6 pounds annually, and grow approximately 4 to 5 inches annually. The pulse of a toddler remains steady at 100 beats per minute, and the typical respiratory rate is 26 breaths per minute. At eighteen months of age the anterior fontanel closes to form a solid cranial structure. At approximately 18 months the toddler will begin to have control of his/her bowels. At approximately 2 years of age the child will begin to control his/her bladder during waking hours. Typically a child will gain control of his/her bladder at night at approximately 36 months.

Motor development
At approximately fifteen months the child will be walking steadily on his/her own and be able to ambulate slowly up stairs with much assistance from hand rails, a banister or may crawl up stairs. At eighteen months a child is capable of climbing stairs with the use of one hand for support, the child is clumsy when he/she attempts to run, and the child can stand in one position and jump up and down, and will be able to hold, push or pull a toy as he/she ambulates. At age 24 months the child will ambulate up and down steps without difficulty or support, is able to take steps and walk from side-to-side and backwards, run and does not appear clumsy, and is able to kick objects such as a ball or toy. At the age of 30 months a child is able to stand on one foot momentarily, and ambulate on his/her tip toes.

Fine motor development

At approximately fifteen months of age a child is able to stack 2 blocks, scribble, open packages, and use a cup without difficulty. At approximately eighteen months a child is capable of using a spoon with little or no difficulty, build a tower with several blocks, and turn pages. At 24 months a child can manipulate 6 or 7 blocks, copy lines, open doors by turning a knob, open lids with a twist motion, and use scissors. A child of 30 months can build a tower with eight or greater blocks, and copy pictures such as arrows, crosses or large outline prints.

Language

At fifteen months a child can express, say approximately 5 words, point to show wants and needs, and has a tendency toward negativism or saying no even if they mean yes. At age 18 months a child has a vocabulary of 10 words and can identify and name at least two body parts. At age 2 years a child has an active vocabulary of 300 words, uses phrases that have two or three words in them, uses pronouns, and can obey simple commands. At thirty months a child can recite his/her first and last name, use plurals, and should be able to name at least one color.

Personal and social development

The fifteen month old child tolerates periods of separation from the mother without difficulty, may imitate the parent, might have episodes of temperament or unwanted behavior, and may chose to not us a bottle. At eighteen months the child will designate items as belonging to them or use the word mine, may develop a need for security objects such as blankets, bottles, and special toys, and may begin to test his/her limit of actions. At twenty-four months the child will begin to separate from the mother and display attributes of independence. At 24 months a child might have an imaginary play mate, help undress themselves, realize right from wrong, and begin to ritualize events such as bedtime, nap time or story time.

Play

Children ages 12 to 36 months prefer to play with pull or push toys, enjoy parallel play, and demonstrate continuous motor development and skills. At age 1 to 3 years the child will display excessive energy, enjoy playing beside other children (not with), and begin to demonstrate moral value with actions. The child of age 12 to 36 months will be learning colors, textures, shapes, and size. Toys that are the most productive and popular for the toddler are various, bright colored blocks. Puzzles that the toddler can manipulate to either take apart or put together, and telephones. Other toys for the toddler include dolls, hammers, finger puppets, clay, play dough, crayons, markers, paints, and small, simple musical toys or instruments. A tricycle may be utilized by some children of this age group. Wagons and trucks are toys toddler boys enjoy. Toddlers enjoy being read to, listening to musical stories and stories on tape as well as looking at pictures.

Terrible two's

The terrible two's:

- Age 12-36 months, Intense period of exploration, Temper tantrums/obstinacy occur frequently
- Biologic Development - Weight gain slows to 4-6 lbs/year, Birth weight should be quadrupled by 2 1/2, Height increases about 3" per year, Growth is "step like" rather than "linear", Visual acuity of 20/40 acceptable, Hearing, smell, taste, and touch increase in development

- Uses all senses to explore environment
- Maturation of Systems
- Most physiologic systems relatively mature by the end of toddlerhood
- Upper respiratory infections, Otitis Media, and Tonsillitis are common among toddlers
- Voluntary control of elimination
- Sphincter control—age 18-24 months
- Locomotion- improved coordination—between age 2-3, Fine motor development
- Improved manual dexterity age, Throw ball—by age 18 months
- Cognitive Development - Piaget: sensorimotor and preconceptual phase, Awareness of causal relationships between two events, Learn spatial relationships

Preschool aged children

The following are the general characteristics of a preschool aged child:
- The preschool period—age 3-5 years
- Preparation for most significant lifestyle change: going to school.
- Experience brief and prolonged separation
- Use language for mental symbolization
- Increased attention span and memory
- Physical growth slows and stabilizes
- Average weight gain remains about 5 lbs/year
- Average height increases 2½" to 3"/year
- Body systems mature and stabilize; can adjust to moderate stress and change
- Gross motor: walking, running, climbing, and jumping well established
- Refinement in eye-hand and muscle coordination, Drawing, art work, skillful manipulation
- Poorly defined body boundaries. Fear that if skin is "broken" all blood and "insides" can leak out
- Intrusive experiences are frightening
- Associative play, Imitative play, Imaginative play—imaginative playmates, Dramatic play
- Caloric requirements approximately 90 kcal/kg
- Fluid requirements approximately 100 mL/kg depending on activity and climate.

Growth and development
The child who is three to five years old will typically gain four to five pounds annually. The child who is three to five years old will typically grow 2 to 3 inches in height annually. Normal vital signs for the three to five year old will include a pulse rate of approximately 90 beats per minute, and a respiratory rate of 20 respirations per minute. The three to five year old child will have a normal systolic blood pressure of 90 and a normal diastolic blood pressure of 60. By five years of age the child will have chosen his or her dominant hand.

Fine motor development
A child age three can build a block tower using approximately ten blocks. The three year old can copy circles. A three year old can string beads, can undress, can assist in dressing him or herself and use the bathroom without help. A three year old can wash his/her own hands. A three year old is beginning to brush his/her own teeth and may begin to do simple chores around the house. A four year old will cut out photographs, shapes, copy squares, lace

his/her shoes, and can button clothes in the front and on the side. A four year old child may begin to draw a stick figure that has three body parts. Five year-old children can copy diamond shapes, will begin to print letters, words, and numbers. A five year old child can dress alone.

Gross motor development
At three years of age a child can ride a tricycle, make broad jumps, walk backward, walk up and down stairs without any difficulty, and begins to dance. At age four a child can jump and climb without difficulty. At age four a child can skip and hop on one foot. At age four the child will be able to catch a ball. At age four the child can throw a ball over handed. At age four the child will make steps alternating his or her feet. The five year old child jumps rope without difficulty, and can skate while keeping good balance.

Language
Three year old children have a vocabulary of approximately 900 words and may speak in complete sentences using three or four words. The three year-old will use plurals in his/her speech. The three year-old is aware of his/her family name. A three year old will constantly ask questions and may sing simple songs. Four year old children have a vocabulary of approximately 1,500 words. At age four a child may begin to use profane words they have heard and exhibit name calling behavior. The four year-old likes to exaggerate his/her stories. The four year old can understand simple analogies, and will repeat four numbers. Age 4 is the peak questioning age for children. The vocabulary of a five year old child consists of 2,100 words. The five year old speaks in sentences using five or six words, utilizes all parts of speech, and asks relevant questions.

Play
Preschool children are cooperative with play. Preschool children share toys and other items. Preschool children often imitate the dominant adult in their life at play. Preschool play is dramatic and without rules. Preschool children utilize vividness with play and are very active at play. Typical toys of the preschool child include, but are not limited to wagons, and tricycles, and backyard items such as swings, and jungle gyms. Preschool children often use house hold items as toys. Preschool children play dress up, doctor, nurse, and store keeper. Preschool children often play with trucks, trains, cars, and boats. Children of the preschool age use blocks, peg boards, puzzles, musical toys, and simple tools to play.

School age children

Theorists and theories of development
Freud's Psychosexual Theory of Development believes the school age child is in the latest stages of development and has no sexual consciousness or interest.

Erikson's Psychosexual Theory of Development states that school age children are developing feelings of industry vs. inferiority. Erikson feels the school age child is beginning to develop self-worth and engages in meaningful tasks. Erikson sees the school age child as one who compromises, cooperates, and is competitive. Peers form the main relationships of school age children according to Erikson. Erikson feels that school age children should be praised for their accomplishments to avoid feelings of inferiority.

Piaget's Theory of Cognitive Development states that school age children are in the concrete operational stage of development are able to understand the point of view of others, and have obvious problem solving skills. Piaget feels the school age child has the ability to deal with hypothetical situations, can use a system of classification for organization, is conservative, and understands past, present and future.

Growth and development
The child age 6 to 12 typically gains five pounds per year, and grows approximately 2 inches per year. The average pulse of a child age 6 to 12 is 90 beats per minute and the average respiratory rate is 18 breaths per minute. The normal systolic blood pressure of a child age six to twelve ranges from 90 to 110 and the diastolic blood pressure ranges from 60 to 70. The child age six to twelve will begin to get his/her permanent teeth. Girls age 12 will experience a school age growth spurt at approximately age 10, and boys will experience a school age growth spurt at age 12. Children may begin to experience changes in secondary sexual characteristics around age twelve.

Motor development
At age six children use crayons, pencils, scissors, tape and glue without difficulty. Six year olds print letters and numbers, run, jump, climb, hop, and skip. Six year old children can draw a human form that includes limbs, head, and torso. At age seven children are riding a bike, and like quiet time for play. Children age eight enjoy competition, are more careful with work, and detail. Nine year-old children have fully functional eye and hand coordination, control and timing. Ten year olds have total motor control, and increased strength with activities such as running, biking, climbing, and jumping. Eleven year olds are less balanced and are beginning to experience clumsiness. Twelve year old children have defined fine motor skills.

Personal social attributes
Children age six fear ghosts, thunder, large animals, and people under their beds. Six year old children wash and dress primarily on their own. The six year old enjoys winning and will cheat. The six year old enjoys being best and first. The six year old will blame other individuals, tattle, boast, and start fights. The six year old has a short attention span. At seven the child is reasonable, cooperative, and modest. The seven year old complains about parents, and wants parental approval. The eight year old fears loneliness, has a "best" friend, and values secrets. At age nine a child is peer oriented, enjoys pleasing others, is responsible for personal possessions, enjoys being part of the club, has good manners, and accepts blame for his/her own actions. The ten year old is not interested in personal hygiene, and forms good peer relationships. At age eleven the child will take personal responsibility. The twelve year old child enjoys coed play and is sensitive to the feelings of others.

Language
At age six a child has a vocabulary of approximately 2,500 words, reads simple sentences, and is beginning to sound out words. The six year old will count by ones, fives and tens, can distinguish right and left, and knows morning, noon, and night. Children age seven are able to name dates, months, years, and seasons, can tell time, add and subtract and use simple logic. At age eight a child has developed an increased memory, vocabulary and can define words. The nine year old child has an increased attention span, and can use practical knowledge in activities. Ten year olds like memorization, are interested in society, and continue to have difficulty making connections with facts. At age eleven a child wants to know the mechanism of things, and likes to read. The twelve year old may enjoy science and social studies, and can explain abstract thoughts.

Play

School age children enjoy board games, models, arts and crafts, bicycles, sports events, musical instruments, and scientific games and toys. School age children enjoy grooming and grooming devices. School age children like to participate in activities to earn money. The school age child plays most often with the same sex. Children age six to twelve have hobbies, and collections of items such as rocks, pictures, and leaves or favorite toys. The school age child will become involved in school sports, clubs, and participate in after school activities. The school age child enjoys speaking with peers on the phone, via the internet, and after school.

Puberty

Puberty is characterized by events in which children become young adults. Features of puberty in boys include gonadotropin secretion, gametogenesis, and secretion of gonadal hormones. The typical period that marks puberty in boys is age 9 to 18. The development of secondary sexual characteristics occurs during puberty. With girls puberty may begin around age 8 and end around age 16. Girls usually experience breast budding, development of axillary and pubic hair, and develop menarche (the beginning of menstruation). The growth spurt occurs in both males and females during puberty. Puberty is often a time of emotional and social change as well with the development of changes in body image, expectations, and levels of maturity with social actions.

Adolescence

Theorist and theories of development

Freud's Psychosexual Theory of Development states the adolescent is at the genital stage of development, and they rival for the love of the parent of the opposite sex.

Erikson's Psychosocial Theory of Development states the adolescent is in the phase of development known as identity vs. identity diffusion. Erikson sees the period of adolescence as stressful for the individual and the parents. The adolescent is beginning to separate from the parents. Adolescents accept body changes and body image changes. The adolescent characteristically makes plans for the future. During late adolescence the individual may experience intimacy vs. isolation, and the adolescent may struggle with sexual feelings, and emotions.

Piaget's Theory of Cognitive Development states the adolescent is in the formal stage of cognitive development between the ages of eleven and fifteen. The individual at this stage can solve abstract problems, consider multiple points of view, hypothesize, and use both inductive and deductive reasoning.

Growth and development

The adolescent weight gain is approximately 15 to 60 pounds with an expected growth in height of two to twelve inches. The rapid skeletal growth typically appearing in the adolescent leads to clumsiness, poor coordination and poor posture. The pulse rate of the adolescent ranges from 70 to 85, and the expected respiratory rate is 16 to 20 breaths per minute. The normal blood pressure of the adolescent is 120 systolic and 80 diastolic. Both the male and female will begin to experience secondary sexual characteristics. Adolescents will experience an increase in the activity of the sebaceous glands producing acne. The adolescent may have his/her wisdom teeth.

Motor development and language
Early adolescence is described as the thirteenth and fourteenth year. At this age the individual will enjoy being involved in sports, and dance. The adolescent at age 13 and 14 will begin to become more graceful with movement, but continue to have episodes of clumsiness. The term late adolescence is used to describe the years between ages fifteen and eighteen. The adolescent age fifteen to eighteen will have adult levels of motor function and control and be able to move without episodes of clumsiness. The adolescent will experience a very fast increase in vocabulary that will include slang and teenage jargon.

Work and play
Characteristically the adolescent spends more time involved in peer activities and less time involved in family activities or activities with the parents. Adolescents have and enjoy employment. The adolescent is partial to team activities and cooperative play where physical skills are demonstrated and utilized. Adolescents begin to develop an interest in social activities and functions. Adolescents are typically involved in the following activities: clubs, sports (in or out of school), arts, crafts, reading, movies, music, socialization with friends, self improvement activities, and some are involved in religious activities such as church, and youth organizations.

Dietary habits, eating disorders, and obesity
Puberty can as much as double teens need for iron, calcium, zinc and protein
Excess intake of calories- found in all income, racial/ethnic groups and both genders
Girls more susceptible to iron deficiency at menarche
Maximum bone mass acquired as teen, calcium deposited determines risk of osteoporosis

Obesity:
- 1/3 US students thought were overweight
- 7.6% females and 2.2% males reported taking laxatives or vomiting to lose weight
- US 18-22% of all adolescents are obese, 22% girls and 20% boys are overweight based on BMI.

Obesity and eating disorders:
BMI equal to or greater than the 95th percentile for age and gender are overweight, refer for further assessment if wt. Loss greater than 10% of previous wt. Recurrent dieting when not overweight, distorted body image, BMI below the 5th %, use of laxatives, emesis, starvation.

Tanner staging for female breast development

The preadolescent breast (stage 1 per Tanner's ratings) consists of a small elevated nipple with no significant underlying breast tissue.
Stage 2 - Puberty begins (usually between ages of 8 and 13, average age is 11) with the development of breast tissue and pubic hair. With the hormonal changes of puberty, breast buds form. This second stage of breast development is the breast bud stage. Here, there is elevation of the breast and nipple as a small mound; the areola begins to enlarge. Milk ducts inside the breast begin to grow.

In stage 3, there is further enlargement and elevation of the breast and areola (with no separation of their contours). The areola begins to darken in color. The milk ducts give rise to milk glands that also begin to grow.

Next, there is projection of the areola and nipple to form a secondary mound (stage 4). In the mature adult breast (stage 5), there is projection of the nipple only (though in some woman the areola continues to form a secondary mound).

Tanner staging for pubic hair development

The stage 1 preadolescent has no pubic hair except for a fine "peach fuzz" body hair.
In stage 2, there is sparse growth of long, slightly darkened, downy hair mostly along the labia. This hair is usually straight or only slightly curled. In stage 3, the pubic hair becomes darker, coarser, and curlier. It now grows sparsely over the mons veneris area. In stage 4, the hair grows in more densely. It becomes as coarse and curly as in the adult, but there is not as much of it. The mature adult, stage 5, has the classic coarse and curly pubic hair that extends onto the inner thighs.

Tanner staging for males

Stage 1 - preadolescent phase, genitalia relatively unchanged from childhood

Stage 2 - Testes and Scrotum enlarge

Stage 3 - Penis enlargement

Stage 4 - Enlargement of the glans and increase in the caliber of the penis

Stage 5 - Adult genitalia

Phases of adolescence and sexual maturation in girls

Adolescent phases:
- Early adolescence- ages 11-14
- Middle adolescence- ages 15-17
- Late adolescence- ages 18-20

Biologic changes of adolescence are called puberty.

Sexual maturation in girls:
- Small bud of breast tissue (thelarche) are the earliest, most visible changes of puberty (average age 11, range 9 to 13 ½)
- Appearance of pubic hair (adrenarche) follows by 2-3 months, although sometimes pubic hair precedes breast buds
- Increase in vaginal discharge early in puberty (physiologic leukorrhea)

Menarche occurs approx. 2 years after breast buds, 9 months after peak height and 3 months after peak weight. Mean age of menarche in US 12.8 years with normal range of 10 ½ to 15 years, menarche requires about 17 % body fat and 22% to maintain menstruation,

Pubertal delay if no breast development by age 13 or no menarche within 4 years of onset of breast development.

Sexual maturation in boys

Sexual maturation in boys:
- First changes are testicular enlargement accompanied by thinning, reddening, and increased looseness of the scrotum
- Usually occur between 9 ½ and 14
- Also get initial appearance of pubic hair
- Voice changes, facial hair
- Gynecomastia- breast enlargement and tenderness common in mid puberty 1/3 of boys and temporary (stop 2 years)
- Ejaculation may occur spontaneously as a "wet dream" or self- stimulation, and can be troubling, embarrassing events

Physical growth during puberty:
- Final 20 to 25% of lean body mass occurs during puberty, up to 50% ideal adult body weight is gained as well.
- Growth spurt refers to general increase in growth of skeletal, muscles, and internal organs, which reaches peak age 12 girls and 14 boys

Adolescent pregnancy

Adolescent pregnancy
Rate decreased nationally for all races, and ages-result of drop of repeat pregnancies and increase in use of long term hormonal contraception. Condoms used most frequently at first intercourse, older teens use OCP most often.

Complications of teen pregnancy
Bleeding is common early in the pregnancy. Half of these end in spontaneous abortion. If patient presents with bleeding and abdominal pain, rule out ectopic pregnancy. Teens have highest rate of mortality from this. Risk factors for ectopic pregnancy include previous PID, IUD, history of pelvic surgery, and previous ectopic pregnancy.

Structural factors
Labor may be prolonged in younger teens due to
Fetopelvic incompatibility- that is reflection of teen smaller stature and incomplete growth (esp. age 12-16)
Age 12-13 highest rate of c-sections, ages 15-21 often have labors shorter than average (esp. if 2nd birth).

Growth of STD's and unintended pregnancy in adolescents

Risky sexual behaviors among teenagers contribute to high rates of STD's and pregnancy in this age group. Each year 3 million US adolescents 1 in 6 acquire an STD. About 1 million become pregnant each year: about 1/2 obtain abortions, about 1/2 give birth. Sexually active teens should be screened for gonorrhea, chlamydia, and for females Pap test to detect HPV or other cervical dysplasia. At risk teens should be screened for HIV and syphilis.

All teens should receive health guidance regarding responsible sexual behaviors including abstinence.

Developmental attributes of early adulthood

Erikson's Psychosocial Theory of Development states that the individual will begin to develop a sense of intimacy, begin to form relationships by becoming parents and marriage partners. By early adulthood (19 to 39 years) an individual has a very real expectation and appreciation of who they are and has established an identity. Occupation choice is traditionally made during early adulthood. The young adult feels a sense of commitment in his/her relationships with others. The young adult treasures and enjoys affiliations and partnerships. Erikson's theory of psychosocial development believes the individual with poor interpersonal and communication skills will have difficulty during the period of young adult hood.

Developmental tasks of the middle adult years

Erickson's Psychosocial Theory of Development states that the individual age forty to sixty-four is focused on productivity, creativity, and generativity. The individual age forty to sixty-four traditionally tries to maintain a profitable and enjoyable occupation. The middle-age adult is typically concerned with the amount of time they have left to live. Stagnation vs. self-absorption is the developmental task of the middle-aged adult. If the individual is unable to accept the changes in one's life they may feel sorry for themselves, cease to be productive, become depressed, or become ill with psychosomatic illness.

Developmental tasks of the older adult

Erikson's Psychosocial Theory of Development states that the older adult (age 65 and over) is concerned with maintaining his or her identity or ego integrity. The older adult is adjusting to new situations including economic, social, familial, and sexual changes that occur with age. The older adult may experience a fear of death, as well as fear of becoming an invalid or a burden to their family. Older adults fear loss of self as they age and the ability to function as they once did. The older adult may experience feeling of despair related to the increased age and attributes of his or her increased age and the normal aging process. The older adult may feel apprehension related to body image changes due to age. The older adult often feels worthless, as they are unable to perform tasks as they once did.

Changes in older adults

Cardiovascular system changes
The older adult (age 65 and up) will begin to experience thickening and rigidity of the heart valves, the endocardium will thicken and sclerosis occurs. Contraction and dilatation of the cardiac muscle becomes difficult as a result of loss of elasticity related to age. The older adult will have an increased prevalence for cardiac arrhythmias. The older adult is at an increased risk for decreased levels of circulating hemoglobin. With decreased levels of hemoglobin cardiac oxygen becomes decreased and is less efficient. The older adult will experience a higher systolic blood pressure related to the decrease in elasticity of the peripheral vessels and an increase in peripheral resistance. The older adult will also experience a decrease in sensitivity of the baroreceptors, as well as changes in the EKG that are a reflection of the muscle changes and decreased function of the heart.

Gastrointestinal changes

The gastrointestinal system of the older adult will begin to manifest change in salivary production. The individual will experience a decrease in saliva that will result in dry oral mucous membranes. The older adult will have a decrease in taste buds, especially sweet and salty. The older adult will begin to experience a weakening of the pharyngeal muscles, possible dilatation of the esophagus, and decreased mobility of the esophagus. The older adult will have a decrease in peristalsis. The pancreatic enzyme production of the older adult will decrease, and the older adult will begin to have periods of altered insulin levels.

Normal physiological changes of the pulmonary/respiratory system

The older adult (age 65 and over) will experience a weakness of the connective tissue that is responsible for respiration and ventilation. The older individual will experience a decrease in body fluids that will ultimately result in dry mucous membranes and decrease the ability to remove secretions from the lungs. Barrel chest occurs as a loss of resilience to the thorax. Expiration in the older adult will require active use of accessory muscles. The alveoli of the older adult are less elastic and contain fewer functional capillaries. The normal arterial oxyhemoglobin saturation of the older adult is reduced to approximately 92 to 95 percent.

Normal physiological changes of the genitourinary system

The older adult will have a decrease in bladder capacity that will result in nocturia, and frequency of urination. The older adult will begin to experience weak bladder muscles, poor urinary retention, stress incontinence and dribbling of urine. The older adult will have decreased renal tubular function, and proteinuria may be normal. The female will begin to experience vaginal atrophy, reduction of pubic hair, and a drier, alkaline vaginal flora. The cervix and uterus of the older female may shrink. The fallopian tubes and ovaries will atrophy. The older adult female may experience painful coitus (sexual intercourse). The male will begin to notice a decrease in size and firmness of the testes. The older male may require an increased amount of time to form an erection. The older male will begin to experience slower, less forceful ejaculation, and may experience prostate enlargement.

Normal physiological changes of the nervous system

The nervous system of the older adult age sixty-five and up will begin to experience dilatation of the cerebral ventricles, loss of neurons, and a decrease of 5 to 7 percent in brain weight. The older individual will have impaired vision that includes decreased transparency of the lens, decreased pupil size, and altered vitreous humor. The older adult will have a decrease in the ability to hear high-pitched, high-frequency sounds, as well as a decrease in the ability to smell and distinguish odors. The older individual will have decreased tactile sensation, and slower reaction time related to slower conductivity of impulses. The older adult will begin to experience memory changes such as decreased short-term memory. Many older adults who experience short-term memory loss will retain the long-term memory.

Gametogenesis

Gametogenesis is the creation of gametes (a germ cell: sperm (male reproductive cell) or oocyte (female reproductive cell)). The gametes each contain one-half of the required chromosomes needed to form a zygote (the early embryo that is formed with union of the sperm cell and oocyte). Gametogenesis unites the haploid cells to form a standard human diploid cell. Gametogenesis is the process of creating an embryo with a total of 46

- 64 -

chromosomes with each parent attributing 23 chromosomes via germ cells. The human zygote cannot be produced without gametogenesis as the initial step in fertilization.

Oogenesis

Oogenesis is the method for the creation of the female haploid (oocyte) that contains 23 of the 46 needed chromosomes for a normal human cell to develop. The oocyte develops from the oogonial cells of the ovary. When a female is born she possesses all the female eggs (ova) that she will ever produce. The process of meiosis begins prior to birth and ceases until puberty begins. The process of meiotic division continues in the fallopian tube of the pubescent female. The oocyte undergoes 2 cell divisions, the first produces a microscopic polar body or an X chromosome (female chromosome), and a secondary oocyte. The second cell division occurs at the time of ovulation and completes cell division upon fertilization. The end product is 4 haploid cells, three microscopic polar bodies that will eventually dissipate, and a female egg.

Spermatogenesis

Spermatogenesis is the mechanism for producing male gametes (sperm cells). The process of spermatogenesis has three phases. Phase one is the spermatocytogenesis in which the spermatogonia (spermatoblast) facilitate the formation of spermatocytes or 2 haploid cells that contain 22 autosomal chromosomes and an X (female chromosome) or a Y (male chromosome). The second phase is meiosis in which the formation of 4 spermatids takes place. The third phase is spermiogenesis in which the spermatoblast divides and differentiates into sperm cells. During the third phase of spermatogenesis the cytoplasm is lost, the nucleus of the cell is compounded to form the head of the sperm cell, and a centriole produces the tail.

Cellular division

Cellular division occurs as a mechanism of reproduction of self. Mitosis is the exact replication of a cell that contains DNA identical to the original cell. Mitosis is characterized by 5 stages. The five stages of cellular division are prophase, prometaphase, metaphase, anaphase, and telophase. Mitosis is the body's ability to regenerate its own cells to assist in growth, and maturation. Meiosis is cell division that produces 4 gametocytes, each containing half the DNA required to form somatic (the cells of an organism that are not germ cells) cells. Both the male and female cells produce haploid cells prior to adjoining to become a diploid capable of fetal development.

Fetal development

Fetal development takes 40 weeks from fertilization to birth. During the first stages of development there is rapid growth and cellular replication to form embryonic membranes and germ layers; this is termed the preembryonic phase. During the embryonic phase which begins during the third week of pregnancy and continues until approximately the second month the embryo develops tissue that will distinguish the various organs. External embryonic features also develop during this stage. At week eight the embryo has the appearance of a human. Movement begins between weeks 13 and 16. Quickening is felt by the mother at week 20. At week 20 the fetal heart beat is also audible. Week 24 marks the development of alveoli in the lungs. During weeks 25 to 28 the fetal lungs can facilitate gas

- 65 -

exchange, but are not yet mature; it is unlikely a child would survive if born at this stage of development. Weeks 29 to 32 mark fetal bone development, and a central nervous system that is adequate enough to support respiratory efforts of the fetus. The fetus is considered to be full term at 38 weeks.

Signs of pregnancy

- Delay of Menstruation, During entire pregnancy, Excessive weight gain or loss, tension, stress.
- Nausea and vomiting, 2 - 8 weeks after conception, Food poisoning, stress and variety of other stomach disorders.
- Tender or swollen breasts, 1 - 2 weeks after conception, Impending menstruation.
- Feeling exhausted or "sleepy," 1 - 6 weeks after conception, Stress, fatigue, depression and other physical and mental strains.
- Backaches, During entire pregnancy, A variety of back problems and physical or mental strains.
- Frequent headaches, Sometimes during entire pregnancy. Dehydration, caffeine withdrawal.
- Food cravings, During entire pregnancy, Poor diet, stress, depression.
- Darkening of areola, (breast nipple) First signs 1 - 14 weeks after conceptions and then throughout pregnancy
- Fetal movements, 16 - 22 week after conception, Gas, lower gastrointestinal bowl contractions.
- Frequent urination, 6 - 8 weeks after conception, Diabetes, taking excessive diuretics causing urination.
- Fetal heart beat 10 - 20 weeks and then throughout entire pregnancy.

Chadwick's sign, Hegar's sign, and Goodell's sign

Chadwick's sign--this is an old term meaning a bluish discoloration of the vaginal tissue, caused by venous congestion in the area. (pregnancy)

"Hegar's Sign" is when the uterus becomes so soft, usually at 6 weeks that it is felt separately from the firmer cervix.

Softening of the cervix usually occurs at about the same time. This occurrence is called "Goodell's Sign."

Nagel's rule

Used to calculate EDD- Estimated Date of Delivery

EDD = 1st day of last menstrual period + 7 days - 3 months + 1 year

Placenta

The placenta is a fetomaternal organ that allows for the exchange of nutrients, waste, blood, and oxygen from mother to baby. The placenta is typically 4 centimeters deep, and has a distance of approximately 18 inches. The placenta has a smooth surface that is exposed to the fetus, and a rougher surface that remains attached to the uterine wall until birth. The placenta is approximately 1/6 the weight of the fetus. The placenta is the circulatory mechanism for the fetus while in utero. Fetal respiration takes place via the placenta as well as providing immunological protection.

Variable decelerations

Variable decelerations are characterized by slowing of the FHR with an abrupt onset and return. They are frequently followed by small accelerations of the FHR. They vary in depth, duration, and shape. Variable decelerations coincide with cord compression, and they usually coincide with the timing of the uterine contractions. Variable decelerations are the most common decelerations seen in labor, and they are caused by umbilical cord compression. They are generally associated with a favorable outcome. Persistent, deep, and long lasting variable decelerations are nonreassuring. Persistent variable decelerations to less than 70 bpm, lasting more than 60 seconds are concerning.

Late decelerations

Late decelerations are U-shaped with a gradual onset and gradual return. They are usually shallow (10-30 beats per minute), and they reach their nadir after the peak of the contraction. Late decelerations occur when uterine contractions cause decreased fetal oxygenation. In milder cases, they can be a result of CNS hypoxia. In more severe cases, they may be the result of direct myocardial depression. Late decelerations generally become deeper as the degree of hypoxia becomes more severe. Occasional or intermittent late decelerations are not uncommon during labor.

Weight gain during pregnancy

A proper diet and adequate weight gain during pregnancy are essential for good health of the mother and optimum development of her baby. If a mother doesn't gain enough weight, her baby may be born small. On the other hand, if weight gain is excessive, the baby may grow too large. This could complicate the birth process and increase risk of problems during pregnancy. Pregnant patients should gain five lbs. in the first trimester, and approximately 1lb/wk in the second and third trimesters. The appropriate weight gain during a pregnancy depends on several factors, including mother's pre-pregnant weight and age. A woman who is of average weight is encouraged to gain somewhere between 25-30 pounds during pregnancy. Underweight women need to gain a bit more weight, and high weight women a bit less. No one should ever try to lose weight during pregnancy. Maternal weight loss results in excess blood ketone levels. Ketones are toxic to fetuses.

Placenta Previa

Abruptio placentae (ie, placental abruption) refers to separation of the normally located placenta after the 20th week of gestation and prior to birth. Maternal hypertension is the most common cause of abruption, occurring in approximately 44% of all cases.
- Class 0 is asymptomatic. Diagnosis is made retrospectively by finding an organized blood clot or a depressed area on a delivered placenta.
- Class 1 is mild and represents approximately 48% of all cases. No vaginal bleeding to mild vaginal bleeding, Slightly tender uterus, Normal maternal BP and heart rate, No coagulopathy, No fetal distress

- Class 2 is moderate and represents approximately 27% of all cases. No vaginal bleeding to moderate vaginal bleeding, Moderate-to-severe uterine tenderness. Maternal tachycardia with orthostatic changes in BP and heart rate, Fetal distress
- Class 3 is severe and represents approximately 24% of all cases. No vaginal bleeding to heavy vaginal bleeding. Very painful tetanic uterus, Maternal shock, Coagulopathy, Fetal death

Hazards for an Rh negative woman with an Rh positive partner

An Rh negative woman has no RhD antigen and therefore is capable of generating anti-D antibodies if exposed to Rh positive cells (those which do carrying the RhD antigen). This is known as sensitization. An Rh positive man may have phenotype DD or Dd since the RhD antigen is dominant (the woman is dd). Therefore there is a 50% chance (Dd) or 100% chance (DD) that the baby of an Rh positive man will be Rh positive. If the baby is Rh positive, then the mother will develop anti-D antibodies, due to sensitization, after the birth. Rh positive cells enter the mother's bloodstream at the time of placental separation. The mother would develop memory anti-D antibodies, which would come into play on in second and subsequent pregnancies with an Rh positive fetus. The mother's anti-D antibodies are of the IgG type, which can cross the placenta to the foetal blood and cause agglutination and hemolysis of foetal cells to a varying degree. This could result in death in utero, erythroblastosis foetalis, icterus gravis neonatorum, hemolytic anaemia, kernicterus or liver damage of the fetus.

Diabetes and pregnancy

Diabetes is a disorder of the endocrine system in which there is insufficient production of insulin to maintain metabolism of carbohydrates resulting in an elevated blood glucose level. The production of insulin is from the beta cells of the islets of Langerhans within the pancreas. When a woman becomes pregnant she will have an automatic elevation in serum estrogen, progesterone and many other hormones. These hormones form as a catalyst for insulin production. An increased amount of insulin production causes an increased amount of insulin in the tissues. This increased amount of insulin production characteristically takes place during the early months of pregnancy. During the last months of pregnancy the woman will experience an increase in the circulating amounts of human placental lactogen and prolactin. The woman in her last months of pregnancy will also exhibit a rise in cortisol and glycogen. These elevations in hormone will cause insulin resistance to occur with destruction of tissue related to catabolism (the breakdown of chemical complexes—most often associated with energy production) to maintain energy levels and avoid starvation of the cells.

Risks
Elevated maternal serum glucose levels with increased production of ketones in the mother cause a fifty percent increase in fetal death. Fetal congenital abnormalities include cardiological defects that include septal anomalies, coarctation of the aorta, lesions, and transposition of the great vessels. Hydrocephalus (increased size of the ventricles due to an increased amount of cerebral spinal fluid), meningomyelocele (a protrusion of the spinal cord related to a flaw in the formation of the vertebral column), and anencephaly (absence of portions of the brain). Sacral Agenesis is also a congenital anomaly that is characteristic for diabetic mothers. These babies are born with defects in the lower region of the spinal column. Mother's with diabetes have abnormally large babies. Respiratory distress

syndrome and polycythemia are also seen in babies born to mothers who have diabetes. As nurses it is important to counsel and educate those at risk prior to conception to avoid birth related anomalies as much as possible.

<u>Nursing assessment</u>
The nurse should assess the woman's knowledge and level of understanding of diabetes with routine questions, and non guided explanation. Physical examination should include an assessment of the vascular system, urine glucose testing, and assessment for infectious processes. Prenatal visits usually occur as often as bi-monthly for the first 6 months of pregnancy and then once weekly for the last 3 months of pregnancy. The pregnant diabetic woman will be referred for an ophthalmologic exam, cardiology examination if you cannot perform an electrocardiograph in the office, and a creatinine clearance test should be done. Pregnant women should be offered nutrition education and counseling.

Screening for gestational diabetes

Gestational diabetes (GDM) is defined as glucose intolerance of variable degree with onset or first recognition during the present pregnancy. It can be screened by drawing a 1-hour glucose level following a 50-g glucose load, but is definitively diagnosed only by an abnormal 3-hour OGTT following a 100-g glucose load. The growth and maturation of the fetus are closely associated with the delivery of maternal nutrients, particularly glucose. This is most crucial in the third trimester and is directly related to the duration and degree of maternal glucose elevation. The ADA (American Diabetes Association) recommend that all pregnant women, who have not been identified with glucose intolerance earlier in pregnancy, be screened with a 50-g 1-hour GCT between 24 and 28 weeks of pregnancy. For the mother with GDM there is a higher risk of hypertension, preeclampsia, urinary tract infections, cesarean section, and future diabetes. Many of the problems associated with overt diabetic pregnancies can be seen in infants of gestational diabetic pregnancies, such as macrosomia, neural tube defects, neonatal hypoglycemia, hypocalcemia, Hypomagnesemia, hyperbilirubinemia, birth trauma, prematurity syndromes, and subsequent childhood and adolescent obesity.

Hyperemesis gravidarum

Hyperemesis gravidarum is a severe and intractable form of nausea and vomiting in pregnancy. It is a diagnosis of exclusion and may result in weight loss; nutritional deficiencies; and abnormalities in fluids, electrolyte levels, and acid-base balance. The peak incidence is at 8-12 weeks of pregnancy, and symptoms usually resolve by week 16. Interestingly, nausea and vomiting of pregnancy is generally associated with a lower rate of miscarriage. Extreme nausea and vomiting may be related to elevated levels of estrogens or human chorionic gonadotropin.

Signs/Symptoms:
- Weight loss
- Dehydration
- Decreased skin turgor
- Postural changes in BP and pulse

Fetal lung maturity

The various assessments of fetal lung maturity are as follows:
- Lecithin to Sphingomyelin ratio (L/S ratio) > 2:1
- Positive Predictive Value: 98% (if no comorbidity)
- Not accurate in Diabetes, fetal asphyxia, Rh Disease
- Phosphatidylglycerol (PG) present >3%
- More reliable than L:S ratio if maternal comorbidity
- Phosphatidylinositol (PI) present
- Desaturated Lecithin (DSL)
- Fetal Lung Maturity Test (TDX-FLM, Abbott Labs) >70%
- Foam Stability Index (Beckman Inst.) >47
- Bedside Tests
- Tap Test, Turbidity Test

Preeclampsia

Preeclampsia is the presence of protein in the urine, and increased BP during pregnancy. It is found in 8% of pregnancies. Symptoms are:
- Abnormal Rapid Weight gain
- Headaches
- Peripheral edema
- Nausea
- Anxiety
- Htn
- Low urination frequency

PRE is a mnemonic to help remember the main signs of Pre-eclampsia.
Proteinuria
Rising blood pressure
Edema

Tests include:
- Proteinuria
- BP check
- Weight gain analysis
- Thrombocytopenia
- Evidence of edema

Treatment includes:
- Deliver the baby
- Bed rest
- Medications

HELLP is an acronym that refers to the OB syndrome that is thought to be a severe form of preeclampsia. The acronym describes the main symptoms of this disorder:
Hemolysis
Elevated
Liver function tests
Low
Platelet count

Eclampsia

Seizures occurring during pregnancy, symptoms of pre-eclampsia have worsened. Factors that cause eclampsia vs. pre-eclampsia relatively unknown.
Symptoms:
- Weight gain sudden
- Seizures
- Trauma
- Abdominal pain
- Pre-eclampsia

Tests:
- Check liver function tests
- Check BP
- Proteinuria presence
- Apnea

Treatment:
- Magnesium sulfate
- Bed rest
- BP medications

BURP is a helpful mnemonic to assist you to remember the symptoms of magnesium sulphate toxicity, a common treatment for eclampsia.
Blood pressure decrease
Urine output decrease
Respiratory rate decrease
Patellar reflex absent

High risk factors related to maternal conditions

High risk related to maternal conditions:
Diabetic Mothers-severity of affects on infant affected by severity of disease
Hypoglycemia can occur in infant after birth within 1.5-4 hrs
Drug exposed-narcotics readily cross placenta;
Mothers who Smoke-Significant birth weight deficit and lower APGAR
Developmental delays, Passive smoking at home increases SIDS, respiratory infections, deficits in learning
Caused by maternal infection (especially viral during early gestation) TORCH

TORCH is a helpful mnemonic to assist you to remember the infections that can be vertically transferred from mother to fetus/embryo.

Toxoplasmosis
Other viruses
Rubella
Cytomegalovirus
Hepatitis A and B

Fetal alcohol syndrome (FAS)
Fetal Alcohol Effects – show cognitive, behavioral, and psychosocial problems without facial dysmorphia and growth retardation. It is the leading cause of intellectual disability. Early diagnosis and treatment are beneficial.

Cocaine/crack and pregnancy

Cocaine and/or crack have a systemic effect on the nervous system which blocks the use of dopamine and norepinephrine. The result of a lack of dopamine and norepinephrine is noted with vasoconstriction, causing elevated blood pressure (hypertension), and elevated heart rate (tachycardia). Vasoconstriction is a narrowing of any artery or vessel. The umbilical cord that supplies nutrients and oxygen to the fetus via the blood is made of arteries and vessels that are a direct route from mother to fetus. A natural constriction of the umbilical cord takes place with ingestion of crack/cocaine resulting in a decreased supply of blood to the fetus. A decreased blood supply decreases the amount of nutrients and oxygen to the fetus causing growth retardation and intellectual disability. Women who continue to abuse crack/cocaine during pregnancy have an increased risk for abruptio placenta, abortion in the first trimester, growth limitations, premature, and non-living births. Babies who are born to mothers who ingest crack/cocaine have a tendency to have lower APGAR scores, neurological problems, irritability, increased startle reflexes, altered emotions (labile-easily altered), intellectual disability, and an increased risk for sudden infant death syndrome (SIDS).

Anemia and pregnancy

Anemia is a decreased amount of circulating hemoglobin (Hb). Anemia is diagnosed with a hemoglobin level below 12g/dl in women who are not experiencing pregnancy, and below 10 g/dl in women who are pregnant. The hemoglobin level is affected by the altitude an individual resides in, the medications they take on a daily basis, and the race of the individual. African American individuals have normal hemoglobin 1 g/dl lower than Caucasian Americans. Women who smoke or live at a greater altitude seem to require more red blood cells to provide adequate amounts of oxygen. The smoker who lives at a greater distance above sea level may appear to be anemic by normal standards when in-fact she is within normal limits for her life-style and location. The most common anemia's associated with pregnancy include nutritional deficits of folate and iron. Sickle cell anemia and thalassemia also seems are inherited diseases that cause anemia among pregnant women.

Amniotic fluid

Amniotic fluid--greatest at 34 weeks gestation.

Functions:
- Allows normal lung development
- Freedom for movement
- Fetus temperature regulation
- Trauma prevention

Oligohydramnios and Polyhydramnios

Oligohydramnios: Low levels of amniotic fluid that can cause: fetal abnormalities, ruptured membranes and fetus disorders.

Polyhydramnios: High levels of amniotic fluid that can cause: gestational diabetes and congenital defects.

Polyhydramnios Causes:
- Beckwith-Wiedemann syndrome
- Hydrops fetalis
- Multiple fetus development
- Anencephaly
- Esophageal atresia
- Gastroschisis

Chorionic villus sampling

Removal of placental tissue for analysis from the uterus during early pregnancy. US helps guide the procedure. 1-2 weeks get the results. Can be performed earlier than amniocentesis.

Used to check for:
- Tay-Sachs disease
- Down syndrome
- Other disorders

Monitor the patient for:
- Infection
- Miscarriage
- Bleeding

Fetal tachycardia

Causes of fetal tachycardia:
- Fetal hypoxia
- Maternal fever
- Hyperthyroidism
- Maternal or fetal anemia

- Parasympatholytic drugs
- Atropine, Hydroxyzine (Atarax)
- Sympathomimetic drugs, Ritodrine (Yutopar)
- Terbutaline (Bricanyl),
- Chorioamnionitis
- Fetal tachyarrhythmia
- Prematurity

Fetal bradycardia

The causes of severe fetal bradycardia:
- Prolonged cord compression
- Cord prolapse
- Tetanic uterine contractions
- Paracervical block
- Epidural and spinal anesthesia
- Maternal seizures
- Rapid descent
- Vigorous vaginal examination

Impending labor

The signs and symptoms of impending labor are as follows:
- Lightening: The phase of fetal progression into the pelvis (engagement). Once lightening has occurs the mother-to-be might breathe more comfortably as the fundus is no longer pressing on the diaphragm. Other symptoms include lower extremity pain, pressure and leg cramping, a noted increase in the amount of pelvic discomfort and pressure felt, bilateral lower extremity edema related to the decreased return of blood flow to the heart.
- Braxton Hicks Contractions: Consist of the irregular, discontinuous contractions that have been happening all the way through the pregnancy. Most pain with Braxton Hicks contractions is located in the abdomen, and is uncomfortable. Pregnant women are said to be in false labor if the contractions are consistent and strong enough. Vaginal examination will determine false labor.
- Cervical changes: Include rigidity and firmness at the onset of pregnancy. As the cervix ripens it becomes soft enough to form the birthing canal allowing the fetus to exit the pelvic cavity and pass into the vagina and out.
- Bloody Show: The mucous plug that develops over the length of the pregnancy. Once the presence of bloody show is evident labor will proceed within 24 to 48 hours. Bloody show does not occur related to a routine vaginal exam it is a mucous plug that is released as the cervix ripens and thins out to form an opening and facilitate the birth canal.
- Rupture of membranes: When the bag of amniotic fluid that contains the fetus ruptures labor traditionally results within 24 hours.

It's Not My Time is a helpful mnemonic to assist you to remember the Uterine Relaxants (Tocolytics).

Indomethecin (NSAID)
Nifedipine (CA channel blocker)
Magnesium Sulfate
Terbutaune (adrenergic agonist)

Stages of labor

- Stage 0 Occurs until the cervix is 4 cm.
- Stage 1 During this stage, the woman should prepare herself to push the baby out from the uterus and into the world. Stage 1 signals labor and concludes at the time the cervix reaches a dilatation of 10 cm. Stage 1 labor consists of the latent phase, the active and the transition phases. The latent phase is characterized by routine contractions, and rupture of the membrane releasing the amniotic fluid. Normal cervical dilatation is 1 to 3 cm. The active phase of labor is characterized by a cervical dilatation of approximately 5 cm, increased anxiety and a sense of helplessness. The transition phase is characterized by a cervical dilatation from 8 to 10 cm. Over stage 1 labor the contractions become more frequent and intense, propelling the fetus down the birthing canal at approximately 1 cm per hour.
- Stage 2 During this stage, the uterus has opened completely and expelled the fetus through the birth canal. Stage 2 begins with complete dilatation and concludes with the birth of the baby. Fetal descent continues during stage 2. Crowning takes place during stage 2. Crowning occurs when the head of the fetus is visible at the vaginal opening. As stage 2 progresses the fetus changes position to accommodate birth. Flexion, internal rotation, extension, restitution, external rotation, and expulsion all occur as part of the transition of birth.
- Stage 3 includes placenta parting form the intra uterine wall, and delivery of the placenta.
- Stage 4 This stage describes the hour after the placenta is delivered; it is an important time, because there could be bleeding. Stage 4 includes the first 4 hours post labor in which the mother's body begins to return to its pre-pregnant state.

Induced labor

Induced labor may occur with the following criteria:
- Eclampsia
- HELLP syndrome
- High serum creatinine levels
- Prolonged elevated diastolic blood pressure >100mmHg
- Thrombocytopenia
- Abnormal fetal growth

Umbilical cord and problems

Umbilical cord has two arteris and one vein. Arteries carry deoxygenated blood and veins carry oxygenated blood.

The umbilical cord is the pathway for oxygen, nutrients, blood products, properties of the mother's immunity and other protective mechanisms to be passed between the fetus and mother during the intrauterine period. During birth the umbilical cord may appear prior to the presenting fetal part, this is termed a prolapsed cord. Cord compression will cause a cease in flow of blood and oxygen between the mother and fetus. The umbilical cord has the potential to have missing vessels. The nurse has the responsibility to determine if the cord has the correct vessels and evaluate the fetus if not. Congenital artery absence can cause fetal anomalies and problems with gestational age. Fetal heart rate irregularities result when the vessels of the umbilical cord become torn, or ripped during labor due to lack of Wharton's jelly (the natural protective mechanism of the cord). Rips or tears in the cord cause hemorrhages and are termed velamentous insertion with succenturiate placenta. Asphyxia of the fetus is the result of hemorrhage. The umbilical cord should measure 55 cm in length. Abnormal length of the umbilical cord may lead to umbilical hernia (if the cord is to short), abruptio placenta with a short cord, and cord rupture if the length is short. Potential problems of an extensive cord include transient deceleration variations, and knots in the cord that decrease blood and oxygen supplies.

Possible problems with the placenta during birth

The placenta continues to act as the source of oxygen for the fetus throughout the birthing process. Vascularity with the placenta places the mother and fetus at an increased risk for demise, and hemorrhage. Sources of hemorrhage include, but are not limited to:
- Abruptio placenta: Abruptio placenta occurs as often as four in every five hundred births. Abruptio placenta is an early, unexpected, unexplained break of the placenta from the intrauterine wall during pregnancy, or labor. The exact cause of abruptio placenta is not known, potential causes include smoking, ingestion of alcohol, increased amounts of intrauterine pressure, multiple pregnancies, and maternal hypertension.
- Placenta previa: Placenta previa is an altered position of the placenta, traditionally on the lower uterine wall or covering the cervical os (opening).

Meconium Aspiration Syndrome

Meconium Aspiration Syndrome (MAS) is caused when fetal asphyxia or intrauterine stress causes relaxation of anal sphincter and passage of meconium into amniotic fluid.
- Infants stained green if exposed long before birth
- Tachypneic; hypoxic; depressed; grunting; retractions; nasal flaring; hypothermic; hypoglycemic; hypocalcemic
- Quickly leads to respiratory failure.
- Prevention-suctioning as soon as head is through birth canal and chest still compressed; tracheal suctioning based on assessment at birth

Birth injuries

Some of the more common problems with birth injuries and newborns are:
- Soft tissue injuries
- Caput succedaneum
- Cephalhematoma
- Subgaleal hemorrhage

- Fractures (clavicle)
- Facial paralysis
- Brachial palsy
- Phrenic nerve paralysis
- Erythema toxicum neonatorum
- Candidiasis
- Birthmarks

Apgar score

The Apgar score is a determination of the condition of the fetus at the time of birth. The Apgar score is taken one minute and five minutes after birth. The Apgar score ranges from 0-10. Factors of the Apgar rating include:
- Activity (Muscle Tone)
    - Absent - (0)
    - Arms & legs extended - (1)
    - Active movement with flexed arms & legs - (2)
- Pulse (Heart Rate)
    - Absent - (0)
    - Below 100 bpm - (1)
    - Above 100 bpm - (2)
- Grimace (Response Stimulation or Reflex Irritability)
    - No Response - (0)
    - Facial grimace - (1)
    - Sneeze, cough, pulls away - (2)
- Appearance (Skin Color)
    - Blue-gray, pale all over - (0)
    - Pink body and blue extremities - (1)
    - Normal over entire body – Completely pink - (2)
- Respiration (Breathing)
    - Absent - (0)
    - Slow, irregular - (1)
    - Good, crying - (2)

The Apgar score is universal in health care and was developed by Dr. Virginia Apgar. The test is administered at one minute and five minutes after birth. If there are problems with the infant, an additional score may be repeated at a 10-minute interval. For a Cesarean section the baby is additionally assessed at 15 minutes after delivery.

Initial newborn exam

The attributes of an initial newborn exam are:
- Respiratory status: The nurse should expect a respiratory rate of 36-60 and irregular. Red flags for respiratory distress include retractions, and grunting to get air in.
- Apical Pulse: The nurse should expect a pulse rate of 120-160 beats per minute and may be slightly irregular.
- Temperature: The nurse should expect a temperature of the skin to be greater than 97.8/F.

- Skin Color: The nurse should expect the body of the infant to be pink. The extremities of a new born may be cyanotic in appearance.
- Umbilical cord: The nurse should expect the umbilical cord to appear with 2 arteries and 1 vein.
- Gestational age is 38 to 40 weeks
- Sole creases should involve the heels of the foot

Theory and theorists of the postpartum phase of labor

Reva Rubin discusses and theorizes the biopsychosocial experience of childbirth. The postpartum phases according to Rubin include:
- Taking in or the first 2 to 3 days following labor. This is a time in which the mother begins to claim her baby, and regenerate herself from childbirth. This is a period of rest and acquaintance for the neonate and the mother. The nurse should encourage the mother to reflect and verbalize her labor and delivery experience during this time.
- Taking hold begins on day 3 following delivery and may extend for several weeks. The taking hold phase states that the mother will begin to feel more autonomous and require less assistance from those around her, she will dominate the care of the infant. The mother's own bodily functions should be returning to normal during this period. Mothers in the taking hold phase are very sensitive to the care of the infant and insist they want everything to be done right. The nurse should praise the mother during this phase if they have the opportunity, and should educate the family on offering praise to new mothers.
- The letting go phase begins approximately the second week following delivery. The mother begins to see the infant as a separate entity from self. Until this point the mother may have felt guilt when separated from her infant and may grieve over this separation. The letting go phase is a time of returning to pre-pregnancy norms.

Lochia

A period-like discharge from the vagina that occurs after delivery. The discharge will probably be exceptionally heavy at first and may last five to six weeks.
Rubra phase: 1-3 days postpartum (bloody)
Serosa phase: 3-10 days postpartum (brown-pink colored)
Alba phase: 2-6 weeks (yellow)

Birth rate, infant mortality, and maternal mortality

Birth rate describes the number of babies born alive per 1,000 individuals in a population during a specific period of time (normally 1 year). Infant mortality describes the number of babies who die per 1,000 live births in a population during a specific period of time (normally 1 year). Maternal mortality describes any death that occurs during pregnancy per 100,000 live births.

Fetal lung development, respiratory mechanisms, respiratory function, and the first breath of life

Lung development begins upon life of the zygote and continues throughout pregnancy and into infancy. During the initial weeks of fetal development the lungs are forming into pulmonary, lymphatic, and vascular structures. The presence of alveolar ducts begins between weeks 20 and 24. Alveoli in the basic form are present during weeks 24 to 28. Alveoli are the grape like structures within the lungs that facilitate gas exchange (oxygen and carbon). Surfactant is housed within the alveoli and consists of lipoproteins, lecithins and sphingomyelins that are the mechanism of stabilization and reduce surface tension upon alveoli opening and closing. During the fetal period the fetus is routinely breathing amniotic fluid in preparation for extrauterine life in which the neonate is ready to breathe air immediately upon birth. The initial breath of the infant is taken in reaction to the changes that occur from intrauterine life and extrauterine life. The gasp or startle in response to mechanical (decreased lung fluid production the few days prior to birth), chemical (an elevation in carbon and a decreased PH), thermal (a constant temperature of amniotic fluid of thirty seven degrees Celsius to a temperature drop to 23 degrees Celsius), and sensory (a change from a comfortable protective environment to bright lights, loud voices, environmental air and smells) change is the trigger for the alveoli to open and begin to facilitate gas exchange.

Newborn period of life

The period termed newborn begins at birth and continues for the twenty eight days following birth. The terms neonate (a neonate is an infant under one month of age) and neonatal period are also interchangeable with newborn. The newborn period is a period of adjustment from intrauterine to extrauterine life. It is the responsibility of the nurse to understand what normal physiology is for the newborn and to recognize abnormalities and problems and bring these to the attention of the primary care provider. During the period of neonatal transition (the first hours after birth) the newborn must become adept to breathing on its own.

Changes in the cardiovascular system of the neonate

The increased pulmonary blood flow at birth is a facilitator of newborn circulation. During fetal development phases the blood is routed thru the placenta with blood containing increased amounts of oxygen going to the heart and brain. Upon birth and the inflation of the lungs a resistance develops that stimulates increased blood flow to the pulmonary veins. As blood begins to return from the veins of the pulmonary system the left atrium begin to feel more pressure, at the same time the pressure in the right atrium is decreased related to the umbilical cord being clamped. The neonate will experience an elevation in aortic pressure and a decreased amount of venous pressure as the umbilical cord becomes clamped. The vascular bed that supported function is no longer viable and decreases the amount of intravascular support and space available. As the arterial pressures change the foramen ovale closes within the first 2 hours following birth. The ductus arteriosus closes as the flow of blood is routed thru the aorta to the pulmonary artery. The ductus venosus closes when as the umbilical cord is clamped and cut causing the circulatory pattern of blood to enter the liver.

Times of newborn assessment

Neonates should have routine physical exams upon birth with the first one being the initial Apgar score followed by a full body exam immediately upon completion of the birthing process. A 5 minutes post birth exam to determine the second Apgar score. An assessment should be performed within the first four hours post birth. The nurse should provide the baby and parents ample time to bond following birth. This assessment should include adaptation to extrauterine life, gestational age determination, and assessment of any high-risk problems. During the first 24 hours period of life the newborn should have a total physical examination, a physician, midwife, or nurse practitioner exam, and an assessment of nutritional stability and function.

Neurological functions of neonate

Neonates are born with unmyelinated nerve fibers and have a brain size that is 33 percent less than that of an adult. The behavior of the mother during pregnancy will determine the reaction to various stimuli the neonate will have. Research has also noted that newborns of higher birth weight have experienced better maternal nutrition and are more responsive to visual and auditory stimuli. Higher birth weight babies have increased motor maturity as opposed to those with low birth weight and poor maternal nutrition. Newborns will often experience non-purposeful extremity movements with resistance to flexion, follow objects with their eyes and maintain a stare on faces or other objects. Growth of the neonate is cephalocaudal or in a head-to-toe fashion. Normal reflexes for the neonate are brisk knee jerk, ankle clonus with 3 or 4 beats, plantar flexion, Moro reflex, grasp, and rooting reflexes, Babinski, and sucking reflexes. These reflexes indicate normal neurological function of the newborn.

Current prophylactic measures used with newborns

Newborns are required by law to be given a prophylactic intramuscular injection of vitamin K. This initial injection of vitamin K will provide a mechanism of prevention for the possible hemorrhages that can occur immediately following birth when the prothrombin time is elevated. At birth the infant has little or no bacterial flora within the gastrointestinal tract. Newborns are also given prophylactic eye ointment as a preventive mechanism for Neisseria gonorrhoeae. This preventive mechanism is most effective when the eye ointment is deposited directly in the lower conjunctival sac of both eyes.

Attributes of newborns skin

All newborns that are considered to be healthy have a characteristic pink flush to the skin. Those born with ruddy hues have had an increase in red blood cell concentration to the area and have decreased amounts of subcutaneous fat. Newborns that appear cyanotic at rest and pink during activity may have a congenital defect known as choanal atresia (a blockage between the nose and pharynx). Crying with cyanosis may signal cardio or pulmonary problems. Anemic newborns and those with decreased fluid volumes may appear pale. Acrocyanosis is a term used to describe a newborn with bluish hands and feet. Harlequin sign is a change that appears only on one side of the newborns body, and is the result of vasodilatation. Jaundice is the yellowish color noted at birth; this should dissipate within the first 24 hours of birth and should be reported to the practitioner if it doesn't. Facial milia are the raised white cysts that are present on the skin of the newborn.

Babinski's reflex

Babinski's reflex occurs when the great toe flexes toward the top of the foot and the other toes fan out after the sole of the foot has been firmly stroked. This is normal in younger children, but abnormal after the age of 2. Babinski's reflex is one of the infantile reflexes. It is normal in children under 2 years old, but it disappears as the child ages and the nervous system becomes more developed. In people more than 2 years old, the presence of a Babinski's reflex indicates damage to the nerve paths connecting the spinal cord and the brain (the corticospinal tract). Because this tract is right-sided and left-sided, a Babinski's reflex can occur on one side or on both sides. An abnormal Babinski's reflex can be temporary or permanent.

Topics of education for nurse and new mother

Nurses are the primary educators of new mothers. To ensure infant safety it is important for the nurse to review the following topics with new mothers. Choking, gagging, safety, cord care, skin care, recognition of signs and symptoms of illness, care of a circumcised neonate, recognition of abnormal skin colors and what to do, use of a thermometer, use of the bulb syringe, how, why and when to burp the infant, feeding and positioning, breast feeding education and benefits, formula preparation, stools, emesis, sleep patterns, car safety, hygiene, care of bottles, education and prevention of sudden infant death syndrome.

Benefits of breastfeeding

Health Benefits for Mom and Baby:
- Enhanced Immune System and Resistance to Infection
- Breast milk has agents (called antibodies) in it to help protect infants from bacteria and viruses.
- Because breastfed babies are sick less often they have fewer visits to health care providers.
- Breastfed infants' immune systems (the system that helps fight infection) have a better response to immunizations like polio, tetanus, diphtheria, and Haemophilus influenzae, and to respiratory syncytial virus infection, a common infant respiratory infection.
- Human milk straight from the breast is always sterile (or clean).
- A mother's milk has just the right amount of fat, sugar, water, and protein that is needed for a baby's growth and development. Most babies find it easier to digest breast milk than they do formula.
- Nursing uses up extra calories, making it easier to lose the pounds of pregnancy. It also helps the uterus to get back to its original size and lessens any bleeding a woman may have after giving birth.
- Breastfeeding lowers the risk of breast and ovarian cancers.

Attributes of early attachment

A large part of the postpartal period is the initial mother baby attachment that should begin to take place immediately upon birth. The nurse should monitor if the mother is involved with her newborn, the level of involvement, what is the body language of the mother toward the infant. The nurse should be aware of the mothers actions, is she stable. Does the mother ask or seek out information in providing care for her infant? Does the mother see to the needs of the newborn immediately or does she hesitate. Do the mother and father appear to be pleased with the newborn? Are the interactions with the mother frequent and pleasurable? The nurse should be aware of social and cultural factors that are present within the family dynamic of the neonate.

Stress incontinence

Stress incontinence: A laugh, sneeze or activity that causes involuntary urination. Urethral sphincter dysfunction.

Tests:
- Rectal exam, X-rays, Pad test
- Urine analysis, PVR test
- Cystoscopy, Pelvic exam

Treatment:
- Surgery
- Medications (pseudoephedrine/phenylpropanolamine)
- Estrogen
- Pelvic floor re-training
- Fluid intake changes

Urge incontinence

Urge incontinence is urine loss caused by bladder contraction.
Symptoms:
- Frequent urination
- Abdominal pain/distention

Tests:
- Pelvic exam
- X-rays
- Cystoscopy
- EMG
- Pad test
- Urinary stress test
- PVR test
- Genital exam-men

Treatment:
- Surgery
- Medications-(tolterodine, propatheline, imipramine, tolterodine, terbutaline)
- Biofeedback training
- Kegel strengthening

Ovarian cycle

The ovarian cycle occurs on a regular basis and is considered a normal part of the sexual reproductive activities of the female. The ovarian cycle occurs every 28 days. The ovarian cycle consists of the follicular phase or day one to day fourteen. The follicle stimulating hormone and luteinizing hormone are present and assist in the development of the graafian or ovarian follicle. The ovarian follicle ruptures and expels the ovum or female egg into the fallopian tube. Upon discharge of the ovum there is formation and regression of the corpus luteum. The ovarian cycle continues until a female has an artificial surgical procedure to disrupt the cycle, begins menopause, or controls the cycle with methods such as estrogen, progesterone containing birth control.

Cycles involved with menstruation

Ovulation and the menstrual cycle are characterized by the menstrual phase which occurs from day one to day six of the menstrual cycle. During the menstrual cycle the woman experiences decreased levels of estrogen, endometrial tissue detaching, and small amounts of tenacious cervical mucus. During the proliferation phase or day seven to day fourteen the woman will experience endometrial thickening, peak levels of estrogen, decreased body temperature, and has the potential for scant amounts of blood production. The secretory phase of the menstrual cycle consists of a decline in estrogen, increased uterine vascularity, and preparatory signs of implantation. The ischemic phase of the menstrual cycle is characterized by decreased estrogen and progesterone levels, pale endometrial tissue, vasoconstriction of the spiral arteries, rupture of the blood vessels and the stromal cells of the uterus become filled with blood.

Irregularities associated with menses

The following are irregularities associated with menses:
- Amenorrhea is characterized by a lack of or uncharacteristic pause of menses.
- Dysmenorrhea is characterized by painful menses.
- Hypomenorrhea is characterized by a limited period or period of short duration.
- Hypermenorrhea is characterized by an extensive menses.
- Oligomenorrhea is characterized by irregular menses.
- Polymenorrhea is characterized by abnormally frequent menses.
- Anovulatory cycle is characterized by a menstrual cycle in which a woman does not ovulate.

PMS

Premenstrual syndrome occurs in women during the age of reproduction. Premenstrual syndrome is characterized by emotional, physical, and behavioral symptoms that occur during the luteal or premenstrual phase of the menstrual cycle and cease to exist upon menstruation. Signs and symptoms include swelling (bloating), and weight gain due to the retention of fluid, breast soreness or tenderness, irritability, anxiety, obvious mood changes, fatigue, lack of concentration, appetite changes, and altered libido. Premenstrual syndrome (PMS) occurs in women at any age during the reproductive years. Premenstrual syndrome may continue well into the late forties or early fifties, but will cease upon menopause.

Dysmenorrhea

Dysmenorrhea: painful menses.
Symptoms: Constipation, Nausea, Vomiting, Diarrhea

Primary dysmenorrhea- painful menses without a disorder- most common cause painful menses in teens

Secondary dysmenorrhea- painful menses with a disorder such as endometriosis, congenital abnormalities

Incidence is as high as 92%, with 15% experiencing pain that inhibits daily activities

Relationship between uterine contractility and secretion of prostaglandins. Prostaglandins also responsible for N,V, D, HA, emotional changes

Menopause

Menopause is the permanent termination of the menstrual cycle. Menopause may be caused by ovarian failure or surgical procedures to stop ovulation from occurring. Menopause traditionally ceases on its own around age 50 for most women. Menopause is the end of the reproductive phase for women. Signs and symptoms of menopause include, but are not limited to hot flashes and night sweats or vasomotor instability, mood changes such as nervousness, irritability, anxiety, and depression. Women who are experiencing menopause often experience insomnia. Due to the lack of estrogen production women often experience atrophy of the urogenital epithelium and surrounding skin. Follicle Stimulating Hormone (FSH) is greater than or equal to 40 IU/l in menopausal women.

Mammogram procedure

Mammography is a specific type of imaging that uses a low-dose x-ray system for examination of the breasts. The images of the breasts can be viewed on film at a view box or as soft copy on a digital mammography work station. Current guidelines from the U.S. Department of Health and Human Services (HHS), the American Cancer Society (ACS), the American Medical Association (AMA) and the American College of Radiology (ACR) recommend screening mammography every year for women, beginning at age 40. The test should be performed yearly in women 51 and older. The National Cancer Institute (NCI) adds that women who have had breast cancer and those who are at increased risk due to a genetic history of breast cancer should seek expert medical advice about whether they should begin screening before age 40 and about the frequency of screening.

Mastitis

Breast infections/Mastitis: Infection or inflammation due to bacterial infections

Symptoms: Fever, Nipple pain/discharge, Breast pain, Swelling of the breast

Tests: Physical examination

Treatment: Antibiotics, Moist heat, Breast pump

Pap smear

The Pap test (also called a Pap smear) checks for changes in the cells of your cervix. The cervix is the lower part of the uterus (womb) that opens into the vagina (birth canal). The Pap test can tell if you have an infection, abnormal (unhealthy) cells, or cancer. It is important for all women to make pap tests, along with pelvic exams, a part of their routine health care. You need to have a Pap test if you are over 18 years old. If you are under 18 years old and are or have been sexually active, you also need a Pap test. There is no age limit for the Pap test. Even women who have gone through menopause (the change of life, or when a woman's periods stop) need to get Pap tests.

Atrophic vaginitis

Atrophic vaginitis- low estrogen levels cause inflammation of the vagina. Most common after menopause.

Symptoms:
- Pain with intercourse
- Itching pain
- Vaginal discharge
- Vaginal irritation after intercourse

Tests: Pelvic examination

Treatment:
- Hormone therapy
- Vaginal lubricant

Trichomoniasis

Trichomoniasis is a vaginal infection cause by a species of the genus Trichomonas that thrives in an environment that is non-acidic and most often transmitted sexually. Trichomoniasis can be found in both women and men. Signs and symptoms include vaginal discharge that may be clear, vaginal discharge in large quantities, genital irritation, difficult urination (dysuria), odor, painful sexual intercourse, suprapubic pain and discomfort. Those at highest risk for trichomoniasis are those with multiple sexual partners and those who have unprotected sexual intercourse with infected individuals. Treatment for Trichomonas includes Metronidazole (Flagyl); treat all sexual partners, discuss abstinence from sex to deter transmission, and sex education.

Bacterial vaginosis

Bacterial vaginosis is a bacterial infection of the vagina characterized by a disproportionate amount of malodorous discharge. Bacterial vaginosis occurs when hydrogen peroxide producing lactobacilli of the normal flora of the vagina are replaced by anaerobic bacteria. The major causes of bacterial vaginosis include multiple sexual partners and the use if intra-uterine devices to avoid pregnancy. Organisms known to cause bacterial vaginosis include Candida Albicans, Trichomonas vaginalis, and Gardnerella vaginalis. Microscopic exam reveals the presence of clue cells, scant leukocytes, no lactobacilli and mixed flora. Bacterial vaginosis is treated with Metronidazole (Flagyl), or 2% Clindamycin cream.

Pelvic structures

The various types of pelvic structures a woman may possess are:
- Gynecoid pelvis: A Gynecoid pelvis is characterized by a round inlet, and is the most often seen type of pelvic structure.
- Android pelvis: An Android pelvis is characterized by a heart shaped inlet, and is the normal male pelvis.
- Anthropoid pelvis: The Anthropoid pelvis is characterized by an oval shaped inlet.
- Platypelloid pelvis: A Platypelloid pelvis is characterized by a transverse oval inlet, and is often noted as a flat pelvis.

Nutrition and the cardiovascular system

The cardiovascular system entails the heart, blood vessels, arteries and veins. Diets that assist in controlling and decreasing consumption of cholesterol, fats (total fat, saturated fat, unsaturated fat, and trans fatty acids), and alcohol, along with simple and complex carbohydrates are all part of a regimen that will potentially lower the risk for cardiovascular disease. By controlling the amount of fats ingested the client is potentially lowering their cholesterol levels, decreasing their risk of blockage, and fat emboli that cause ischemic damage to the heart and/or myocardial infarction (MI/heart attack). Often diet changes are accompanied my medications to lower triglyceride or lipid levels, and exercise is also prescribed.

Pressure ulcers

Pressure ulcers are a chronic ulcer that appears in an area of pressure on the human body. Pressure ulcers are the end result of pressure on overlying skin of bony prominences in patients who are debilitated, have restricted or limited motion, are confined to bed or chair, or are immobilized for any reason. Circulatory compromise or deficiency is a leading contributor of pressure ulcers. Pressure ulcers are also termed bedsores, decubital gangrene, pressure sores, and hospital gangrene. The most frequent location of pressure ulcers is the occiput at the base of the skull, the scapula, the sacrum, the elbows, the ischial tuberosity, the trochanter, the calcaneous, and the lateral malleolus.

Treatment of infectious mononucleosis

Treatment of infectious mononucleosis includes rest (especially during the initial phase of the disease). The individual should be educated to avoid contact sports, strenuous lifting, and any other rigorous activity. Antipyretics may be utilized to reduce temperature. Mild analgesics are often used to assist with pain and discomfort associated with infectious mononucleosis. The nurse should educate the client on rest periods, adequate sleep, quiet activities that require little activity, and the use of salt water gargles for sore throat irritation. The nurse should educate the individual that milk shakes or cool liquid may assist in the throat discomfort associated with infectious mononucleosis. The nurse should encourage the intake of fruit juices and soft foods. The nurse should stress periods of rest and relaxation. Antibiotics are normally used, steroids may or may not be utilized depending upon the provider, and antiviral therapies may be included in the treatment regimen. The nurse should educate the individual on mode of transmission.

Iron deficiency anemia

Diagnosis-changes in RBC, decreased serum iron concentrations, decreased MCV, stool for blood, total iron binding capacity elevated.

Prevention
- Use only breast milk or iron fortified formula for first 12 months,
- Iron supplements (cereal) at 4-6 months in term and 2 months in preterm
- Iron drops to breast fed preemies after 2 months until cereal intro
- Limit formula to 1L/d to encourage iron rich foods

Treatment
- Increase dietary iron (formula, foods, not cow' milk if under 1y/o)
- Iron supplements
- Counseling

Monitor for side effects-nausea, gastric irritation, diarrhea, constipation, anorexia,
Transfusion only for severe
Monitor Vit B12 def (develops when mucosa cannot secret enough intrinsic factor

Acne

More common in boys than girls and peak ages is 16-17 F, and 17-18 M

Disease that involves the pilosebaceous unit which is the sebaceous glands and hair follicles.

Excessive sebum production, Comedogenesis, Overgrowth of Propionibacterium acnes

Management of Acne
Combined approach most effective, General- well balanced diet, rest, decrease stress

Cleansing-acne not caused by dirt or oil on the skin. Gentle cleansers QD to BID sufficient.
Antibacterial soaps are ineffective. Keep hair off the forehead

Scoliosis

Scoliosis is an abnormal curvature of the spine to one side. The curvature varies from slight to severe. The spine can bend either way at any point along the spine. The chest area (thoracic scoliosis) and the lower part of the back (lumbar scoliosis) are the most common regions. Scoliosis can develop at any time during childhood and adolescence. It is more common in girls than boys, most commonly occurring at the start of adolescence. Scoliosis is rarely present at birth, however it can develop in infancy or early childhood.

Signs/Symptoms:
- Spinal curvature
- Sideways curvature of the spine
- Sideways body posture
- One shoulder raised higher than the other
- Clothes not hanging properly
- Local muscular aches
- Local ligament pain

Cognitive impairment

- Mild retardation: Those with an IQ of 52 to 69 are believed to have educable mild retardation. This individual will achieve a mental age of 8 to 12 years, can learn daily living activities, communication skills that will resemble a grade school student, and be able to function with minimal vocational skills to provide self-care and maintenance.
- Moderate retardation: An IQ of 36 to 51 designates moderate retardation. This individual will achieve a mental age between 3 and 7 years, has noted developmental delay, shows simple communication skills, and can learn self-help skills.
- Severe retardation: Severe retardation is determined with an IQ of 20 to 35. Individuals with severe retardation will have the mental age of a toddler, have marked developmental delay, has little or no communication ability, and can learn repetition related to activities. This individual must be supervised continuously with self-protective mechanisms in place.
- Profound retardation: The individual with an IQ of less than 19 is profoundly retarded. A profoundly retarded individual will have the mental age of an infant, have obvious developmental delays in all aspects of life, and require total care.

IQ definition and classifications of intellectual disability

Intellectual Disability (ID) – IQ less than 70
Problems in day to day functioning, difficulty securing or maintaining employment, inadequate self-care, impaired social skills.

Classification of ID:
- Mild – (IQ of 50-70)
- Moderate (IQ of 35-49)
- Severe (IQ of 20-34)
- Profound (IQ below 20) – usually other severe problems as well

Down syndrome

Down syndrome is an abnormality with chromosome 21. Down syndrome may also be referred to as trisomy 21 syndrome. Chromosome 21 may have a triplication, or variation that causes Down syndrome. The individual with Down syndrome will have 47 chromosomes instead of 46. Down syndrome occurs most often in babies born to mother's age thirty-five and over. Down syndrome is a disorder that causes intellectual disability, growth retardation, flat face, short nose, small low-set ears, thick, fissured tongue, laxness in joints and ligaments, pelvic dislocation, wide hands and feet, and short, fat fingers. Individuals with Down syndrome characteristically have Brushfield's spots on the iris. Infants with Down syndrome will have difficulty feeding, may experience intestinal obstruction, and frequent respiratory infections. Those with Down syndrome will almost always develop Alzheimer's disease by age 40, and have an increased risk for Leukemia.

Treatment of hypoglycemia and hyperglycemia in newborns

Hypoglycemia
Plasma glucose<45mg/dl(2.5mmol/L) requires intervention
At risk-maternal illness (diabetes, HTN, terbutaline administration) or newborn factors (hypoxia, infection, hypothermia, polycythemia, congenital malformations, hyperinsulinism, SGA, fetal hydrops), Interventions-breast/bottle feed, oral D5W, IV dextrose

Hyperglycemia
Glucose>125 in full term or >150 in preterm infant
At risk-SGA, with decreased insulin sensitivity (transient DM), receiving methylxanthines, infants that are stressed (respiratory, surgery)
Usually asymptomatic, Treat by reducing glucose intake or insulin in very SGA

Hemolytic-Uremic Syndrome in children

Sickle cell anemia:
- Occurs primarily in African Americans
- Occurrence 1 in 375 infants born in US
- 1 in 12 have sickle cell trait
- Occasionally also in persons of Mediterranean descent
- Also seen in South American, Arabian, and East Indian descent

Etiology of sickle cell:
- Autosomal recessive disorder
- Partial or complete replacement of normal Hgb with abnormal hemoglobin S (Hgb S)
- Hemoglobin in the RBCs takes on an elongated "sickle" shape
- Sickled cells are rigid and obstruct capillary blood flow
- Microscopic obstructions lead to engorgement and tissue ischemia
- Hypoxia occurs and causes sickling

Response to pain with infants and children

Young infant's response to pain:
- Generalized response of rigidity, thrashing
- Loud crying
- Facial expressions of pain (grimace)
- No understanding of relationship between stimuli and subsequent pain

Older infant's response to pain:
- Withdrawal from painful stimuli
- Loud crying
- Facial grimace
- Physical resistance

Young child's response to pain:
- Loud crying, screaming
- Verbalizations: "Ow", "Ouch", "It hurts"
- Thrashing of limbs
- Attempts to push away stimulus

School-age child's response to pain:
- Stalling behavior ("wait a minute")
- Muscle rigidity
- May use all behaviors of young child

Adolescent:
- Less vocal protest, less motor activity
- Increased muscle tension and body control
- More verbalizations ("it hurts", "you're hurting me")

Pain assessment with children

Principles of Pain Assessment in Children – QUESTT:
- Question the child
- Use a pain rating scale
- Evaluate behavioral and physiologic changes
- Secure parent's involvement
- Take the cause of pain into account
- Take action and evaluate results

Pain rating scales:
- Not all pain rating scales are reliable or appropriate for children
- Should be age appropriate
- Consistent use of same scale by all staff
- Familiarize child with scale

Pain Scales:
- FACES pain rating scale
- Numeric scale
- FLACC scale:
  - Facial expression
  - Legs (normal relaxed, tense, kicking, drawn up)
  - Activity (quiet, squirming, arched, jerking, etc)
  - Cry (none, moaning, whimpering, scream, sob)
  - Consolability (content, easy or difficult to console)

Loss of control with hospitalization and illness of infants and children

Loss of control:
- Infants' Needs –
  - Trust
  - Consistent loving caregivers
  - Daily routines
- Toddlers' Needs –
  - Autonomy
  - Daily routines and rituals
  - Loss of control may contribute to: Regression of behavior, Negativity, Temper tantrums
- Preschoolers –
  - Egocentric and magical thinking typical of age
  - May view illness or hospitalization as punishment for misdeeds
  - Preoperational thought
- School Age –
  - Striving for independence and productivity
  - Fears of death, abandonment, permanent injury
  - Boredom
- Adolescents - Struggle for independence and liberation
  - Separation from peer group
  - May respond with anger, frustration
  - Need for information about their condition

Newborn seizures

Causes of neonatal seizures:
- Metabolic, Toxic and electrolyte
- Perinatal infections, Postnatal infections
- Trauma at birth, Malformations, Miscellaneous

Neonatal seizure types:
- Clonic
- Tonic
- Myoclonic
- Subtle

Term newborn seizure types:
- Clonic
- Multifocal clonic
- Migratory clonic

Therapeutic management of neonatal seizures:
- Treat underlying cause
- Respiratory support PRN

Medications:
- Phenobarbital (IV or PO)
- Phenytoin (Dilantin)
- Lorazepam
- Diazepam (Valium)

Ways infants lose body heat

The 4 ways infants can lose body heat are as follows:
- Conduction is the flow of heat energy from regions of warmer temperature to regions of cooler temperature.
- Convection is the movement of heat by currents in the medium, ie. the wind.
- Radiation is the emission of electromagnetic energy (which your body does in the infrared wavelengths).
- Evaporation is of course simply the change of phase of sweat.

Vaccinations for children

The vaccines available for children and the appropriate ages are:
- Hepatitis B vaccine-Newborn, 2 months, 1 year
- DTP vaccine-2,4,6 months and 15 months old
- Polio vaccine 2,4,6 months and 4-6 years old
- Hepatitis B vaccine-Newborn, 2 months, 1 year
- MMR vaccine-1 year and 4-6 years old
- Varicella vaccine- 1 year old
- Polio vaccine 2,4,6 months and 4-6 years old

Neuroblastoma condition in children

Neuroblastoma is a tumor in children that starts from nervous tissue. It is capable of spreading rapidly. The cause unknown.

Symptoms:
- Abdominal mass
- Skin color changes
- Fatigue
- Tachycardia
- Motor paralysis
- Anxiety
- Diarrhea
- Random eye movements
- Bone and joint pain
- Labored breathing

Tests:
- Bone scan
- CBC
- MIBG scan

- Catecholamines tests
- X-ray
- CT scan
- MRI

Treatment:
- Radiation
- Chemotherapy
- Surgery

Monitor the patient for:
- Kidney failure
- Metastasis
- Various organ system failures
- Liver failure

Aortic coarctation

The aorta becomes narrow at some point due to a birth defect. The symptoms are:
- Headache
- Hypertension with activity
- Nose bleeding
- Fainting
- SOB

Tests:
- Check BP
- Doppler US
- Chest CT
- MRI
- ECG
- Chest X-ray
- Cardiac catheterization

Treatment: Surgery

Monitor the patient for:
- Stroke
- Heart failure
- Aortic aneurysm
- Htn
- CAD
- Endocarditis
- Aortic dissection

Childhood and adult immunization schedule

Children should be inoculated to avoid disease processes; mandatory inoculations include:

Birth	2 mos.	4 mos.	6 mos.	9-10 mos.
HBV-B	DTP	DTP	DTP	HBV-B
	HIB	HIB	HIB	
	IPV	IPV	PCV	
	PCV	PCV		
	HBV-B			

12-14 mos.	15-24 mos.	4-6 yrs.	11-12 yrs.
HIB	DTP	DTP	Tetanus Booster
IPV		IPV	
MMR		MMR	
VAR			

HBV-B—Hepatitis B Vaccine
DTP---Diphtheria, Tetanus, Pertussis
HIB---H-Influenza Type B, IPV---Inactivated polio vaccine
MMR---Measles, mumps, rubella
VAR---Varicella (Chickenpox)
PCV---Pneumococcal conjugate vaccine

Adults and children can obtain an annual flu inoculation. Pneumonia vaccinations should be given every 5 years and only once past the age of 50 years. (Some recent studies discuss one pneumonia vaccination prior to age 50 and one after age 50)

Rh system (Rh blood group) and hemolytic disease of the newborn

The Rh system is the second most complex blood group and is derived of a protein antigen system. The Rh system is named for the Rhesus monkey related to the increased levels of polymorphism. The Rh factor D is responsible for maternal-fetal blood compatibility with potential for newborn hemolytic disease. Erythrocyte development begins at approximately two weeks following gestation. Hemolytic disease is the end product of incompatible fetal antigens of erythrocytes and maternal antigens of erythrocytes. Antigens are genetic formations that may include A, B, AB, and O; Rh antigen D may or may not be included. Differences that occur most often include a mother that has a different blood type than that of the fetus, or a mother that has a positive Rh antigen and a fetus that does not or is Rh negative. On smear the blood cells will include immature red cells not traditionally found in the blood.

Clinical manifestations of Rh system incompatibility and treatment

Signs and symptoms of Rh incompatibility include healthy appearing neonates or neonates who are slightly pale in appearance. Minimal hepatomegaly and splenomegaly is apparent in the neonate. If the neonate has an enlarged liver or spleen this is an indicator of anemia and places the neonate at an increased risk for cardiovascular disease and shock. Hyperbilirubinemia and icterus neonatorum (neonatal jaundice) may appear following birth related to the destruction of erythrocytes and maternal antibodies that remain in the circulatory system of the neonate for several weeks post birth. This neonate will require transfusion with the needed Rh factor antibodies. If no antibodies are transfused bilirubin will deposit in the brain of the neonate causing kernicterus and cerebral damage. Neonates with incompatibility issues are given Rh immune globulin or RhoGAM which is an antibody that works against Rh antigen D; this immune globulin should be given within the first 3 days (72 hours) of exposure to Rh positive erythrocytes.

Blood compatibility and blood transfusion reactions

RBC Compatibility

RECIPIENT				DONOR				
	AB+	AB-	B+	B-	A+	A-	O+	O-
AB +	YES	YES	YES	YES	YES	YES	YES	YES
AB-	NO	YES	NO	YES	NO	YES	NO	YES
B+	NO	NO	YES	YES	NO	NO	YES	YES
B-	NO	NO	NO	YES	NO	NO	NO	YES
A+	NO	NO	NO	NO	YES	YES	YES	YES
A-	NO	NO	NO	NO	NO	YES	NO	YES
O+	NO	NO	NO	NO	NO	NO	YES	YES
O-	NO	NO	NO	NO	NO	NO	NO	YES

AFH is an mneumonic to help you remember the signs of a blood transfusion reaction.
Allergic- facial flushing, hives, rash, anxiety, wheezing, decrease bp
Febrile- headache, tachycardia, tachypnea, fever/chills
Hemolytic- decreased bp, increased rr, hemoglobinuria, chest pain, anxiety, lower back pain, fever, tachycardia, chills

Treatment of hypocalcemia in newborns

Hypocalcemia- Normal range 7.0-8.5 mg/dl

Early-onset hypocalcemia- appears in 1st 24-48 hrs.; generally temporary and resolves
Most common in preterms/SGA with hypoxia or to diabetic mother
Jittery, long QT interval, apnea, cyanosis, high pitched cry, abdominal distension

Late-onset hypocalcemia (cow's milk-induced hypocalcemia/neonatal tetany)
After 3-4 days of life, Common with intestinal malabsorption, hyperinsulinemia, hypoparathyroidism, hypomagnesemia, or with phosphate enemas, Neuromuscular irritation, Rare in industrial countries with commercial formula and use of mother's milk
Treat with early feedings, correction of hypoparathyroidism, and sometimes calcium supplements

IV calcium gluconate 10%-very slowly monitoring heart and BP; constant surveillance of IV site due to necrotic affects; incompatible with lots of drugs; monitor for seizures
Monitor for signs of hypercalcemia-vomiting, bradycardia

Lymphomas

Lymphomas - Hodgkin disease
More prevalent in 15-19 yrs of age

Non-Hodgkin lymphoma (NHL)
More prevalent in children <14 yrs of age
Approximately 60% of pediatric lymphomas are NHL

Classifications of Hodgkin Disease:
- Classification A: asymptomatic
- Classification B: temperature of 38 or higher for three consecutive days, night sweats, unexplained wt loss of 10% or more over previous 6 months, signs - enlarged, firm, nontender, movable nodes in supraclavicular or cervical area (sentinel node L clavicle); systemic symptoms

Therapeutic management:
- Radiation
- Chemotherapy (alone or with radiation)
- Prognosis varies

Immune system of the neonate

Newborns are traditionally born with decreased levels of immunoglobulins and a decreased reaction of the complement system. The alterations of the newborns immune system make him/her vulnerable to infection and disease processes because the immune system does not readily recognize insidious bacteria resulting in lack of recognition of signs of infection or infectious processes. The most reliable sign of infection or an infectious process in the neonate is hypothermia or an abnormally low body temperature. When the neonate is born he/she has only had the protective immunity of IgG as it is the only immunoglobulin that crosses the placental blood barrier causing acquired passive immunity to occur. If the pregnant female has experienced a disease process or infection during her pregnancy and developed antibodies this is termed active acquired immunity. The majority of maternal immunity takes place during the final trimester of pregnancy. Preterm infants have little or no passive acquired immunity increasing their vulnerability to infection.

Circumcision

Circumcision is the act of removing the foreskin from the penis of infant males. Circumcision is a sterile surgical procedure that removes the prepuce (epithelial tissue) from the tip or head of the penis. Circumcision is a choice made by the parents of the male infant and is not an automatic practice of the hospital. The nurse has the responsibility of educating the parents on the procedure of circumcision, the benefits and potential risks. Circumcision of females is practiced in many countries and involves the removal of female genitalia, prepuce and/or other parts of the external female genitalia.

Health promotion in infancy

Health promotion of infants includes meeting the physiological needs of the infant. These physiological needs include sleep, fresh air, and adequate amounts of natural sunlight, skin care, appropriate dress, and promotion of regular elimination patterns. Solid foods should be added to the diet slowly during infancy. Finger foods at approximately six months, soft table foods at 12 months, whole milk at 3 to 5 months, diluted juices at 6 months, new foods one at a time, and avoid egg whites until 12 months related to the potential for allergic reactions. Safety issues of infants include accident prevention mechanisms. Immunizations begin during infancy as a prevention mechanism. And routine practitioner visits are done during infancy to monitor health status, growth and development.

Kawasaki disease

A disease that primarily affects young children, Kawasaki is an autoimmune disease of unknown origin. It attacks the heart, blood vessels, and lymph nodes.

Symptoms:
- Fever
- Joint pain
- Swollen lymph nodes
- Peripheral edema
- Rashes
- Papillae on the tongue
- Chapped/Red lips

Tests:
- CBC
- Presence of pyuria
- Chest X-ray
- ECGH
- ESR
- Urine Analysis

Treatment:
- Gamma globulin
- Salicylate treatment

Monitor the patient for:
- Coronary aneurysm
- MI
- Vasculitis

Phases of wound healing

The following are the four phases in the process of wound healing:
- Phase 1: inflammation - edema, angiogenesis, phagocytosis
- Phase 2: granulation/proliferation - Lasts 5-30 days
- Phase 3: contraction - Fibroblasts bring wound edges closer together
- Phase 4: maturation - Scar forms and changes over time

Factors influencing healing:

- Moist crust-free environment enhances wound healing
- Nutrition
- Stress
- Infection
- Diseases
- Circulation

Sample patient care outcomes for diabetic patient with known knowledge deficit

The care plan for a diabetic patient should show patient education to include the family. The learners should be able to describe signs and symptoms of hypoglycemia as well as hyperglycemia. The patient and the family should be able to demonstrate the correct procedure for giving insulin injections, the proper site for injections, the proper use of the syringe, and the proper storage methods for medications. The education should also include preventive measures for avoiding hyperglycemia, diet knowledge, and the proper care of skin and feet.

Assessing readiness for change in morbidly obese patient

A nurse may need to assess readiness for change in a multitude of patient care situations, depending on the population of patients he/she works with. A nurse who works with a patient who is morbidly obese may need to provide instruction and guidance to foster weight loss in order to reduce the incidence of complications associated with this situation. Weight loss in a morbidly obese patient involves making changes in diet and lifestyle, and the nurse must assess the patient's readiness for change. This may involve asking the patient to consider future health outcomes, goals for weight and activity levels, or ideas about how best to provide self-care. Once the nurse determines that the patient is ready to change, the nurse works as a change agent to provide resources and support to the patient during the change process.

Role in population screening

Depending on the type of screen being performed, the nurse plays a pivotal role when working with groups of people being screened for disease. The nurse may provide education to patients about the reasons for the screen and potential outcomes of the testing. The nurse can also educate the patients if their screens return as positive, giving them instructions for self-care or helping them to make decisions about treatment. In some cases, the nurse may care for the patients who are receiving the screening by drawing blood or assisting with the screening exam. Finally, the nurse may also administer treatments to those clients who have decided to pursue preventive measures to reduce their risks.

Learner readiness

Learner readiness is the term used to describe and measure whether the person being educated is ready to learn. In the case of a terminal diagnosis or an injury which has reduced a client's attention and cognitive abilities, learner readiness may be minimal or non-existent. This is documented in the patient care plan, and a family member or other support person is then brought in to be a learner too. The client, family, or support person will not learn, retain, or be able to repeat the material if they are not at a point in the care where they are ready to learn. The nurse may have to be encouraging in some instances to get the teaching started and to get the family or client to accept responsibility for the learning process. The nurse may also assist in identifying barriers to learning and addressing those barriers to enhance the learning process.

Learning styles

The nurse may need to assess the learning styles of the client and the family when doing patient teaching to make the process more effective. Some clients will learn easily with verbal instruction and no visual aids. Others may need to see pictures or printed words to understand what is being taught. Families may need to be taught concepts several times and in several different ways before the material sinks in because of stress, different learning styles, and level of comprehension. The nurse may teach material herself, or she may delegate or supervise the teaching. The teaching methods used may be verbal, visual, return demonstration, or a combination of the three. The material may need to be repeated more than once before the client and family fully understand the scope of what is being taught.

Strategies for effective teaching

Here are some effective methods to increase client and family learning:
- Use visual aids, videotapes, written brochures, and clearly written handouts.
- Assess the need for low-level reading material to make learning easier for clients who have a low reading level.
- Encourage family participation.
- Limit what is taught during each session.
- Put special emphasis on the needs of the patient after the patient goes home, rather than just focusing on the here and now.
- Allow time for questions and answers.

Patient education regarding coronary artery disease

A nurse doing a care plan for a chronic condition like coronary artery disease would discuss the definition of CAD and its causes with the client and his or her family. The signs and symptoms of exacerbation of CAD should also be discussed. An explanation of the treatment measures and complications can be part of the education, as can skin care, assessment edema, and skin color and temperature. The education also includes presenting information about any prescribed regimens the physician has ordered, any medications, and any associated side effects of those medications. Teaching about chronic conditions may need to be done in small segments so the patient is not overwhelmed. Too much information presented in too short of a timeframe will not be absorbed by the patient, and will lead to noncompliance.

Psychosocial Integrity

Maslow's hierarchy of needs

Maslow's hierarchy of needs describes a theory of basic needs for each person set up in the style of a pyramid. In order to move upward, a person's basic needs must first be met. The lowest portion of the pyramid is physiological needs, including needs for food, sleep, and clothing. Unless these basic needs are met, trying to meet other needs, such as a sense of belonging, is irrelevant. The next level is safety, in which a person must feel secure psychologically; this may involve feelings of security for the future or freedom from uncertainty. Love and belonging is the next level, which involves feelings of being accepted and cared for by others and establishing rewarding relationships. Self-esteem makes up the next level, in which a person feels good about himself and his choices. Finally, self-actualization crowns the top of the pyramid, which involves a secure individual allowing himself to be challenged in new ways and finding satisfaction in new pursuits.

Physiological needs - Physiological needs are the very basic needs such as air, water, food, sleep, sex, etc. When these are not satisfied we may feel sickness, irritation, pain, discomfort, etc.
Safety needs - Safety needs have to do with establishing stability and consistency in a chaotic world. These needs are mostly psychological in nature.
Love needs - Love and belongingness are next on the ladder. Humans have a desire to belong to groups: clubs, work groups, religious groups, family, gangs, etc.
Esteem Needs - There are two types of esteem needs. First is self-esteem which results from competence or mastery of a task. Second, there's the attention and recognition that comes from others.
Self-Actualization - The need for self-actualization is "the desire to become more and more what one is, to become everything that one is capable of becoming."

Dementia

Dementia is really a (chronic) syndrome that encompasses any disorder characterized by multiple cognitive deficits that include memory impairment. For example: Alzheimer's type; vascular; other general medical conditions such as HIV, head trauma, Parkinson's disease; substance induced; or those of indeterminate origin. An essential feature of a dementia is the development of cognitive deficits that include memory impairment and at least one of the following problems: aphasia, apraxia, agnosia, or a disturbance in executive functioning.

Delirium

Delirium is an acute alteration in consciousness that cannot be explained by a pre-existing or evolving dementia. It tends to fluctuate over the course of the day and attention span is impaired. Delirium is often accompanied by a disturbance in the sleep-wake cycle and psychomotor behavior. However, it's very important to realize that the latter can be either increased OR decreased. It's easy to overlook a quietly delirious older person, but delirium has to be considered a RED FLAG, because it can indicate many underlying pathological processes (such as a UTI, MI, or pneumonia). It also can be superimposed upon an existing dementia; thus any sudden change in cognition in a person with dementia has to be evaluated for an underlying physiological cause (including pain).

Schizophrenia

Schizophrenia symptoms:
- Social withdrawal
- Depersonalization (intense anxiety and a feeling of being unreal)
- Loss of appetite
- Loss of hygiene
- Delusions
- Hallucinations (e.g., hearing things not actually present)
- The sense of being controlled by outside forces.

A person with schizophrenia may not have any outward appearance of being ill. In other cases, the illness may be more apparent, causing bizarre behaviors. For example, a person with schizophrenia may wear aluminum foil in the belief that it will stop one's thoughts from being broadcasted and protect against malicious waves entering the brain.

Treatment for schizophrenia, psychotic disorders, and developmental disorders

Such dysfunctions as delusions, hallucinations, inappropriate emotions, disorganized speech and inappropriate behavior make up the category of mental illness called schizophrenia. Persons with schizophrenia may suffer from disrupted or disturbed thought processes, perceptions, speech, and movement. The types of schizophrenia include schizophreniform, schizoaffective, and delusional. Schizophrenia is usually treated with medication, but psychotherapy may be necessary to help the patient continue to take the medicine and also to help him or her deal with social situations. Such developmental disorders as intellectual disability, attention deficit/hyperactivity, dyslexia and other learning disorders, autism, and Asperger's start while the patient is a child or at birth and continue through life. The presence of a developmental disorder may delay or disrupt the development of other skills in the child. Brain functions cause many of the developmental disorders, but the interaction with psychosocial influences creates a complex situation. Treatment varies according to the disorder and may include a combination of medication, education, and training in daily living skills.

Manic depression disorder

Depressive symptoms associated with manic depression disorder may include:
- Chronic pain
- Sad mood
- Decreased energy
- Loss of interest in activities
- Weight and/or appetite changes due to over- or under-eating
- Excessive crying
- Increased restlessness and irritability
- Decreased ability to concentrate and make decisions
- Suicidal thoughts and/or attempts
- Feelings of helplessness

- Changes in sleep patterns
- Social withdrawal

Manic symptoms associated with manic depression disorder may include:
- overly inflated self-esteem
- decreased need for rest and sleep
- increased distractibility and irritability
- increased physical agitation
- excessive involvement in pleasurable activities that may result in painful consequence; this may include provocative, aggressive, or destructive behavior
- increased talkativeness
- excessive "high" or euphoric feelings
- increased sex drive
- increased energy level
- uncharacteristically poor judgment
- increased denial

Anxiety, somatoform, dissociative, and mood disorders

Anxiety is a state of uneasiness or apprehension, which can cause physical tension. The tension of looking forward to an event can be positive. Severe anxieties or multiple anxieties, especially when they have comorbidity with another disorder are abnormal behavior. Panic disorder, phobias, posttraumatic stress, and obsessive-compulsive behavior are examples of anxiety disorders. Medication, relaxation techniques, cognitive behavioral therapy, and exposure exercises are acceptable treatments for anxiety disorders. Somatoform disorders involve physical symptoms for which no specific physical cause is present. The disorders include hypochondrias, somatization disorder, conversion, and pain disorder. Treatment is more management than cure and may or may not include medication. Dissociative disorders involve the breakdown of a person's perceptions of his environment, his memory or identity. Dissociative disorders include dissociative amnesia, dissociative fugue (flight), dissociative identity disorder (multiple personality) and depersonalization disorder. Psychotherapy and sometimes hypnosis are among the treatments for dissociative disorders. A mood disorder is a condition in which the person's prevailing mood is disturbed or inappropriate. The disorders include depression, anxiety, and bipolar syndrome. The mood disorders are the most common psychological illnesses and are increasing worldwide in both the adult and child populations.

Anxiety disorders
Anxiety is a normal reaction to stress. It helps one deal with a tense situation in the office, study harder for an exam, and keep focused on an important speech. In general, it helps one cope. But when anxiety becomes an excessive, irrational dread of everyday situations, it has become a disabling disorder. Five major types of anxiety disorders are:
- Generalized Anxiety Disorder
- Obsessive-Compulsive Disorder (OCD)
- Panic Disorder
- Post-Traumatic Stress Disorder (PTSD)
- Social Phobia (or Social Anxiety Disorder)

Goals and interventions for potential anxiety or depression

The goal for a patient with the potential for anxiety or depression should be to reduce the signs and symptoms of anxiety or depression and the associated thought processes by replacing them with effective coping mechanisms. The nurse will instruct the patient and family on the disease process, medications, and safety in the home. The care plan would give interventions like giving positive feedback and encouragement and allowing the patient to vent concerns. The client will develop a rapport with the nurse, identify signs of anxiety, and demonstrate compliance with medications. The client will be able to verbalize alternative ways to cope with and prevent anxiety and give feedback when those methods have been used effectively.

Cognitive disorders and treatment

The cognitive disorders are impairment of such functions as memory, perception, and attention. They usually affect persons at least forty years old and become more common in the over-seventy population. They can be caused by diseases such as Alzheimer's and Parkinson's; brain injury, including damage from stroke; and changes brought on by aging. The disorders include delirium, dementia, and amnesia. Treatment includes medication and psychosocial interventions for delirium, and the prevention of further damage for conditions resulting from injury. Persons with a cognitive disorder require the assistance of a caregiver and may need institutional care.

Eating disorders

Eating disorders are most often caused by emotional trauma or stressors the individual may possess; these emotional ideations are symptomized by disturbed eating patterns. Anorexia is a mental illness in which the affected individual displays periods of self-inflicted starvation and/or periods of bulimic episodes, excessive exercise may accompany anorexia nervosa especially in teens. Bulimia is also a mental illness in which the individual will consume a diet and then purge to not allow the ingested food into the system. Bulimic individuals experience episodes of consuming large amounts of foods only to self-inflict vomiting post food consumption.

Rape

The following are various types of rape:
- Date rape: Date rape is a term used to describe rape that occurs between individuals who are acquainted with one another.
- Virgin rape: Rape of a person thought to be virginal or pure; this person is often unable to offer resistance related to physical or mental disabilities.
- Blitz rape: Blitz rape is violent between strangers, is unforeseen and abrupt, and often involves a weapon.
- Acquaintance rape/confidence rape: Acquaintance or confidence rape is characterized by a deceptive trusting relationship that is violated and ends in sexual assault.
- Power rape: Power rape is a form of dominance in which the attacker renders the victim helpless to assume control over the victim.

- Anger rape: Anger rape involves cruelty and humiliation. Anger rape is seen most frequently with older women.
- Sadistic rape: Sadistic rape involves disfigurement and torment of the victim.
- Gang rape: Gang rape is characterized by men who feel pressured to commit acts of sexual assault as a group to show masculinity or prove themselves equal to or better than their peers; gang rape often is associated with violence as the involved individuals try to perform at a superior level than their peers with no regard to the victim.

Battered women

Women who have experienced abuse will often feel they themselves have failed as a mother, wife, or caregiver and accept the abuse as a normal healthy relationship. Often abused women do not have close family relationships or friendships. Abused women display low self-esteem, prefer isolation, show lack of independence in decision making skills, and express fear or anxiety related to confronting or upsetting the abuser. Battered women often are abusers themselves of their children, and exhibit risqué behaviors. Women who suffer abuse may feel shame and deny any abuse has occurred. Conflicting stories related to injuries, the spouse who dominates the questioning and unexplained injuries are all red flags for abuse. (Clinical note: It is very appropriate for the nurse to first interview a couple, and then do a single interview with the individual they feel is being abused.)

Behavioral indicators of sexual assault

The following are behavioral indicators that sexual assault may be occurring:
- Detailed and overly sophisticated understanding of sexual behavior (especially by young children).
- Regressive behavior, e.g. excessive clinginess in pre-school children or the sudden onset of soiling and wetting when these were not formerly a problem.
- A child may appear disconnected or focused on fantasy worlds.
- Sleep disturbances and nightmares.
- Marked changes in appetite.
- Fear states, e.g. anxiety, depression, phobias, obsession.
- Overly compliant behavior, as often young people who have been abused have experienced extensive grooming behaviors.
- Parentified or adultified behavior, e.g. acting like a parent or spouse.
- Delinquent or aggressive behavior.
- Poor or deteriorating relationships with peers.
- Increased inability to concentrate in school and/or sudden deterioration in school performance.
- Unwillingness to participate in physical/recreational activities, especially if this is due to symptoms of physical discomfort.
- Truancy/running away from home.
- Drug/alcohol abuse.

Somatic symptoms of child abuse

Somatic is a term used to describe the trunk or the body in general. Somatic symptoms of child abuse include, but are not limited to any dislocation of muscle, bone or tissue. Pain that is continuous, constant nausea and vomiting, abdominal edema, tenderness, rigidity, and shock can all be associated with signs of somatic child abuse. Somatic child abuse may be manifested in various hematomas found on the body with no explanation. Often children who suffer somatic child abuse do so for several months or years before they are diagnosed, and treated. Somatic child abuse often results in permanent damage and death. Somatic symptoms are often unrecognizable as child abuse upon initial examination; this is a reason for detailed and accurate assessment.

Signs and symptoms of child abuse

The nurses' role is to identify, assist with treatment, and prevention of child abuse and neglect. The most common signs and symptoms of child abuse include, but are not limited to bruises that can be found on any location of the body. Burns of the hand or foot are most often immersion burns (the limbs of these children are submersed into boiling liquid). Pattern burns can be identified with branding marks such as circles, cigarette burns or any object used to burn the skin of a child in which a certain burn pattern remains. Fractures may occur in any part of the body. Lacerations and abrasions may appear on the mouth, gums, around the eye area, and in the genital region. Often the abuser attempts to force objects into the mouth of an infant or child causing tears in the mouth, vaginal or anal area. Bite marks, fingernail scratches and puncture wounds may also be found on any part of the body. Head trauma may present with bulging fontanelle, and cranial suture separation. Head trauma may also consist of hematomas and broken vessels in the eyes that reveal bleeding. Children exposed to head trauma may experience bleeding from the ears and decreased or impaired hearing.

Behavior of abused children

Children who have experienced abuse may exhibit behaviors such as aggression, and/or pulling back. Abused children often express fright with the home environment and/or the individual who is abusing them. Abused children display apprehensive behavior when they witness episodes of weeping among other children. Abused children often display no emotion with parents. With any display of affection the abused child may become friendly, and interested in the individual. Abused children often avoid eye contact. Children who are abused will also show signs of rigidity when they are approached, and may have inappropriate responses to painful procedures.

Suicide

Suicide is among the ten most frequent causes of death in the United States with approximately 30,000 recorded each year. The actual number is estimated to be closer to 75,000. The suicide rate increases with age. Among 15-24 year olds, suicide is the third most frequent cause of death with about 4,000 each year. Males are more likely to commit suicide than females, but the attempt rate is higher among females. Groups at greatest risk include Native American and Alaska Native adolescents and gay and lesbian youth. No differences in the profiles of suicidal and non-suicidal individuals are revealed by such standard personality tests as the MMPI and Rorschach. Indications that a person may make

- 105 -

a suicide attempt include depression and anger, experiencing loss or rejection, talking about suicide, planning and securing the means to commit suicide, and giving away possessions. Counselors should be aware of support groups, have a crisis plan, and involve the community when working with at-risk clients.

Suicide precautions:
Windows locked
Breakproof glass and mirrors
Plastic flatware
No phone cords, extension cords, curtain cords, or equipment cords
No belts, sharps, razors, matches or cigarettes
Frequent observation or 1 to 1 care
Communicate therapeutically
Make a behavior contract
Restraints if ordered
Meds if ordered
Monitor and restrict visitors

Alcohol and substance abuse and associated counseling techniques

Substance abuse, which includes the abuse of alcohol, prescription drugs, and illegal drugs, is a major problem in the United States. Of the fourteen percent of adults who admit to dependence at sometime in their life, half have experienced the problem during the last year. More than three million teenagers have a problem with alcohol. There is a strong connection between drinking and such teenage problems as suicide, early sexual activity, and driving accidents. Abuse of alcohol and drugs affects not just the abuser, but family members, friends, and coworkers as well. Characteristics of substance abusers include low self-esteem, anxiety, sexual problems, suicidal impulses, fear of failure, and social isolation. Since addictions are both physical and mental, successful treatment must involve both. The Substance Abuse Subtle Screening Inventory (SASSI) can be used to detect indications of addiction. One effective treatment method is a Twelve-Step Program coupled with individual, group, and family counseling. It is especially important that counseling involve the family. Behavior modification and social learning theory can be used effectively in a residential program.

Good communication

Excellent communication requires active listening, appropriate choice of time and place, and adequate self-expression. Active listening involves watching for non-verbal communication and observing underlying meaning. Choice of time and place sued to communicate will vary from client to client. Children tend to communicate better during play rather than when being expected to sit still. Adult clients typically demand a high level of privacy and calm surroundings in order to be open to communication. It is the job of the counselor to assess each client as to the good timing of communication. Adequate self-expression is about more than just word choice. The counselor should be careful with their tone of voice, facial expressions and body language.

Active listening

Attributes of active listeners include conveying warmth and respect, and offering acceptance of the client. The nurse must acknowledge all behavior of the client and realize it has meaning. The nurse must set boundaries and abide by them when taking part in a conversation. Do not lead the client in a direction; allow ample time for expression making head gestures, and using body language. The nurse should ask questions related to the topic of discussion, maintain eye contact with the client, and face the client, lean in as listening intently, nod, smile, and frown to show agreement or disagreement. The nurse must be aware of his or her own experiences and how they can alter the relationship with the client.

Feedback

Feedback is the important final step in the communication process. With all the problems inherent in communication with other people, the receiver of the message should to let the sender know what was actually heard. Feedback is always given in the form of non-verbal responses. These responses are extremely useful for the perceptive person as a guide as to whether or not the message made it through the obstacles all people have in place. Verbal feedback is usually in the form of continued conversation. Sometimes this can indicate whether or not there is something in the message that is unclear to the receiver. The sender can also specifically ask for a restatement of what was heard if the receiver does not offer feedback unsolicited. Restatements are probably the most reliable indicators of successful communications.

Empathy

Empathy is the process of understanding another person by identifying with his/her situation, rather than seeing it from an outside perspective. Empathy involves putting oneself into another's shoes and seeing the situation as the affected person does. When used in a helping relationship, the counselor can utilize empathy by trying to see the client's viewpoint and consider the situation from the client's perspective, rather than the counselor's. Empathy comprises two stages. The first stage is experiencing the same emotions as the affected person. An example of this might be when a counselor cries with a client who is experiencing significant emotional pain. Stage two of empathy involves realistically looking at the situation from the other person's point of view. An example of this situation might be when a counselor listens to the client and examines his own reaction by considering how he might feel in the same situation.

Contract

A contract is a type of agreement drawn up between two people that is done to promote action and possible reward. A counselor may use a contract with a client who wants to change a behavior; for example, a client may express frustration about making rash decisions that significantly affect his personal life. As part of a contract, a counselor may require that the client agree to consult with a family member or professional before making any decisions that will affect his finances, family life, or health. The contract is drawn up with specific terms and signed by the client. Characteristics of a contract include feasibility—the contract should be written in such a way that the client can actually perform the terms. A contract should also be specific, leaving little room for interpretation. Finally, the contract should be retractable, in that the client can decide that he/she does not want to perform the terms.

Addressing the issue of death with patients and families

The nurse may initiate discussions and be part of the end of life presentation to the patient and their family. The nurse may provide support and assist the patient and their family through the grieving process. With the help of the social worker and case managers, the nurse makes the family aware of support services, can coordinate pastoral care support, and can assist the family in coming to grips with the possibility of death. The nurse may also help the family and patient work through the details of an Advanced Directive or Do Not Resuscitate order. The nurse may provide resources and educational material on end of life issues so the family and patient can make informed decisions regarding how they want end of life issues handled.

Phases of grief

The phases of grief as defined by Kubler-Ross are:
- Denial
- Anger
- Bargaining
- Depression
- Acceptance

(DABDA)

Cultural influences on learning

Cultural influences can make the learning process difficult because of the language barrier. Although a client and family may say they understand, being aware of different cultures and how they view pain, disease, and illness will help the case manager look for clues as to their actual level of comprehension. Using an interpreter and material written in the appropriate language with clear pictures may enhance the case nurse's ability to teach. It is also important to understand that, in some cultures, pride keeps the client or family from admitting that they do not understand something, and fear may keep them from seeking a clear answer to their questions. When teaching procedures, a return demonstration will ensure the client and family have learned the technique or task. When verbal instruction alone is used, care must be taken to ensure that no misunderstanding has occurred.

Physiological Integrity

Basic Care and Comfort

Nutrition

Nutrition involves the recognition and realization of nutrients and how they are utilized in the body for proper homeostasis and normal bodily functions on a daily basis. Nutrition affects bodily functions as they relate to decision making processes, functional ability, cognitive processes, our social abilities to interact, form, and maintain relationships as well as cultural beliefs that guide our daily decision making. Without proper nutritional intake muscles will not function to support daily activities, the brain and neurological system will not have the required nutrients to function in decision making and provide proper neurological functioning mechanisms needed for normal activity. Our emotions are guided by balanced or homeostatic nutritional balance that maintains proper functioning of hormone levels such as insulin.

Dietary standards

Dietary standards are a set of guidelines in which an individual can understand essential nutrients, food consumption and the relationship they possess. Not only do dietary standards increase understanding of foods and their nutritional values they offer a mechanism of comparison. Recommended Dietary Allowances (RDA) is a set of standards the federal government mandates each individual needs on a daily bases to maintain balanced and adequate nutrition. Reference Dietary Intake (RDI) is a combination of recommended daily allowances and mechanisms of risk reduction for diseases such as coronary artery disease, obesity, cancer, and osteoporosis. Dietary standard of RDA, and RDI are used today with meal preparation for our military personnel, groups such as WIC (Women, Infants, and Children), and meals on wheels programs throughout the country.

Food groups and recommended servings

The following are the five food groups and recommended servings on a daily basis:
- Breads and Cereals (6-11 servings) - Foods in this category include rice, cereals, breads and pasta.
- Fruits and Vegetables (3-5 vegetable/2-4 fruit servings) - Foods in this category include tomatoes, green beans, bananas and oranges.
- Meat (2-3 servings) - Foods in this category include beef, chicken, fish, turkey and pork - plus eggs and nuts.
- Milk/Dairy (2-3 servings) - Foods in this category include milk, cheese, yogurt and ice cream.
- Other Foods/Fats - Foods in this category include soda, butter, margarine, candy and processed snack foods.

USDA's MyPlate

The USDA's Food Pyramid was heavily criticized for being vague and confusing, and in 2011 it was replaced with MyPlate. MyPlate is much easier to understand, as it consists of a picture of a dinner plate divided into four sections, visually illustrating how our daily diet should be distributed among the various food groups. Vegetables and grains each take up 30% of the plate, while fruits and proteins each constitute 20% of the plate. There is also a representation of a cup, marked Dairy, alongside the plate. The idea behind MyPlate is that it's much easier for people to grasp the idea that half of a meal should consist of fruits and vegetables than it is for them to understand serving sizes for all the different kinds of foods they eat on a regular basis.

Most experts consider MyPlate to be a great improvement over the Food Pyramid, but it has still come under criticism from some quarters. Many believe too much emphasis is placed on protein, and some say the dairy recommendation should be eliminated altogether. The Harvard School of Public Health created its own Healthy Eating Plate to address what it sees as shortcomings in MyPlate. Harvard's guide adds healthy plant-based oils to the mix, stresses whole grains instead of merely grains, recommends drinking water or unsweetened coffee or tea instead of milk, and adds a reminder that physical activity is important.

USDA dietary guidelines

The dietary guidelines made by the United States Department of Agriculture (USDA) for Americans are as follows:
- To maintain or improve weight, individuals need to preserve a balance between exercise and food consumption.
- Individuals should choose to consume a diet with minimal fats, and cholesterol.
- Individuals should choose to consume a diet high in grains, fresh fruits and vegetables.
- To maintain a nutritional balance individuals should maintain diversity with food choices.
- Diets that minimize the consumption of sodium are recommended by the USDA.
- Diets with sensible use of sugars should be utilized.
- Alcohol consumption should be minimal and controlled.

Nutritional assessment

When attempting to determine the nutritional status of an individual a nutritional assessment is performed. Nutritional assessments identify areas of insufficiency or surplus. Nutritional assessments estimate dietary intake as well as nutrients consumed as they relate to RDA, and RDI. Nutritional assessments provide information on the amount of vitamins and minerals an individual is consuming on a routine basis, this information is then evaluated and compared with what is required to function with or without disease processes. Nutritional assessments provide a way of including nutrition in the healing process as well as in the mechanisms of prevention. Nutritional assessments are the first step in determining a well balanced diet and/or diet that will promote optimal nutrition, body function, and healing processes. Nutritional assessments are done by reviewing a history of the clients/individuals dietary intake over a period of several days.

The 4 areas of the nutritional assessment are as follows:

- Take a history of the dietary intake over the past several days to ensure the period extends beyond 24 or 48 hours. The diet assessment history gives insight into the individuals' daily routine, dietary habits, and patterns. Evaluate the diet to note areas of deficiency.
- Perform a physical examination of the individual to determine height, weight, BMI, overall hydration status, and general condition.
- Anthropometric (comparing measurements of the individual from previous exams) examination will establish normal growth and alert the health care provider to abnormalities in growth.
- Biochemical analysis or evaluation of the individual's molecular findings.

BMI

The body mass index (BMI) is a method of measurement that includes the height and weight of an individual to determine body fat as it relates to nutritional status. The body mass index is determined by dividing the weight in kilograms by the height in meters squared. The preferred range for BMI for the adult is 18-25 kg/m2. A body mass index of less than 18 is considered malnourished. A body mass index of greater than 25 designates the individual as overweight. A body mass index of greater than 30 is considered obese. Body mass index is calculated by dividing the weight in kilograms by the height in meter squared.

Diets

The following are types and attributes of various diets:
- Clear Liquid Diet: A clear liquid diet is made up of items that remain clear and in liquid form at room temperature or body temperature. Clear liquid diets are used primarily with surgical patients or patients who may be experiencing nausea and vomiting.
- Full Liquid Diet: Food that is liquid at room temperature makes up a full liquid diet. Full liquid diets can and do provide total nutrition to individuals who have swallowing or chewing difficulties.
- Pureed Diets: A pureed diet consists of foods that are smooth in consistency; any food item that can be processed into a smooth consistency can be part of a pureed diet. Pureed diets are for individuals with swallowing deficits such as dysphagia (difficulty swallowing). Those individuals who are edentulous (toothless) may benefit from a pureed diet as they do not have the ability to chew food items.
- Mechanical Soft Diet: A mechanical soft diet provides nutrition in the form of foods that require only a nominal amount of chewing.
- Soft Diet: The soft diet provides adequate nutrition by providing foods that are whole, with decreased amounts of fiber and minimal seasoning. Soft diets are utilized when a patient is progressing from a clear to a regular diet.
- Regular Diet: The term regular diet describes a diet that has no limits or needed modifications.
- Diet as tolerated allows for the progression of a very restrictive diet to one that has no dietary restrictions as the healing process or recovery period takes place.

Nutrients

Six categories of nutrients exist and are discussed in society today when we discuss diet and nutrition; these include carbohydrates, vitamins, protein, minerals, water, and lipids (fat). Nutrients are essential or nonessential these refer to the body's ability to produce specific nutrients. Essential nutrients are required by the body on a daily basis for basic functions such as growth or maintenance of health; the body must gain these nutrients through nutrition in order to maintain homeostasis, promote cell growth and function, and promote healing. Nonessential nutrients are produced by the body. Energy providing nutrients include lipids (fats), protein, and carbohydrates. Vitamins and minerals perform in a catalytic fashion to promote the use of nutrients for energy. Tissue repair, growth, and body regulation are the main functions of water and minerals.

Vitamin	Major Functions	Found in
A	Eyes, Skin, Immune System	Dark Green or Orange Fruits and Vegetables, Milk
B6	Producing RBC, Brain/Nerve Function	Spinach, Beans, Nuts, Eggs, Red Meat, Fish
B12	Producing RBC, Nerve Function	Eggs, Milk, Chicken, Red Meat, Fish
C	Teeth, Bones, Skin	Spinach, Tomatoes, Berries, Citrus Fruits
D	Bones, Absorbing Calcium	Milk, Egg Yolk, Sunlight
E	Protects cells from damage, some RBC fx	Nuts, Grains, Oils, Green Vegetables
Folic Acid	Protects against heart disease, Essential for cell health.	Fruits, Dark Green Vegetables

Water-soluble vitamins

Water-soluble vitamins are routinely excreted by the body and need replenished on a daily basis. Water-soluble vitamins include vitamin C, vitamin B1 (thiamine), vitamins B12, and B6 (pyridoxine), vitamin B2 (riboflavin), niacin, folic acid. Water-soluble vitamins can be ingested in the daily diet or with supplementation. Foods containing water-soluble vitamins include citrus, tomatoes, cantaloupe, potatoes, green leafy vegetables, pork, liver, and enriched breads and cereals. Water soluble vitamins dissolve in water or fluid and are discarded by the body via the kidney by way of urine or the bowel by way of fecal matter.

Nutritional requirements of the elderly

The elderly have the following nutritional requirements:
- Protein: 1.0 g Pro /kg body weight for healthy elderly, about 12-14% of total calories.
- Fat: A small amount of fat is necessary for life. They transport fat-soluble vitamins (A, D, K, E), add flavor to food, and enhance its satiety value. Fat digestion is inhibited with aging. No more than 30% of total calories.
- Carbohydrates: Minimum recommended daily intake is 50-100 g/day. At least 50% of total calories should come from complex carbohydrate sources. Daily recommended fiber intake is 20-35 grams.
- Vitamin A needs: Decreases

- Vitamin D needs: Increases; get exposure to sunlight when possible and include vitamin D-rich foods, such as fish and vitamin D fortified skim milk, in the diet. Vitamin B12 needs: Increases; eat vitamin B12-rich foods, such as lean red meat, chicken, and skim milk
- Folate needs: Decreases; no recommended changes.

The calorie content of protein, carbohydrate, and fat are as follows.
Each gram of Protein = 4 calories
Each gram of Carbohydrate = 4 calories
Each gram of Fat = 9 calories

Sodium and sodium restricted diet

Sodium occurs naturally in most foods. The most common form of sodium is sodium chloride, which is table salt. Milk, beets, and celery also naturally contain sodium, as does drinking water, although the amount varies depending on the source. Some of these added forms are monosodium glutamate, sodium nitrite, sodium saccharin, baking soda (sodium bicarbonate), and sodium benzoate. These are ingredients in condiments and seasonings such as Worcestershire sauce, soy sauce, onion salt, garlic salt, and bouillon cubes. Processed meats, such as bacon, sausage, and ham, and canned soups and vegetables are all examples of foods that contain added sodium. Fast foods are generally very high in sodium. In addition, sodium may lead to fluid retention in patients with congestive heart failure, hypertension, liver disease, cirrhosis, or kidney disease. These patients should be on strict sodium-restricted diets as prescribed by their doctor.

Potassium

Potassium is a mineral that is involved in both electrical and cellular functions in the body. (In the body it is classified as an electrolyte). It has various roles in metabolism and body functions:
- It assists in the regulation of the acid-base balance and water balance in the blood and the body tissues.
- It assists in protein synthesis from amino acids and in carbohydrate metabolism.
- It is necessary for the building of muscle and for normal body growth.
- It is needed for the proper functioning of nerve cells, in the brain and throughout the body.

Fish such as salmon, cod, flounder, and sardines are good sources of potassium. Various other meats also contain potassium. Vegetables including broccoli, peas, lima beans, tomatoes, potatoes (especially their skins), and leafy green vegetables such as spinach, lettuce, and parsley contain potassium. Fruits that contain significant sources of potassium are citrus fruits, apples, bananas, and apricots.

Lipids

Nearly all of the energy needed by the human body is provided by the oxidation of carbohydrates and lipids. Whereas carbohydrates provide a readily available source of energy, lipids function primarily as an energy reserve. The amount of lipids stored as an energy reserve far exceeds the energy stored as glycogen since the human body is simply not capable of storing as much glycogen compared to lipids.

Lipid reserves containing 100,000 kcal of energy can maintain human body functions without food for 30-40 days with sufficient water. Lipids or fats represent about 24 pounds of the body weight in a 154 pound male. Fortunately, lipids are more compact and contain more energy per gram than glycogen, otherwise body weight would increase approximately 110 pounds if glycogen were to replace fat as the energy reserve.

Digestion

The digestive system is a sequence of organs that function to breakdown ingested nutrients for digestion and absorption. Digestion is a method of altering foods into smaller and smaller particles until the nutrients are absorbed into the body via the stomach, and small or large intestine. The digestion system is considered a protective mechanism for the body as it relates to absorption of microorganisms and/or noxious substances that are found in foods that are consumed on a daily or routine basis. The digestive system includes the mouth (oral cavity), the esophagus, the stomach, the small intestine, and the large intestine.

Organs involved in digestion
Oral cavity (mouth) facilitates chewing to breakdown ingested materials. The Salivary glands are located in the oral cavity; the salivary glands produce saliva that functions to lubricate ingested materials. Amylase is an enzyme found in the saliva of the oral cavity. Amylase is responsible for the initial stages of carbohydrate breakdown. Swallowing is facilitated by the pharynx. Food is moved from the oral cavity into the stomach via the esophagus. The stomach stores and maintains motion to break down foods. The gall bladder concentrates and facilitates the storage of bile. The liver is responsible for destruction of molecules, aged red blood cells, and toxins. The liver also functions to store vitamins and minerals, and production of digestive bile. The pancreas produces bicarbonate (a base) that assists in the regulation of stomach acid and the production of insulin (a hormone) to regulate blood glucose levels. The small intestine is responsible for the absorption of water, and nutrients once food has been broken into particles small enough to cross the cell membrane of the digestive mucosa. The large intestine also is responsible to absorb water, but in small amounts; by the time food reaches the large intestine it is a mass that is known as feces. The large intestine also reabsorbs small amounts of vitamins and ions. The rectum is the distal portion of the large intestine and stores feces. The anus serves as the outlet for fecal material.

Digestive process terms

The six terms associated with the digestive process are described below:
- Ingestion is the initial step of placing food in the oral cavity (mouth).
- Digestion takes place by mechanical digestion as with chewing, or chemical digestion as with the process of digestive enzymes mixing with foods to form altered compounds that facilitate passage thru the digestive tract, and absorption into the walls of the stomach, and intestines.
- Motility is the way foods are transported through the digestive system; terms associated with motility include peristalsis and segmentation and refer to the musculature of the digestive tract.
- Secretion occurs when digestive liquids are excreted during the digestive process.

- Absorption occurs when nutrients are broken down into particles small enough to move through the intestinal mucosa, and into the blood stream.
- Elimination is the formation of feces in the rectum, and defecation of stool via the anal canal and anus.

Absorption

Absorption is the process of nutrients that have been digested into microscopic particles moving through the walls of the digestive mucosa of the small intestine into the blood stream or lymph (fluid). Passive diffusion occurs when molecules are transported from areas of high to areas of low concentration (lack of resistance with transfer related to the area of decreased concentration they are migrating to allow passive mobility to take place. The nutrition molecules automatically move to a less dense environment from one that is packed or concentrated). Facilitated diffusion is the process of nutrient molecules (or any molecule) being transported through the cell membrane via transporter proteins from areas of high concentration to areas of low concentration. Active transport takes place when cellular energy is used to transfer molecules into areas of high pressure via transporter proteins. Pinocytosis occurs when molecules are enveloped by the membrane of a cell, forming a separate vesicle inside the cell.

Metabolism and nutrition

Metabolism occurs within the cells when nutrients previously absorbed are utilized by the body to maintain proper function, energy levels, and maintenance. Metabolism occurs in two forms. When food particles are minimized into particles of small molecular structure this is known as catabolism. Catabolism is the main form of chemical and heat energy. The introduction of new substance formation via synthesis is known as anabolism. Anabolism is responsible for the production of new tissue. To maintain proper metabolic function and decrease the chance of obesity we must be aware of what our body requirements are for daily functional needs and maintain this balance without consuming an over abundance of calories that produce excess fat that is not utilized and in turn deposits itself within the body.

Nutrition and disease prevention and health

Nutrition to enhance wellness is a form of food consumption to nourish the body by a positive behavior. Providing an organized lifestyle that allows for a pattern of eating that enhances the status of health is an example of maintaining nutritional wellness. Nutritional wellness also includes factors such as consumption of a high fiber, low-fat diet in moderation. Following a desired or prescribed diet is affirmation of self-control and personal competency toward nutritional health and wellness. Disease prevention through proper nutrition includes limiting the intake of certain foods (salt for example in those with hypertension, or consuming a low fat diet for weight reduction) and maintaining an adequate amount of vitamin and mineral intake for the body to function properly through food consumption.

Primary prevention

Primary prevention mechanisms attempt to prevent the primary development of a disease process. Primary prevention of disease through nutrition includes consumption of the recommended daily amounts of food as determined by the American Dietetic Association to avoid disease, and disease processes. Primary Prevention mechanisms may include low fat diets to prevent obesity, consumption of a diet high in fiber to decrease the risk of cancer, and/or consumption of a variety of fruits and vegetables to maintain adequate vitamins and minerals lost on a daily basis. Primary prevention may also include the consumption of at least six 8 ounce glasses of water daily to avoid dehydration, and maintain fluid and electrolyte balance.

Tertiary prevention

Methods of tertiary prevention occur once the disease is established in the body. Mechanisms of prevention at this stage are aimed at decreasing further complications as well as production of the best possible outcome. Education on disease processes and treatment are part of tertiary prevention. Maintaining a diet that will produce the most effective outcome of the treatment prescribed is a mechanism of tertiary prevention. Nutritional therapy is often a main prevention mechanism with disease processes such as gastric ulcer, ulcerative colitis, diverticulitis, and coronary artery disease (CAD). Tertiary prevention is relevant with cancer patients that may no longer be able to tolerate foods they once chose to consume, and need to be reeducated (counseled) on the benefits of a well balanced diet and their disease process.

Dehydration and the gastrointestinal tract

Dehydration occurs when the body loses an excessive amount of fluid. Imbalances of electrolytes needed for daily homeostasis and function are the result of dehydration and excessive fluid loss. Dehydration of cells is possible and often occurs although the patient presents with edema. Keep in mind intracellular fluids are inside the cell and extracellular fluids are outside the cell. The proper amount of the nutrient water promotes functionality of cells. Dehydration is a potential any time the body is experiencing vomiting or diarrhea. Terms associated with dehydration include, anhydration or the absence of water, exsiccation or the removal of water crystallization, and desiccation. Absolute hydration is a deficit of water in relation to solutes. Voluntary dehydration occurs when an individual does not have a thirst.

Nutrition and the immune system

When the body is deprived of adequate nutrients the immune system (the body's own natural mechanism of resistance) does not function to protect the body from disease and disease processes or may be slowed enough to allow microorganisms to invade and cause infectious processes to begin. The immune system activates a response to infectious organisms as a measure of protection for the body. If the immune system is compromised defense mechanisms such as the skin, oral mucous membranes, gastrointestinal tract, t-lymphocytes (blood cells formed in bone marrow that are responsible for cell mediated immunity), granulocytes (mature white blood cells), macrophages, and antibodies (immunoglobulin molecules that respond to foreign antigens) may be slow to respond or may not have enough energy to mount a cell mediated immune response allowing invasion, and growth of organisms. Malnutrition causes the microvilli of the mucous membranes to level decreasing the amount of nutrient absorption and antibody excretion. With malnutrition the skin becomes elastic and healing is delayed.

Iatrogenic malnutrition

Iatrogenic malnutrition may occur with prolonged hospitalization, surgical procedures, and/or prescribed treatments. When an individual is unable to take in the proper nutrition required for normal bodily functions they may suffer from iatrogenic (unfavorable) responses and become malnourished causing delayed healing responses. Patients are at risk for malnutrition when they are hospitalized. Monitoring of diet, hydration status, and level of consciousness, alertness, fatigue, and overall state are all ways nurses can prevent iatrogenic malnutrition from taking place while patients are hospitalized. Iatrogenic malnutrition often occurs with diseases such as cancer, fractures in the elderly, pulmonary disorders, and Alzheimer's disease. Medications prescribed to individuals often include iatrogenic side effects.

Medical nutrition therapy

Medical nutrition therapy is a mechanism to maintain a balance with blood pressure and control elevations in blood pressure with a low-sodium diet. Medical nutrition is also used to decrease the amount of edema an individual may be experiencing by decreasing the daily intake of salt/sodium. Medical nutrition therapy uses a formula to maintain adequate levels of functioning protein so the body does not break down lean body tissue and cause malnutrition. Medical nutrition therapy provides nutrients for energy while decreasing disease progression rates. Ultimately medical nutrition therapy is a form of diet maintenance to control disease processes and disease progression.

MODS and nutritional requirements

Multiple organ dysfunction syndrome (MODS) is the progressive malfunction of two or more organ systems within the body occurring consecutively. Patients who suffer multi-organ failure require an increased number of kilocalories to maintain the high rate of metabolism (hypermetabolic state) needed to produce the required amounts of energy for cell function to take place. An individual with multiple organ dysfunction syndrome may exhibit symptoms such as lethargy, altered level of consciousness, an elevated body temperature, have lower than normal lymphocyte counts, lack energy, experience ascites, and may experience an alteration in bowel pattern or decreased peristalsis.

COPD and medical nutrition therapy

Chronic obstructive pulmonary disease (COPD) is an umbrella term for diseases of the respiratory tract that act to constrict bronchi and decrease airflow into the lungs and expulsion of carbon from the lungs. Diseases that fall under the COPD umbrella include asthma, chronic bronchitis, and emphysema. Medical nutrition therapy for those individuals affected with COPD is designed to improve respiratory functionality, and quality. Hypermetabolic states often accompany disease processes and the goal is to increase the nutrient intake to meet the metabolic demands placed on the body to avoid tissue damage or total destruction.

Gastroparesis and nutritional medical therapy

Gastroparesis is characterized by decreased peristalsis. As a result of gastroparesis delayed gastric emptying occurs. Signs and symptoms of gastroparesis include bloating, feelings of fullness and/or nausea, vomiting, gastric pain, and heartburn. Patients who have been diagnosed with diabetes have and increased risk of gastroparesis related to diabetic neuropathy of the vagal nerve that innervates the stomach area. The diet of an individual who suffers gastroparesis is as tolerated with few carbohydrates included. Small, frequent meals will replace the normal daily three meals most often eaten. Low-fat, soft or liquid diets may also assist with food toleration.

African American diet

The most commonly consumed foods among the African American population include flour and lard biscuits, a variety of breads made of cornmeal, grits, greens, multiple pork products, organ meats along with a variety of fish, and legumes. Traditionally the African American diet does not include a multitude of milk products; buttermilk has been viewed as the main dairy product of the African American culture. The traditional African American diet includes increased amounts of pork fats and lard for frying, and baking. Sugary products are not a major factor in the African American diet.

Native American diet

Some of the most frequently utilized dishes among the Native American population include a variety of breads made from blue corn flour, mush, fried bread, corn tortillas and cornbread. Other bread products include dumplings, wheat and rye breads, and acorns. A variety of vegetables are also utilized on a regular basis by the Native American population; these include corn, onion, potatoes, greens, squash, and pumpkin. Among fruits most frequently consumed by the Native American there are wild cherries, bananas, grapes, and yucca. Native Americans traditionally have a diet very low in dairy products, or oils, fats and sugars. The main source of protein for the Native American population comes from a variety of poultry, eggs, legumes, nuts, venison, and rabbit. The nurse should be aware that there is a high rate of alcohol use and abuse among the Native American population as well as an increased incidence of diabetes.

Chinese diet

Traditionally the Chinese diet consists of a variety of rice, corn and wheat products. Among the vegetables consumed by the Chinese most often are roots, bamboo shoots, cabbage, Chinese celery, green leafy vegetables and other leaves such as the amaranth green, chard, okra, peas, and the white radish. The Kumquat is the major fruit consumed among the Chinese culture. The Chinese consume fair amounts of fat and oils such as peanut, soy, sesame, rice and lard. Among the meats consumed are fish, seafood, legumes, nuts, pork, and organ meats. Traditionally the Chinese culture does not have an increased amount of dairy products in their diet.

Japanese diet

The traditional diet of the Japanese culture consists of a variety of rice, and rice products, fish, nasi, persimmons, soybeans, bean sprouts, tofu, and red beans. Traditionally the Japanese culture does not include an increased amount of dairy products in the daily diet. The Japanese diet consists of increased amounts of fresh fish and seafood, with little of the diet being cooked in any type of fat or lard product. The Japanese diet is proven with research to provide protection against multiple cancers; this can be attributed to the decreased amounts of fat and dairy in a traditional Japanese diet.

Mexican diet

The Mexican culture consumes a moderate amount of corn products for tortillas and white flour products. Traditionally the Mexican culture utilizes a variety of fruits and vegetables consisting mainly of peppers, yucca, avocado, and papaya. Among the foods containing protein are beans (black and pinto), beef, poultry, and eggs. Cheese and sour cream are among the two most frequently consumed dairy products. The Mexican culture uses a moderate amount of bacon fat, salt pork and lard. The Mexican diet traditionally contains multiple peppers and spices as part of each dish. Increased amounts of tomato are part of the Mexican diet.

Vegetarian diet

The vegetarian diet consists of primarily fruits, and vegetables and no meat. Among the various types of vegetarian diets is the lacto-ovovegetarian diet in which the individual does allow for the consumption of dairy and eggs in their diet. Lactovegetarians on the other hand do not allow egg in the diet but do consume dairy products. The vegan diet does not allow for the consumption of animals. Ethnic vegetarians do not include any products that have any association with animals, animal by-products or that have been tested on animals. A fruitarian vegetarian consumes only fruits, nuts, berries and seeds. A living food diet vegetarian consumes only fruits and vegetables that are raw. A semi-vegetarian consumes dairy, eggs, poultry, and fish.

Nutrition terms

- Malnutrition - Malnutrition is inadequate nutritional intake that can be the result of improper food consumption and/or an inability of the body to absorb nutrients.
- Dehydration - Dehydration is a lack of or loss of significant amounts of water from the body.
- Undernutrition - Undernutrition is a decreased amount of nutrient intake as stated by the recommended daily allowances.
- Overnutrition - Overnutrition is the increased consumption of nutrients.

Pharmacological and Parenteral Therapies

Pharmacokinetics

Pharmacokinetics includes the absorption, distribution, and elimination of drugs/medications. Absorption, distribution, and elimination all take place with the passage of cell membranes. Determinants of metabolism include molecular size, shape, ionization, and solubility of the drug. Drugs must permeate the cell membrane to become active within the blood stream or specific target organ. Absorption is the rate a drug leaves the site of administration and the extent of the drugs entrance into the cells. Bioavailability is the amount of drug available when it reaches its target destination or organ system. Distribution involves the mechanism of distribution into interstitial and intracellular fluids. Excretion is the way drugs are eliminated from the body.

Routes of administration, oral medication abbreviations, and major injection sites

Routes of Administration
- Sublingual
- Buccal
- Parenteral
- Topical
- Inhalation
- Intraocular

Oral medication abbreviations
- CR: Controlled release
- CRT: Controlled release tablet
- LA: Long acting
- SA: Sustained action
- SR: Sustained release
- TR: Timed release
- XL: Extended length
- XR: Extended release

Four major injection sites
- Subcutaneous (SQ)
- Intramuscular (IM)
- Intravenous (IV)
- Intradermal (ID)

ID, SQ, and IM injections

Intradermal injections (ID) can also be termed intracutaneous. Intradermal injections are given within the dermal layer of the skin. An example of an intradermal injection is the mantoux given to screen for Tuberculosis exposure or disease. They are most often given in the forearm, chest, and back. Twenty-seven to thirty gauge needles are used for intradermal injections; the needle length is 1/4th to 3/8th of an inch. The angle used for intradermal injections is ten to fifteen degrees. Subcutaneous injections (SQ) are given beneath the skin normally given in an area that has more adipose (fat) tissue. Subcutaneous injections are traditionally given in the upper, outer arm, the anterior thigh, and the abdomen. Subcutaneous injections use a 25 to 28 gage needle, and go into the skin at a ninety degree angle; very thin individuals may require a forty-five degree angle. The needle length is 5/8th of an inch long. The normal volume of a subcutaneous injection is 0.5 to 1ml of fluid. Intramuscular injections (IM) are given within the muscle. Intramuscular injections are traditionally given in the gluteus, thigh, or deltoid muscle. The gauge of an IM injection 23; the needle length is 1-1.5 inches. The angle of an IM injection is 90 degrees. Up to 3ml of fluid can be given in one IM injection. The small individual may only be able to tolerate an IM injection of one milliliter. Aspirate for blood prior to giving an IM injection.

Problems maintaining intravenous access site

The most common problems with maintaining an intravenous access site are:
- Infiltration - Infiltration occurs when a substance is penetrated into a cell or tissue. The nurse should assess an IV site for infiltration with each assessment. Common signs and symptoms of infiltration include swelling, tenderness at site, decreased or no infusion rate, blanching of the skin at the IV site and surrounding tissue, and the site of an infiltration may be warm to touch. Treatment of an infiltration includes discontinuing the IV, and application of warm compresses to the area.
- Phlebitis - Phlebitis is inflammation of a vein. The nurse should assess an IV site for phlebitis with each assessment. Common signs of phlebitis include a red line of irritation along the course of the vein. Additional signs of phlebitis include erythema (redness), heat, swelling (edema), and tenderness. Treatment of phlebitis includes discontinuation of the IV, and application of warm compresses.

Types of IV solution

Carbohydrate solutions are utilized to provide calories to individuals. Common types of carbohydrate solutions include, but are not limited to 5 or 10% in saline solution or water. Electrolyte solutions include sodium chloride that is used for the treatment of dehydration, shock, and hydrogen ion imbalances. Common fluid in this category are 0.45% (half-strength saline solution), 0.9% normal saline (what is normally found within the body), 3% normal saline for those individuals with elevated sodium levels who need fluid replacement and for women who have hypernatremia following surgical procedures. Normal saline also comes in 5% solution. Lactated Ringer's or Hartmann's solution has an electrolyte concentration that is comparable to extracellular fluid. Protein hydrolysate solutions supply protein to the body. The most common types of protein hydrolysate solutions are Amigen, and Aminosol. Plasma volume expanders are glucose solutions that draw interstitial fluid into the bloodstream to restore blood volume. Common types of plasma volume expanders include Dextran 70, and Gentran 75. Clinical note: Nurses should be aware of the increased risk of hypernatremia in post-surgical females of younger ages.

Calculations of drip rates

A micro drip is normally 60 gtts (drops)/cc of fluid. The formula to determine drops (gtt) per minute is:

$$\frac{\text{Total volume infused} \times \frac{\text{drops}}{\text{cc}}}{\text{Total time of infusion in minutes}} = \text{drops per minute}$$

Example: The order is for one liter (1000 cc) of Normal Saline (NS) to be administered over 8 hours, with the use of an administration set that will deliver ten (10) drops (gtts)/cc. What will the drip rate be for this fluid?

$$\frac{1000 \times 10}{8 \times 60} = \frac{10,000}{480} = 20.8 \ \frac{gtt}{min}$$

Example: The order is for two liters (2000 cc) of 5% Dextrose to be administered over 12 hours, with the use of an administration set that will deliver fifteen (15) drops (gtts)/cc. What will the drip rate for this be?

$$\frac{2000 \times 15}{12 \times 60} = \frac{30,000}{720} = 41.7 \ \frac{gtt}{min}$$

Insulin for the type I diabetic

Stabilization of blood glucose levels is the priority of care with the type I diabetic patient. Blood glucose levels considered within normal range is 70 to 110 mg/dl. Insulin therapy is initiated to maintain the blood glucose levels within this range. Insulin therapy is the only course of medications that can be utilized with the Type I diabetic patient; insulin injections serve to replace what is not being produced by the body. Clinical note: Oral diabetic agents supplement, and stimulate insulin production in the pancreas and its efficiency, with the type I diabetic the pancreas is not producing insulin so a medication to enhance function is not effective for these individuals. Diabetics are educated on food exchanges to maintain the proper carbohydrate, protein, and fat ratios that promote normal blood glucose levels. Carbohydrates represent 50% of the diabetic diet, protein represents 20%, and fat represents the remaining 30% of the diabetic diet.

Mixing insulin

Insulin should be drawn up in the appropriate subcutaneous needle depending on dose in units. Insulin is ALWAYS dosed in units. Steps to drawing up insulin include:
   1.) Mix the insulin by gently rolling in back and forth in ones hands. Do not shake insulin or insulin products.
   2.) Obtain syringe of appropriate size, draw up the same dose of air as insulin to be given.
   3.) Inject the cloudy insulin with the air equal to the dose of insulin to be given.
   4.) Inject the clear insulin with air equal to the dose of insulin to be given.
   5.) Insert the needle into the clear insulin and draw the desired dose.
   6.) Insert the needle into the cloudy insulin and draw the desired dose.

Remember to always draw clear insulin before cloudy insulin. Shaking will cause air bubbles and may alter the insulin dose that is given. Insulin should be checked by two nurses prior to injection.

Diabetes type II

The following are medications most often used to treat Diabetes type II:

- Chlorpropamide (Diabinese), Tolazamide (Tolinase), Tolbutamide (Orinase) are second generation sulfonylureas that target the beta cells of the pancreas to stimulate insulin production. Clinical note: The sulfonylurea drugs end in mide (ase).
- Glipizide (Glucotrol, and Glucotrol XL), Glyburide (Glynase, Micronase, and DiaBeta) are first generation sulfonylureas that target the beta cells of the pancreas to stimulate insulin production.
- Metformin (Glucophage) is a Biguanide which lowers the level of glucose produced in the liver as well as reducing the amount of glucose that is absorbed in the intestinal tract.
- Clinical note: Metformin is the drug of choice for obese diabetic patients related to properties that promote weight loss.
- Acarbose (Precose) is an alpha-glucosidase inhibitor that slows the absorption of glucose in the intestinal tract.
- Repaglinide (Prandin) is classified as a meglitinide and functions to increase insulin production in the pancreas.
- Troglitazone (Resulin) is a Thiazolidinedione that functions to facilitate glucose clearance.

Clinical Note: Diabetes Type II can be treated with oral and/or injectable medication.

Otitis media

Treatment of otitis media includes antibiotics, traditionally amoxicillin. Tylenol or aspirin are used to treat pain and fever. Monitor dose with children, and do not give aspirin to children who are susceptible to rye syndrome. Antihistamines may reduce erythema, itching, and decongestants will assist with swelling and congestion to facilitate drainage of fluid from the middle ear. Steroids treat inflammation. Fluids and rest should be utilized in the treatment of otitis media. The client or parent should be educated on the effects of smoking as a causative agent for otitis media. Local heat compresses may assist in alleviating pain and discomfort associated with otitis media. Children with otitis media should be positioned on the affected side to facilitate drainage.

Acne treatment

Medications for acne:

- Tretinoin (Retin-A) - only drug that effectively interrupts abnormal follicular keratinization that produces microcomedones. Use at HS approx. 30 min. after cleansing, and use a sunscreen SPF at least 15 daily
- Topical benzoyl peroxide- antibacterial that inhibits the growth of P. Acnes . Less likely to result in antibiotic resistant strains.
- Clindamycin, erythromycin metronidazole, azelaic acid.
- Retin-A improves the penetration of these products and is the only way to address the 3 pathogenic causes of acne

- OCP (oral contraceptive) may help by reducing endogenous androgen production (Ortho Tri-Cycle) acne indication for over age of 14
- Accutane (Isotretinoin 12-cis-retinoic acid) - Very potent and effective oral agent.

Asthma and status Asthmaticus

Drug therapy for asthma:
LT control meds, Quick relief meds
MDI, Corticosteroids, Cromolyn sodium NSAID, Albuterol, metaproterenol, terbutaline (beta adrenergic agents)
LT bronchodilators (Serevent), Theophylline—monitor serum levels, Leukotriene modifiers- Singulair

Asthma Interventions: Exercise, Chest physiotherapy (CPT), Hyposensitization - allergy shots

Status Asthmaticus - Respiratory distress continues despite vigorous therapeutic measures. Emergency treatment—epinephrine 0.01 mL/kg SQ (max dose 0.3 mL)

Goals of asthma management:
- Avoid exacerbation, Avoid allergens, Relieve asthmatic episodes promptly, Relieve bronchospasm
- Monitor function with peak flow meter, Self-management of inhalers, devices, and activity regulation

Hypnotics and sedatives and insomnia management

Sedatives are medications that decrease activity, moderate excitability, and calm the recipient. They are considered hypnotics when given in large doses. Hypnotics are medications that produce drowsiness and facilitate the onset and maintenance of sleep. Three main classes of synthetic drugs include: benzodiazepines, barbiturates, and nonbenzodiazepine-nonbarbiturate drugs. Benzodiazepines are sedative-hypnotics that produce central nervous system depression. Examples of benzodiazepines include temazepam, diazepam, alprazolam, and chlordiazepoxide. Barbiturates are sedative-hypnotics that function to cause depression of the central nervous system. The most common barbiturates used are butabarbital, aprobarbital, phenobarbital, and secobarbital. Miscellaneous sedative-hypnotic drugs include paraldehyde, chloral hydrate, ethchlorvynol, and meprobamate. Insomnia is managed with sedative-hypnotics. Insomnia is treated with hypnotics that attempt to mimic natural sleep. Transient insomnia is sleeplessness lasting less than 3 days. Short term insomnia is sleeplessness lasting 3 days to 3 weeks and long-term insomnia is sleeplessness lasting more than 3 weeks. Sedatives and hypnotics also include alcohol and OTC sleep aids.

Generalized seizures

There are 3 types of generalized seizures. The three types of generalized seizures are absence, myoclonic, and tonic-clonic seizures. Absence seizures have abrupt onset with impaired consciousness that is characterized by episodes of staring, cessation of activities and the absence seizure typically lasts approximately 30 seconds. Absence seizures are treated with valproate, and ethosuximide. Myoclonic seizures have a brief shock-like contraction of muscles. This muscle contraction may be limited to a certain limb or area or the muscle contraction may be generalized to include the entire body. Normal treatment for myoclonic seizures is valproate. Tonic-clonic seizures are described as simple or complex partial seizures that involve loss of consciousness and sustained muscle contraction that is generalized to the entire body. Tonic (contraction) movements are alternated with clonic (relaxation) movements, and this typically lasts one to two minutes. Tonic-clonic seizures are treated with carbamazepine, phenobarbital, phenytoin, primidone, and/or valproate.

Heart failure

Heart failure encompasses ventricular dysfunction, ischemic cardiomyopathies, systolic and diastolic dysfunction. The goal of treating heart failure is to treat the symptoms. Symptom treatment will increase hemodynamic function. Treatments for heart failure include low sodium diets, loop diuretics such as lasix, bumex, and demadex. Thiazide diuretics utilized include hydrochlorothiazide, and metolazone. The nurse should remember that diabetic patients who experience heart failure are often placed on drug therapy that consists of an ACE inhibitor. Vasodilators used to treat heart failure include nitroglycerine, nipride, captopril, losartan, hydralazine, and labetalol. The nurse should consider the decreased amount of oxygen the individual has related to heart failure and allow for extra time with medication administration and treatments.

Pulmonary Edema

Pulmonary edema is fluid in the lung, most often caused by ineffeciency of the left ventricle of the heart. MAD DOG is a helpful mnemonic to assist you to remember the treatment for Pulmonary Edema.
Morphine
Aminophylline
Digitalis
Diuretics
Oxygen
Gases (ABGs)

Dyspnea

Dyspnea is a feeling of difficulty breathing. Common causes include pneumonia, asthma, congestive heart failure, COPD, and anxiety. The 6ps are a helpful mnemonic to assist you to remember the causes of dyspnea.
Pump failure
Pulmonary embolus
Pulmonary bronchial constriction
Possible obstruction from a foreign body
Pneumonia
Pneumothorax

HTN

Hypertension (HTN) is the most commonly diagnosed cardiovascular disease. Hypertension is a leading cause of cerebral vascular accidents (stroke) among American adults. Hypertension is a blood pressure of greater than or equal to systolic 140 over a diastolic of

90. Severe levels of blood pressure are systolic greater than or equal to 210 and a diastolic greater than or equal to 120. The nurse should be aware of organ changes that occur with hypertension such as stenosis, peripheral vascular disease, and increased vascular resistance. The alteration of sodium balance with low sodium diets and diuretics is a management technique of hypertension. Hydrochlorothiazide is a diuretic used for hypertension. Sympatholytic agents used to control HTN include methyldopa, and clonidine. These medications reduce vascular resistance.

Blood Pressure: BP = CO x SVR
Blood **P**ressure
Cardiac **O**utput
Systemic **V**ascular **R**esistance

Peptic ulcers and gastroesophageal reflux disease

Both peptic ulcers and Gastroesophageal reflux disease are acid-peptic disorders. Treatment for peptic ulcers and gastroesophageal reflux disease include proton pump inhibitors that act to suppress gastric acid production and secretion from within the stomach. The most commonly utilized proton pump inhibitors include prilosec (omeprazole), prevacid (lansoprazole), and protonix (pantoprazole). Histamine H2-receptor antagonists used to treat peptic ulcers and gastroesophageal disease include tagamet (cimetidine), zantac (ranitidine), pepcid (famotidine) and axid (nizatidine). Prostaglandin analogs are used to treat peptic ulcer disease and gastroesophageal reflux by inhibition of acid production. The most commonly used prostaglandins include cytotec, and misoprostol.

Antimicrobial agents

Antimicrobial (antibiotics) agents are used to treat a variety of infectious disease process. Antimicrobials originate from bacteria, fungi, and actinomycetes. Antimicrobial agents stifle the growth of microorganisms. Antimicrobial agents are classified as to the pharmacological action they produce. Agents that inhibit bacterial cell wall synthesis include the penicillins and cephalosporins. Antimicrobial agents that act upon the cell membrane to cause destruction include polymyxin, nystatin, and amphotericin B. Bacteriostatic medications that affect the function of ribosomal subunits include chloramphenicol, and the tetracyclines including erythromycin and Clindamycin. Do not tetracycline at bedtime. When patients lie down it often causes gastric reflux. Aminoglycosides bind to the ribosomal subunit and alter protein synthesis causing cell death. The quinolones alter bacterial nucleic acid metabolism. The sulfonamides and trimethoprim block folate metabolism. Antiviral agents function to reverse transcriptase inhibitors.

The sulfonamides are primarily used to treat urinary tract infections, otitis media, bronchitis, sinusitis, and Pneumocystis carinii pneumonia. The Quinolones are used primarily to treat urinary tract infection, prostatitis, sexually transmitted diseases, osteomyelitis, and bacterial diarrhea. The Penicillins are used for the treatment of Pseudomonas aeruginosa, are used to treat disease processes that are caused by gram-positive cocci, and certain Neisseria species. Penicillins are useful in the treatment of syphilis, actinomycosis, diphtheria, anthrax, clostridial infection, and Lyme disease. Penicillins are used as prophylactic measures for the treatment of rheumatic fever, and sickle cell anemia. The Aminoglycosides are used in the treatment of aerobic gram-negative bacterial infections. Aminoglycosides are used to treat strep infections, and infectious processes of the ear and kidney.

Anticoagulants, thrombolytics, and antiplatelets

Antiplatelet agents include aspirin (ASA), and function to control blood fluidity. Other antiplatelet medications include persantine, ticlid, and plavix.

Coumadin anticoagulants act to block coagulation. The most widely utilized anticoagulant is warfarin. Warfarin therapy is monitored with Pt Inr, and aPTT. Anticoagulants are antagonists of vitamin K. Coumadin/warfarin is monitored closely and dosed per the Inr (International normalized ratio).

Heparin derivatives stimulate natural inhibitors of coagulant proteases. Heparin is found in mast cells and is a glycosaminoglycan. Heparin is used to treat venous thrombosis and pulmonary embolism. Heparin is monitored using the aPTT.

Fibrinolytic agents lyse pathological thrombi. Thrombolytic agents dissolve intravascular clots.

Immunomodulators and immunosuppressive agents

Immunosuppression is caused by medications that decrease the response of the immune system. Immunosuppressive agents are utilized with organ transplants to halt negative organ reactions, and with autoimmune disorders. Classes of immunosuppressive agents include glucocorticoids, calcineurin inhibitors and antiproliferative agents. The immunosuppressive agents are very successful in the treatment of immune rejection of organs, and autoimmune disorders, but require life-long treatment. The overuse of glucocorticoids may result in toxicity of the individual. Immunomodulators work to stimulate the immune responses to microorganisms. Immunomodulators restore a depressed immune system and allow normal function in fighting infectious processes. Types of immunomodulators include thalidomide, levamisole, and interferons. Vaccinations are a provider of immunization, along with immune globulins.

Insulin

Prior to 1921 insulin dependent diabetes was a fatal disorder. Individuals with type 1 diabetes cannot survive without insulin. Insulin is the treatment of diabetes mellitus. Diabetes is a group of disorders that encompass hyperglycemia, alteration of lipid metabolism, and altered carbohydrate and protein metabolism. Type I diabetes is insulin dependent diabetes. Type II diabetes is non-insulin dependent diabetes. Insulin works to lower concentrations of glucose within the blood by inhibition of hepatic glucose production and stimulation of metabolism of glucose in muscle and adipose (fat) tissue. Regular (rapid) insulin is clear in appearance, has an onset of thirty to forty-five minutes after injection, peaks at ninety minutes to 4 hours post injection and lasts 5-8 hours post injection. Types of rapid acting insulin include regular or lispro. Some forms of rapid acting insulin may begin to act within the first 15 minutes following injection. Intermediate insulin is cloudy in appearance, has an onset of 1-2 hours, peaks in 6-12 hours, and has duration of 18-24 hours. Types of intermediate acting insulin include NPH (isophane), and Lente (lente is often considered a long acting insulin). Slow (long-acting) insulin is cloudy in appearance, has an onset of 4-6 hours, peaks in 16-18 hours, and has duration of 20-36 hours. Types of slow or long-acting insulin include ultralente, protamine zinc, and glargine.

Thyroid and antithyroid drugs

The thyroid hormones are thyroxine (T4), and triiodothyronine (T3). Thyroid hormones contain iodine compounds that are crucial to normal development. In the adult the thyroid hormones act to maintain metabolic homeostasis. Thyroid hormones are synthesized by iodine reuptake, oxidation, coupling, proteolysis and the conversion of thyroxine to triiodothyronine. Thyroid hormones are used for the treatment of hormone replacement in patients with hypothyroidism. The most commonly utilized drugs include synthroid, levoxyl, levothroid and levothyroxine. Myxedema coma is a rare syndrome that occurs from long term untreated hypothyroidism. Antithyroid medications interfere with the mechanism of action of thyroid hormones and are utilized in the treatment of hyperthyroidism. The most commonly utilized medications for the treatment of hyperthyroidism include propylthiouracil, and methimazole. Graves's disease is synonymous for hyperthyroidism.

Dermatology and dermatological pharmacology

The skin functions to protect, regulate temperature, offer immune responses, biochemical synthesis, and sensory detection. Topical treatments involve applying medication directly on the site of inflammation. Oral steroids are often given to assist in the treatment of dermatological conditions. Ultraviolent radiation is used as a treatment method for psoriasis. Sunscreens are prophylactic treatments for dermatological conditions. The most recent forms of skin treatment include vitamin D-analogs, retinoids, and anthralin. Topical glucocorticoids are often used as dermatologic treatments for inflammatory conditions such as rash, pruritus, bullous disorders (pemphigus vulgaris, bullous pemphigoid, and herpes gestationis), collagen diseases such as systemic lupus erythematosus, and vasculitis.

Oral hypoglycemic agents

Sulfonylureas are one type of oral hypoglycemic agent. The sulfonylureas act to decrease glucose within the blood stream by stimulation of pancreatic B cells. Sulfonylureas are mainly used to treat type II diabetes mellitus. Types of sulfonylureas include orinase, diabinese, tolinase, diabeta, and glucotrol. Biguanides are oral antihyperglycemic not hypoglycemic agents. The most commonly used biguanide is metformin (glucophage). Biguanides assist in control of diabetes and lipid concentrations in diabetic patients. Metformin is commonly given to individuals who are overweight. The nurse should be aware of contraindication of giving metformin and elevations in the client's creatinine levels. Thiazolidinediones such as avandia (rosiglitazone) require the presence of insulin, therefore they are not indicated for individuals with type I diabetes who produce no insulin. Alpha-glucosidase inhibitors reduce the amount of intestinal absorption of starch, dextrin and disaccharide. This type of diabetic agent is often utilized with the elderly patient or the client who has problems controlling the post-prandial blood glucose. Acarbose (precose) is the most commonly used a-glucosidase inhibitor.

Decongestants

Classified as systemic or topical.

Systemic decongestants stimulate the sympathetic nervous system to reduce swelling of the respiratory tract's vascular network.

When applied directly to swollen mucous membranes of the nose, topical decongestants provide immediate relief from nasal congestion.

These drugs include: ephedrine, epinephrine, phenylephrine, Prototype: naphazoline (Afrin), oxymetazoline, tetrahydrozoline, and xylometazoline.

Pharmacotherapeutics: Used to relieve the symptoms of swollen nasal membranes resulting from: hay fever, allergic rhinitis, vasomotor rhinitis, acute coryza, sinusitis, and the common cold.

Systemic decongestants are frequently given with: antihistamines, antipyretics-analgesics, antitussives, and expectorants.

Drug interactions: Because of vasoconstriction, topical drug interactions seldom occur. Increased CNS stimulation may occur when taken with other sympathomimetic drugs. Taken with MOA inhibitors may cause severe hypertension or a hypertensive crisis. Alkalinizing drugs may increase the effects of pseudoephedrine.

Adrenergic receptors

Adrenergic receptors are the sites where adrenergic drugs bind and produce their effects. Adrenergic receptors are divided into alpha-adrenergic and beta-adrenergic receptors depending on whether they respond to norepinephrine or epinephrine. Both alpha- and beta-adrenergic receptors have subtypes designated 1 and 2. Alpha-blockers and beta-blockers bind to the receptor sites for norepinephrine and epinephrine blocking the stimulation of the SNS. Drugs that stimulate the parasympathetic nervous system are called cholinergics.

Alpha1-adrenergic receptors are located on the postsynaptic effector cells. Alpha2-adrenergic receptors are located on the presynaptic nerve terminals. Both beta-adrenergic receptors are located on the postsynaptic effector cells. Beta1-adrenergic receptors are primarily located in the heart. Beta2-adrenergic receptors are primarily located in the smooth muscle of bronchioles, arterioles, and visceral organs.

Antiviral drugs

Antiviral drugs are used to prevent or treat viral infections. Drugs include: acyclovir, ganciclovir, famciclovir, foscarnet, amantadine hydrochloride, nelfinavir, zidovudine, didanosine, and zalcitabine. Antiherpes drug, acyclovir, is used to treat infections caused by herpes viruses and varicella-zoster virus by disrupting viral replication. Foscarnet is used to treat cytomegalovirus (CMV) retinitis in patients with AIDS. Amantadine and rimantadine hydrochloride are used to prevent or treat influenza A respiratory infections by inhibiting the early stage of viral replication. Ribavirin, administered by nasal or oral inhalation, is used to treat respiratory syncytial virus (RSV) infections in children. Protease inhibitors act against an enzyme, HIV protease, preventing the enzyme from dividing a larger viral precursor protein into the active smaller enzymes the virus needs to fully mature. The result is an immature, noninfectious cell.

Cephalosporins

Cephalosporins are grouped into generations according to their effectiveness against different organisms, their characteristics, and their development (first through fourth generation). Loracarbef (Lorabid) is a synthetic beta-lactam antibiotic that belongs to a new class of drugs called the carbacephem antibiotics. It is similar to the second generation cephalosporins, and therefore is classified as such.

Pharmacotherapeutics:
- First-generation - act primarily against gram-positive organisms and used as an alternative to penicillin.
- Second-generation - act primarily against gram-negative bacteria.
- Third-generation - act primarily against gram-negative organisms and are the drug of choice for anaerobic organisms.
- Fourth-generation - active against a wide range of gram-positive and negative bacteria.
- Drug interactions:
- Mixing cefamandole, cefoperazone, or moxalactam with alcohol (up to 72 hours after taking a dose) may lead to acute alcohol intolerance.
- Taking with uricosurics may reduce kidney excretion.
- Adverse reactions – hypersensitivity (hives, itching, rashes), N, V, D.

Glucocorticoids

Glucocorticoids are used for the:
- Prevention of leakage of plasma from the capillaries.
- Suppression of the migration of polymorphonuclear leukocytes.
- Inhibition of phagocytosis.
- Decreased antibody formation in injured or infected tissues.

Pharmacotherapeutics:
- Used as replacement therapy for patients with adrenocortical insufficiency.
- Used for immunosuppression and reduction of inflammation and for their effects on the blood and lymphatic systems.
- Drug interactions: Barbiturates, phenytoin (Dilantin), rifampin, and aminoglutethimide (antineoplastic) may reduce effects.
- Potassium-wasting effects may be enhanced by amphotericin B, chlorthalidone (Hygroton), ethacrynic acid (Edecrin), furosemide (Lasix), and thiazide diuretics. Reduce the serum concentration and effects of salicylates.
- Increased risk of peptic ulcers when taken with nonsteroidal anti-inflammatory drugs and salicylates.
- May reduce the response to vaccines and toxoids.
- Effects are increased by estrogen and oral contraceptives.

Aspirin

Aspirin prevents platelets from sticking together and forming blood clots. On the one hand, this effect can be used beneficially, for example, to prevent the blood clots that cause heart attacks or strokes. On the other hand, by preventing blood clots, aspirin can have the detrimental effect of promoting bleeding. Therefore, aspirin should not be used by people who have diseases that cause bleeding (e.g., hemophilia, severe liver disease) or diseases in which bleeding may occur as a complication (e.g., stomach ulcers). Because aspirin causes Reye's syndrome (a potentially fatal liver disease that occurs almost exclusively in persons under the age of 15 years), aspirin should not be given to children when a viral infection is suspected. High doses of aspirin can increase the activity of valproic acid (Depakene; Depakote), an effect which can cause drowsiness or behavioral changes. High doses of aspirin also can enhance the effect of some sugar-lowering medications used in diabetes.

Side effects of chemotherapy

Normal cells usually recover when chemotherapy is over, so most side effects gradually go away after treatment ends, and the healthy cells have a chance to grow normally:
- Fatigue
- Pain-Chemotherapy drugs can cause some side effects that are painful.
- Hair Loss-Hair loss (alopecia) is a common side effect of chemotherapy, but not all drugs cause hair loss.
- Anemia
- Infection Prone
- Blood Clotting Problems
- Mouth and Throat sores
- Diarrhea
- Constipation

Cholinergic drugs and the Autonomic Nervous System

The receptors that bind the acetylcholine and mediate its actions are called cholinergic receptors. These receptors consist of nicotinic receptors and muscarinic receptors. Cholinergic drugs can be direct-acting (bind to and activate cholinergic receptors) or indirect-acting (inhibit cholinesterase which is the enzyme responsible for breaking down acetylcholine). Cholinergic blockers, anticholinergics, parasympatholytics, and antimuscarinic agents are all terms for the class of drugs that block the actions of acetylcholine in the PSNS. Cholinergic blockers allow the SNS to dominate and, therefore, have many of the same effects as the adrenergics. Cholinergic blockers are competitive antagonists that compete with acetylcholine for binding at the muscarinic receptors of the PSNS, inhibiting nerve transmission. This effect occurs at the neuroeffector junctions of smooth muscle, cardiac muscle, and exocrine glands. Have little effect at the nicotinic receptors.

Opioid analgesics

Opioid analgesics include drugs such as heroin, and morphine. Opioids are derived from opium and opium is harvested from poppy. Opioids are highly addictive, cause emotional lability and decrease the ability to learn and memorize. The most common opioids used today are morphine, methadone, fentanyl, naloxone, and butorphanol. The effects of opioids include pain relief (analgesia), elevated mood, and euphoria, decreased respiratory status, decreased cardiovascular status, and altered gastrointestinal and endocrine function. Opioids act in the forebrain to cause an analgesic effect. Respiratory depression that often accompanies opioid use involves a reduction of responses from the brainstem or respiratory center. Morphine an opioid is often used in treating pain accompanying an MI. The action of morphine is treating angina pectoris by decreasing preload, inotropy and chronotropy relieving ischemia and allowing oxygen to return to the myocardium.

Opioids and potential side effects

Opioids are powerful narcotic drugs that have been used for centuries to relieve pain. Those opioids that are derived from the seedpod of the poppy plant (papaver somniferum) are referred to as opiates. Morphine and codeine are commonly known opiates derived from opium. Other opioids include synthetics such as meperidine (Demerol) and chemicals naturally found in the body, such as endorphin. Opioids work to relieve pain in two ways. First, they attach to opioid receptors, which are specific proteins on the surface of cells in the brain, spinal cord and gastrointestinal tract. These drugs interfere and stop the transmission of pain messages to the brain. Second, they work in the brain to alter the sensation of pain. These drugs do not take the pain away, but they do reduce and alter the patient's perception of the pain. Common side effects include euphoria, drowsiness, nausea, vomiting, constipation, dilated pupils and respiratory depression.

Opioids and opioid antagonist

The following are four opioids:
- Morphine
- Hydromorphone (Dilaudid®)
- Meperidine (Demerol®)
- Fentanyl

The term "opioid" refers to all natural and synthetic medications with morphine-like properties. Morphine, hydromorphone, meperidine, and fentanyl are agonists at the opioid receptor. The effects of these agonists are blocked by antagonists such as Naloxone.

Thyroid and antithyroid drugs

Thyroid and antithyroid drugs function to correct thyroid hormone deficiency (hypothyroidism) and thyroid hormone excess (hyperthyroidism). Natural or synthetic and may contain triiodothyronine (T3) and/or thyroxine (T4).
Natural - animal - thyroid and thyroglobulin
Synthetic - sodium salts of L-isomers of the hormones - levothyroxine (Synthroid & Levoxyl), liothyronine sodium, and liotrix.

They act as replacement or substitute hormones in the following situations: to treat hypothyroidism; with antithyroid drugs to prevent goiter formation and hypothyroidism; to differentiate between primary and secondary hypothyroidism during diagnostic testing; to treat papillary or follicular thyroid carcinoma. Levothyroxine is the drug of choice for thyroid hormone replacement and thyroid-stimulating hormone suppression therapy.

Drug interactions: Interact with several common medications.
Adverse reactions: Result from toxicity.

Uricosurics

Two major drugs are probenecid (Benemid) and sulfinpyrazone (Antazone). They are used to prevent or control chronic gouty arthritis by increasing uric acid excretion in the urine.

Pharmacokinetics:
- Absorbed from the GI tract
- Mostly distributed by binding with protein
- Metabolized by the liver
- Excreted by the kidneys and small amount in the feces.

Pharmacodynamics
- Reduce the reabsorption of uric acid at the proximal convoluted tubules of the kidneys resulting in excretion of uric acid in the urine and reducing serum urate levels in the blood.

Pharmacotherapeutics
- Used for treatment of chronic gouty arthritis and tophaceous gout, not for acute gouty arthritis.
- Colchicine is given with both drugs to prevent acute gouty attacks.

Drug interactions
- Probenecid significantly increases or prolongs the effectiveness of cephalosporins, penicillins, and sulfonamides.
- Serum urate levels may be increased when probenecid is taken with antineoplastic drugs.

Antigout drugs

Allopurinol (Zyloprim) is used to reduce the production of uric acid to prevent gouty attacks. Colchicine (Novocolchine) is used to treat acute gouty attacks.

Pharmacokinetics:
- Allopurinol - absorbed in the GI tract; distributed throughout the body as itself or its metabolite oxypurinol; only 50% concentration in the brain; metabolized by the liver; excreted by the kidneys.
- Colchicine - absorbed in the GI tract; partially metabolized in the liver; reenters the GI tract through biliary secretions; reabsorbed from the intestines; distributed to various tissues; primarily excreted in the feces.

Pharmacotherapeutics:
- Allopurinol is used to treat primary gout, hyperuricemia, primary or secondary uric acid nephropathy, recurrent uric acid stone formation, and treat patients who respond poorly to maximum dosages of uricosurics.
- Colchicine is used to relieve inflammation of acute gouty arthritis attacks.

Anticholinesterase drugs

Anticholinesterase drugs block the action of the enzyme acetylcholinesterase, which breaks down acetylcholine, at the cholinergic receptor sites. They are divided into two categories - reversible and irreversible. Reversible have a short duration and include: donepezil (Aricept) and edrophonium (Tensilon). Irreversible anticholinesterase drugs have long-lasting effects. They are used primarily as toxic insecticides and pesticides or as a nerve gas in chemical warfare.

Pharmacotherapeutics:
- Reduce eye pressure
- Increase bladder tone
- Improve GI tone and peristalsis
- Promote muscular contraction
- Diagnose myasthenia gravis
- An antidote to cholinergic blocking drugs
- Treat dementia due to Alzheimer's.

Drug interactions/adverse reactions:
- Taken with other cholinergic drugs can increase the risk of toxicity.
- Nausea, vomiting, diarrhea, respiratory distress, and seizures.

Immunosuppressants

Immunosuppressants include: azathioprine (Imuran), (Prototype) cyclosporine, lymphocyte immune globulin (ATG), muromonab-CD3, and tacrolimus (Prograf). Cyclophosphamide (Cytoxan), an alkylating drug used to treat cancer, also is used as an immunosuppressant. The exact mechanism of action of azathioprine, cyclosporine, and ATG is unknown. What is known is that: Azathioprine antagonizes metabolism of the amino acid purine which may inhibit ribonucleic acid and deoxyribonucleic acid structure and synthesis. Cyclosporine may inhibit helper T cells and suppressor T cells. ATG may eliminate antigen-reactive T cells in the blood and or alter T-cell function. Azathioprine suppresses cell-mediated hypersensitivity reactions and produces various alterations in antibody production in kidney transplant patients. Muromonab-CD3 may block the function of T cells.

Methylxanthines

Methylxanthines are used to treat breathing disorders. Types of methylxanthines include: anhydrous theophylline and its derivative salts, aminophylline, oxtriphylline, and theophylline sodium glycinate.

Pharmacotherapeutics: Used to treat:
- Asthma
- Chronic bronchitis
- Emphysema
- Neonatal apnea.

- 134 -

Drug interactions:
- Smoking increases elimination, decreasing serum concentrations and effectiveness.
- Taking adrenergic stimulants or drinking beverages that contain caffeine may result in additive adverse reactions.
- Phenobarbital, phenytoin (Dilantin), rifampin, and carbamazepine (Tegretol) reduce levels.
- Receiving halothane, enflurane, isoflurane, and methoxyflurane increases the risk of cardiac toxicity.
- May reduce the effects of lithium by increasing its rate of excretion.
- Thyroid hormones may reduce levels.

Antitussives

Antitussives suppress or inhibit dry, nonproductive coughing. They include benzonatate (Tessalon), codeine, dextromethorphan hydrobromide, and hydrocodone bitartrate.

Pharmacotherapeutics:
- Used to treat a serious, nonproductive cough that interferes with a patient's ability to rest and perform ADL's.
- Benzonatate relieves cough caused by pneumonia, bronchitis, the common cold, and COPD.
- Also used during diagnostic procedures.
- Dextromethorphan is the most widely used because of its effectiveness and few adverse reactions.
- Narcotic antitussives (codeine and hydrocodone) are used to treat the intractable cough associated with lung CA.

Drug interactions: Dextromethorphan, codeine and hydrocodone may cause excitation, an extreme elevated temp., hypertension, hypotension, and coma when taken with MAO inhibitors. Codeine may cause CNS depression when taken with other CNS depressants.

Digitalis glycosides

Digitalis glycosides increase the force of the heart's contractions. They are derived from digitalis which is a substance that occurs naturally in foxglove plants and certain toads. Digoxin is the most frequently used. Digitalis glycosides are:
- Used to treat heart failure by increasing intracellular calcium at the cell membrane making the heart contractions stronger.
- Also used to treat supraventricular arrhythmias because it acts on the CNS to slow the heart rate.
- Also used to treat paroxysmal atrial tachycardia. Because of a long half-life, a loading dose must be given in this situation.

Drug interactions: Many drugs can interact with digoxin. Amphotericin B, potassium-wasting diuretics, and steroids taken with digoxin may cause hypokalemia and increase the risk of dig toxicity. Theophylline increases the risk of digitalis toxicity and decreases the effects of lithium and phenytoin.

Adverse reactions: Because of a narrow therapeutic index, monitoring blood levels are required to prevent dig toxicity.

Beta-adrenergic blockers

Beta-adrenergic blockers prevent stimulation of the sympathetic nervous system by inhibiting the action of catecholamines at the beta-adrenergic receptors (beta-blockers). Beta-adrenergic blockers are selective or nonselective. Nonselective beta-blockers affect beta1 receptor sites located mainly in the heart and beta2 receptor sites located in the bronchi, blood vessels, and uterus.
Prototype drug - propranolol hydrochloride (Inderal)
Selective beta-blockers primarily affect beta1 receptor sites only.
Prototype drug - metoprolol tartrate (Toprol)

Pharmacotherapeutics:
- Clinical usefulness is based largely upon how they affect the heart.
- Used to treat heart attacks, angina, hypertension, hypertrophic cardiomyopathy, and supraventricular arrhythmias.

Drug interactions/adverse reactions: Many causing cardiac and respiratory depression, arrhythmia, severe bronchospasm, and severe hypotension.

Anterior Pituitary drugs

The hormones produced by the anterior pituitary gland regulate growth, development, and sexual characteristics by stimulating the actions of other endocrine glands. Anterior pituitary drugs include: adrenocorticotropics (corticotropin & cosyntropin), somatrem (a growth hormone), gonadotropics, and thyrotropics.

Pharmacotherapeutics:
- Corticotropin (ACTH) and cosyntropin (Cortrosyn) are used diagnostically to differentiate between primary and secondary failure of the adrenal cortex. Corticotropin is also used to treat adrenal insufficiency.
- Somatrem (Protropin) is used to treat pituitary dwarfism.

Drug interactions:
When corticotropins are taken with diuretics, an increased potassium loss may occur.

Adverse reactions:
- Hypersensitivity
- Long term use can cause Cushing's syndrome.

Cholinergic agonists

Cholinergic agonists mimic the action of the neurotransmitter acetylcholine. Anticholinesterase drugs inhibit the destruction of acetylcholine at the cholinergic receptor sites.
Mimic the action of acetylcholine.

Include the drugs acetylcholine (rarely used), bethanechol (Urocholine), carbachol (Miostat), and pilocarpine.

Pharmacotherapeutics:
Used to treat: atonic bladder conditions and postop and postpartum urinary retention; GI disorders such as postop abdominal distention and GI atony; reduce eye pressure in glaucoma patients and during eye surgery; and salivary hypofunction.

Drug interactions/adverse reactions: Taken with other cholinergic drugs can increase the effects. Taken with cholinergic blocking drugs can reduce the effects. Can produce adverse effects in any organ innervated by the parasympathetic nerves.

Cholinergic blocking drugs

Cholinergic blocking drugs:
- Interrupt parasympathetic nerve impulses in the central and autonomic nervous systems.
- Also referred to as anticholinergic drugs because they prevent acetylcholine from stimulating the muscarinic cholinergic receptors.
- Drugs include the belladonna alkaloids- the prototype is atropine.

Pharmacotherapeutics:
- Often used to treat GI disorders and complications.
- Atropine is administered preop to reduce GI and respiratory secretions and prevent bradycardia caused by vagal nerve stimulation during anesthesia.
- Other uses include treatment of motion sickness, Parkinson's, bradycardia, arrhythmias, pupil dilation, and organophosphate pesticide poisoning.

Drug interactions/adverse reactions: Many drugs increase the effects: cholinergic agonists and anticholinesterase drugs decrease the effects.

Anticholinergic drugs

Anticholinergic drugs:
- Inhibit the action of acetylcholine at parasympathetic nervous system sites. Anticholinergics used to treat parkinsonism are classified according to two types: synthetic tertiary amines (benztropine - Cogentin) and antihistamines (diphenhydramine).

Pharmacotherapeutics:
- Used to treat all forms of parkinsonism.
- Used most commonly in the early stages.
- Can be used alone or with amantadine (dopaminergic drug) in the early stages. Can be given with levodopa during the later stages.

Drug interactions:
- Amantadine can increase anticholinergic adverse effects.
- Levodopa absorption can be decreased which could worsen parkinsonian signs and symptoms.

- 137 -

Adverse reactions: Drowsiness

A fun way to remember the effects of anticholinergics:
Can't spit: dry mouth
Can't pee: urinary retention
Can't poop: constipation
Can't see: blurred vision

Tetracyclines

Tetracyclines are classified as short-acting, intermediate-acting, and long-acting.

Pharmacokinetics:
- Absorbed from the duodenum when taken orally.
- Distributed widely.
- Excreted primarily by the kidneys.

Pharmacotherapeutics:
- Provide a broad spectrum of activity against: gram-positive and negative aerobic and anaerobic bacteria; spirochetes; mycoplasmas; rickettsiae; chlamydiae; and some protozoa.
- Doxycycline and minocycline provide more action against various organisms than other tetracyclines.
- Used to treat Rocky Mountain Spotted Fever, Lyme Disease, and acne.

Drug interactions:
- Can reduce the effectiveness of oral contraceptives.
- Aluminum, calcium, and magnesium antacids reduce absorption.
- May bind with milk and milk products preventing absorption.

Adverse reactions – superinfection, photosensitivity, N, V, D.

Nitrates

Nitrates:
- The drug of choice for relieving acute angina.
- Include: erythrityl dinitrate, isosorbide dinitrate, isosorbide mononitrate (Imdur), Prototype: nitroglycerin, and pentaerythritol tetranitrate. When the veins dilate less blood returns to the ventricles reducing preload. By reducing preload ventricular size and ventricular wall tension is reduced which reduces the oxygen requirements of the heart.
- Afterload is also decreased by the dilatation of arterioles reducing resistance.
- Used to relieve and prevent angina.

Nitroglycerin is the drug of choice for relief of acute angina (sublingual and transdermal).

Drug interactions: Severe hypotension when taken with alcohol.

Adverse reactions: Headache, hypotension, and increased heart rate.

Antihistamines

Antihistamines are used to treat rash, hives, watery eyes, runny nose, itching, and sneezing due to allergies or the common cold. They may also be used to treat motion sickness, anxiety, or as a sleep aid (for insomnia). They may be taken with food or milk if stomach upset occurs. Sustained-release or long acting tablets and capsules must be swallowed whole. Chewing or crushing the sustained-release/long acting tablets or capsules will destroy the long action and may increase side effects. For chewable tablets, chew thoroughly and swallow. Shake suspensions well before taking.

Antihistamines:
- Primarily act to block histamine effects that occur in an immediate type I hypersensitivity reaction (allergic reaction).
- Histamine-1-receptor antagonists compete with histamine for binding to the H1-receptor sites throughout the body but cannot displace bound histamine.

Include six major classes:
- Ethanolamines – diphenhydramine (Benadryl)
- Ethylenediamines – tripelennamine (Pyribenzamine)
- Alkylamines – chlorpheniramine (Chlor-Trimeton)
- Phenothiazines – prochlorperazine (Compazine)
- Piperidines – loratadine (Claritin)
- Miscellaneous drugs - hydroxyzine hydrochloride (Atarax) and hydroxyzine pamoate (Vistaril)

Pharmacokinetics:
- Absorbed well after oral or parenteral administration.
- Distributed widely throughout the body and CNS, except for fexofenadine (Allegra) and loratadine (Claritin) which minimally penetrate the blood-brain barrier.

Adverse effects of antihistamines:
- May increase the sedative and respiratory depressant effects of CNS depressants such as tranquilizers or alcohol.
- Loratadine (Claritin) may cause serious cardiac effects when taken with macrolide antibiotics (erythromycin), fluconazole (Diflucan), ketoconazole, itraconazole, miconazole, cimetidine (Tagamet), ciprofloxacin (Cipro), and clarithromycin (Biaxin).
- May block or reverse the vasopressor effects of epinephrine resulting in vasodilation, increased heart rate, and very low blood pressure.
- May mask the signs and symptoms of ototoxicity associated with aminoglycosides and salicylates.

Pharmacodynamics: H1-receptor antagonists compete with histamine for H1-receptors on effector cells blocking histamine from causing the allergic symptoms.

Side effects: May cause drowsiness, dizziness, headache, loss of appetite, stomach upset, vision changes, irritability, dry mouth and nose.

Miotic drugs used to treat Glaucoma

Prostaglandin eyedrops include latanoprost (Xalatan), bimatoprost (Lumigan), travoprost (Travatan), and unoprostone (Rescula).
Beta-blocker eyedrops are timolol (Timoptic), levobunolol (Betagan, AKBeta), betaxolol (Betoptic), and carteolol (Ocupress).

Carbonic anhydrase inhibitors include the eyedrops brinzolamide (Azopt) and dorzolamide (Trusopt), and the oral medications acetazolamide (Diamox) and methazolamide (Neptazane, GlaucTabs).

Adrenergic and sympathomimetic eyedrops include brimonidine (Alphagan), apraclonidine (Iopidine), dipivefrin (Propine, AKPro), and epinephrine (Eppy, Glaucon, Epinal, Epifrin). Miotic eyedrops include pilocarpine (Isopto Carpine, Pilocar, Piloptic) and carbachol (Carboptic, Isopto Carbachol).

Antimycotic drugs

Antimycotic drugs:
- Also known as antifungal drugs.
- Are used to treat fungal infections by binding to sterols in fungal cell membranes and altering the permeability of the membranes.
- Amphoceterin B - the most widely used antimycotic drug for severe systemic fungal infections.
- Nystatin - Used only topically or orally to treat local fungal infections.
- Flucytosine - the only metabolite that acts as an antimycotic.
- Ketoconazole - an effective oral antimycotic drug with a broad spectrum of activity.
- Fluconazole - used to treat mouth, throat, and esophageal candidiasis, serious systemic candidal infections, and cryptococcal meningitis.
- Itraconazole - inhibits synthesis of ergosterol, a vital component of fungal cell membranes.

Posterior pituitary drugs

These hormones are synthesized in the hypothalamus, stored in the posterior pituitary, and secreted into the blood. These drugs include:
- Antidiuretic hormone (ADH) - vasopressin (Pitressin), desmopressin, and lypressin
- Oxytocic drugs - oxytocin (Pitocin)

Pharmacotherapeutics:
- ADH is prescribed for hormone replacement therapy in patients with neurogenic diabetes insipidus.
- Desmopressin and lypressin are the drugs of choice for chronic ADH deficiency and are administered intranasally.
- Vasopressin elevates blood pressure for short-term.
- Oxytocics are used to induce labor, treat preeclampsia and eclampsia, control uterine bleeding, contract the uterus, and stimulate lactation.

Typical antipsychotics

Pharmacotherapeutics:
- Used primarily to: treat schizophrenia; calm anxious or agitated patients; improve a patient's though processes; alleviate delusions and hallucinations.
- Many other therapeutic uses have been found.

Drug interactions:
- Interact with many different types of drugs that may produce serious effects.
- Nonphenothiazines interact with fewer drugs than phenothiazines.

Adverse reactions: Neurologic reactions are the most common.

Typical antipsychotics classifications

Typical antipsychotics:
- Include phenothiazines and nonphenothiazines.
- Can be broken down into three smaller classifications:
  - Aliphatics - cause sedation and anticholinergic effects – Prototype - chlorpromazine hydrochloride (Thorazine).
  - Piperazines - cause extrapyramidal reactions - fluphenazine decanoate (Prolixin).
  - Piperidines - cause sedation - mesoridazine besylate (Serentil) and thioridazine hydrochloride (Mellaril).

Nonphenothiazine antipsychotics can be divided into several drug classes:
- Butrophenones - haloperidol (Haldol)
- Dibenzoxazepines - loxapine succinate (Loxitane)
- Dihydroindolones - molindone hydrochloride (Moban)
- Diphenylbutylpiperidines - pimozide (Orap)
- Thioxanthenes - thiothixine (Navane)

Atypical antipsychotics

Pharmacotherapeutics: Indicated for schizophrenic patients who are unresponsive to typical antipsychotics.

Because of the decreased instance of extrapyramidal effects are becoming more widely prescribed.

Drug interactions: Counteract the effects of levodopa and other dopamine agonists.

Adverse reactions: Have less extrapyramidal effects than typical antipsychotics.

Atypical antipsychotics

Atypical anti-psychotics:
- New agents designed to treat schizophrenia.
- Include: clozapine (Clozaril), olanzapine (Zyprexa), and risperidone (Risperdal).

Pharmacokinetics:
- Absorbed after oral administration
- Metabolized by the liver
- Highly protein-bound
- Eliminated in the urine/feces

Pharmacodynamics: Block the dopamine and serotonin receptor activity.

Iron

Iron:
- Used to treat iron-deficiency anemia which is the most common form of anemia.
- Iron preparations include: ferrous fumarate, ferrous gluconate, ferrous sulfate, and iron dextran.
- Transported by blood and bound to transferrin; stored in liver, spleen, and bone marrow; two-thirds is contained in hemoglobin.
- Excreted in urine, stool, sweat, and intestinal cell sloughing; secreted in breast milk.

Pharmacotherapeutics:
- Used to prevent or treat iron deficiency anemia.
- Given to children 6 months to 2 years old and pregnant women.
- Treatment lasts 6 months.

Drug interactions: Absorption is reduced by antacids, coffee, tea, milk, and eggs.

Adverse reactions:
- Most common is gastric irritation.
- Also darkens stool.

Lithium

Lithium carbonate and citrate are the drugs of choice to prevent or treat mania and bipolar disorders.

Pharmacokinetics:
- Absorbed rapidly and completely when taken orally
- Distributed to body tissues
- Not metabolized
- Excreted unchanged

Pharmacodynamics:
- Mania - excessive catecholamine stimulation.
- Bipolar disorder - swings between excessive catecholamine stimulation (mania) and diminished catecholamine stimulation (depression).
- Regulates catecholamine release in the CNS by: increasing norepinephrine and serotonin uptake; reducing the release of norepinephrine from the synaptic vesicles in the presynaptic neuron; inhibiting norepinephrine's action in the postsynaptic neuron.

Heparin

Heparin:
- Prepared commercially from animal tissue.
- Used to prevent clot formation but cannot dissolve already formed clots. Used to prevent deep vein thrombosis in surgical patients.

Pharmacotherapeutics:
- Used to prevent the formation of new clots or the extension of existing clots in the following situations:
  - Venous thromboemboli
  - Disseminated intravascular coagulation
  - Atrial fibrillation
  - Acute MI
- Also used to prevent clotting during use of the cardiopulmonary bypass machine and hemodialysis machine, and during orthopedic surgery.

Drug interactions:
- Increases the effects of oral anticoagulants - monitor PT and INR.
- Risk of bleeding increases when taken with NSAIDS and aspirin.

Folic acid

Folic acid:
- Given to treat folic acid deficiency.
- Preparations include: folic acid and leucovorin calcium.

Pharmacokinetics:
- Absorbed rapidly in the intestine
- Distributed to all body tissues
- Metabolized in the liver
- Excreted in the urine and stool
- Secreted in breast milk.

Pharmacotherapeutics:
- Used to treat folic acid deficiency.
- Patients requiring preventive folic acid therapy include: pregnant women and patients undergoing treatment for liver disease, hemolytic anemia, alcohol abuse, skin disease, or renal failure.

Drug interactions: In large doses may counteract the effects of anticonvulsants potentially leading to seizures.

Adverse reactions: Erythema, itching, and rash.

Vasodilators

Vasodilators:
- Two types: direct vasodilators and calcium channel blockers; both decrease systolic and diastolic blood pressure.
- Direct vasodilators act on arteries, veins, or both and include: diazoxide (Hyperstat), Prototype: hydralazine hydrochloride (Apresoline), minoxidil (Rogaine), and nitroprusside sodium (Nitropress).
- Calcium channel blockers produce arteriolar relaxation by preventing the entry of calcium into the cells.

Pharmacotherapeutics: Are rarely used alone to treat hypertension.

Drug interactions: may produce additive effects when taken with nitrates.

Adverse reactions: compensatory vasoconstriction and tachycardia.

Nicotinic and muscarinic receptors

Nicotinic Receptors:
- Bind nicotine
- Blocked by curare (tubocurarine)
- Linked to ionic channels
- Response is brief and fast
- Located at neuromuscular junctions, autonomic ganglia, and to a small extent in the CNS
- Mediate excitation in target cells Mediate inhibition and excitation in target cells
- Both pre- and postsynaptic

Muscarinic Receptors:
- Bind muscarine
- Blocked by atropine
- Linked to 2nd messenger systems through G proteins
- Response is slow and prolonged
- Found on myocardial muscle, certain smooth muscle, and in discrete CNS regions
- Mediate inhibition and excitation in target cells
- Both pre- and postsynaptic

Macrolides

Macrolides:
- Metabolized by the liver, and excreted in bile.
- Duodenum absorption.
- Can cross the placental barrier.

Types:
- Azithromycin
- Clarithromycin
- Erythromycin derivaties

Drug of choice for legionella pneumophila and mycoplasma pneumoniae infections – Erythromycin.

Drug interactions: Can increase theophylline levels increasing toxicity risk.

Adverse reactions – few but can include N, V, and D.

Oral Anticoagulants

The major oral anticoagulants used in the US are the coumarin compounds warfarin sodium (Coumadin) and Dicumarol.

Pharmacotherapeutics:
- Used to treat thromboembolism and prevent DVT.
- Also prescribed for patients with diseased or prosthetic heart valves.

Drug interactions:
- A diet high in vitamin K reduces the effectiveness of oral anticoagulants. Chronic alcohol abuse increases the risk of clotting; acute alcohol intoxication increases the risk of bleeding.
- Many drugs may increase the risk of bleeding or clotting.

Adverse reactions: Bleeding - may be reversed with the administration of phytonadione (vitamin K1).

Thrombolytic drugs

Thrombolytic drugs:
- Used to dissolve a preexisting clot or thrombus in an acute situation.
- Some of these drugs currently being used include:
  - Alteplase
  - Anistreplase
  - Streptokinase

Pharmacotherapeutics:
- Used to treat certain thromboembolic disorders.
- The drug of choice to break down newly formed thrombi.
- Alteplase is used to treat acute MI, PE, and acute ischemic stroke.
- Anistreplase is used to treat acute MI.
- Streptokinase is used to treat acute MI, PE, DVT, arterial thrombosis, and arterial embolism.

Drug interactions: Interact with anticoagulants, antiplatelets, and NSAIDS increasing bleeding risk.

Alpha-adrenergic blockers

Alpha-adrenergic blockers work by interrupting the actions of the catecholamines norepinephrine and epinephrine at the alpha receptors resulting in: relaxation of the smooth muscle in the blood vessels; increased dilation of blood vessels; and decreased blood pressure.

Prototype drug -prazosin (Minipress)

Pharmacotherapeutics: Used to treat: hypertension; peripheral vascular disorders, and pheochromocytoma (a catecholamine-secreting tumor causing severe hypertension).

Drug interactions/adverse reactions: Many drugs interact producing synergistic effects such as orthostatic hypotension, severe hypotension and vascular collapse.

Antiplatelet drugs

Antiplatelet drugs:
- Used to prevent arterial thromboembolism in patients at risk for MI, stroke, and arteriosclerosis.
- Examples of antiplatelet drugs include:
  - Aspirin, Dipyridamole (Persantine)
  - Sulfinpyrazone, Ticlopidine

Pharmacotherapeutics:
- Used in patients with: a previous MI or unstable angina;
- TIA's
- Post-cardiac valve replacement
- Post-bypass surgery.

Drug interactions: Aspirin taken with heparin, oral anticoagulants, and dipyridamole increases bleeding risk.

Adverse reactions: Hypersensitivity reactions - anaphylaxis.

Mineralcorticoids

Pharmacokinetics:
- Absorbed well and distributed to all parts of the body.
- Metabolized by the liver to inactive metabolites.
- Excreted by the kidneys primarily as inactive metabolites.

Pharmacodynamics: affects fluid and electrolyte balance by acting on the distal renal tubule to increase sodium reabsorption and potassium and hydrogen secretion.

Pharmacotherapeutics: used as replacement therapy for patients with adrenocortical insufficiency; also used to treat salt-losing congenital adrenogenital syndrome.

Monobactams

Monobactams:
- Aztreonam (Azactam) is the first member in the class.
- Has a narrow spectrum of activity that includes many gram-negative aerobic bacteria.

Pharmacotherapeutics:
- Is indicated in a range of therapeutic situations.
- Should not be used alone in seriously ill patients if the infection may be caused by a gram-positive or a mixed aerobic-anaerobic bacteria.

Drug interactions: Synergistic or additive effects occur when used with a variety of other antibiotics.

Adverse reactions – N, V, D, hypersensitivity, hypotension.

Non-catecholamines

Non-catecholamines:
- Local or systemic constriction of blood vessels - phenylephrine (Neo-Synephrine).
- Nasal and eye decongestion and dilation of bronchioles - albuterol (Proventil/Ventolin).
- Smooth muscle relaxation - terbutaline (Brethaire).

Pharmacotherapeutics: Stimulate the sympathetic nervous system and produce a variety of effects in the body. Example - ritodrine (Yutopar) - used to stop pre-term labor.

Drug interactions/adverse reactions: Taken with monoamine oxidase inhibitors can cause severe hypertension and death.

Selective serotonin reuptake inhibitors

Selective serotonin re-uptake inhibitors:
- Developed to treat depression with fewer adverse effects.
- Chemically different from tricyclic antidepressants and MAO inhibitors.

Include: Prototype - fluoxetine hydrochloride (Prozac), paroxetine hydrochloride (Paxil), and sertraline hydrochloride (Zoloft).

SSRIs are Effective for Sadness, Panic and Compulsions is a helpful mnemonic to assist you to remember the purpose for specific SSRIs.
Effective-escitalopram
For- Fluoxetine, fluvoxamine
Sadness- Sertroline
Panic- Paroxetine
Compulsions- Citalopram

Pharmacokinetics: Almost completely absorbed after oral administration; highly protein-bound; metabolized in the liver; excreted in the urine.

Pharmacodynamics: Inhibit neuronal reuptake of the neurotransmitter serotonin.

SSS is a helpful mnemonic to assist you to remember the adverse effects of SSRIs.
Stomach upset
Sexual dysfunction
Serotonin syndrome

Iminostilbenes

Iminostilbenes:
- The most commonly used is carbamazepine (Tegretol).
- Effectively treats: partial and generalized tonic-clonic seizures and mixed seizure types.

Pharmacotherapeutics: Carbamazepine is the drug of choice for treating generalized tonic-clonic seizures, simple and complex partial seizures, and trigeminal neuralgia.

Drug interactions: Can reduce the effects of oral anticoagulants and oral contraceptives.

Adverse reactions: Will affect mood and behavior.

Tegretol is an anticonvulsant that depresses the bone marrow causing TAL:
Thrombocytopenia
Anemia
Leukopenia
*Assess the patient's platelets and hemoglobin

Potassium-sparing diuretics

Potassium-sparing diuretics:
- Have weaker diuretic and antihypertensive effects than other diuretics but conserve potassium.
- Include: amiloride (Midamor), Prototype: spironolactone (Aldactone), and triamterene (Dyrenium).

Pharmacotherapeutics: Used to treat: edema, diuretic-induced hypokalemia in patients with heart failure, cirrhosis, nephrotic syndrome, and hypertension.

Spironolactone is used to treat hyperaldosteronism and hirsutism (excessive hair growth). Commonly used with other diuretics.

PDE inhibitors

PDE inhibitors:
- Used for short-term management of heart failure or long-term management for patients awaiting a transplant.
- Include the drugs inamrinone lactate (Inocor) and milrinone (Primacor).

Pharmacotherapeutics: Used for the management of heart failure when patients haven't responded adequately to treatment with dig, diuretics, or vasodilators.

Drug interactions: Because they reduce serum potassium levels, when taken with potassium-wasting diuretics may cause hypokalemia.

Antacids

Antacids:
- Neutralize gastric pH
- Largely replaced in recent years by other drugs
- Used for fast relief of gastric discomfort, often in combination with other therapies
- Onset: 5-15 minutes
- Duration: 2 hours
- May cause increased acid production, must be used repeatedly to reduce acidity

Key Points:
- Aluminum hydroxide (Amphojel)used in renal failure to reduce phosphorus levels (binds to form aluminum phosphate)
- Calcium carbonate (TUMS) used as calcium supplement to prevent osteoporosis

Clindamycin

Pharmacodynamics:
- Inhibits bacterial protein synthesis.
- Primarily bacteriostatic against most organisms.

Pharmacotherapeutics: Because of its potential for serious toxicity and pseudomembrane colitis, it is limited to a few clinical situations in which safer alternative antibacterials are not available.

Drug interactions: May block neuromuscular transmission and may enhance the action of neuromuscular blockers.

Adverse reactions – pseudomembranous colitis, N, V, D.

MAO inhibitors

Divided into two classifications:
- Hydrazines - phenelzine sulfate (Nardil)
- Nonhydrazines - tranylcypromine sulfate (Parnate)

Pharmacokinetics:
- Absorbed rapidly from the GI tract
- Metabolized in the liver into metabolites
- Excreted mainly by the GI tract

Pharmacodynamics: Appear to work by inhibiting monoamine oxidase, the enzyme that normally metabolizes norepinephrine and serotonin, making these neurotransmitters more available to the receptors.

Bile-Sequestering drugs

Bile-sequestering drugs:
- Include Prototype: cholestyramine (Questran) and colestipol hydrochloride (Cholestabyl).
- Are resins that remove excess bile acids from the fat depots under the skin.

Pharmacotherapeutics: The drug of choice for treating type IIa hyperlipoproteinemia not controlled by diet.

Drug interactions: Absorption of many drugs may be decreased including vitamins, antibiotics, thyroid hormones, and digoxin.

Adverse reactions: Relatively mild GI effects.

Antiarrhythmics

Anti-Arrhythmics are used to treat arrhythmias which are disturbances of the normal heart rhythm.

Categorized into four classes:
- I (A, B, C) - largest group
- II
- III
- IV

Class IB antiarrhythmics

Lidocaine hydrochloride is one of the most widely used for treating acute ventricular arrhythmias.

Pharmacotherapeutics: Used to treat ventricular ectopic beats, ventricular tachycardia, and ventricular fibrillation.

Drug interactions: May exhibit additive or antagonistic effects when administered with other antiarrhythmics.

Adverse reactions: Drug of choice in acute care because usually doesn't produce serious adverse reactions.

Class IC antiarrhythmics

Class IC:
- Used to treat certain severe refractory ventricular arrhythmias.
- Include: flecainide acetate (Tambocor), moricizine (Ethmozine), and propafenone hydrochloride (Rythmol).

Pharmacotherapeutics: Used to treat life-threatening ventricular arrhythmias.

Drug interactions:
- May exhibit additive effects with other antiarrhythmics.
- When used with dig may increase the risk of dig toxicity.

Adverse reactions: Development of new arrhythmias; aggravation of existing arrhythmias.

Class II antiarrhythmics

Class II:
- Composed of beta-adrenergic antagonists (beta-blockers).
- Include: acebutolol hydrochloride (Monitan), esmolol hydrochloride (Brevibloc), and Prototype: propranolol hydrochloride (Inderal).

Pharmacotherapeutics: Slow ventricular rates during atrial flutter, atrial fibrillation, and paroxysmal atrial tachycardia.

Drug interactions: The risk of dig toxicity when taken with esmolol.

Adverse reactions: Arrhythmias, bradycardia, heart failure, hypotension.

Class III antiarrhythmics

Class III:
- Used to treat ventricular arrhythmias.
- Include: amiodarone hydrochloride (Aratac) and bretylium tosylate (Bretylate).

Pharmacotherapeutics:
- Aren't the drugs of choice for antiarrhythmic therapy because of adverse effects.
- Used for life-threatening arrhythmias that are resistant to other antiarrhythmic treatment.

Drug interactions:
- Amiodarone increases the risk of dig toxicity.
- Severe hypotension may result when amiodarone is given with antihypertensive drugs.

Adverse reactions: Aggravation of arrhythmias.

Class IV antiarrhythmics

Class IV:
- Composed of calcium channel blockers.
- Used to treat supraventricular arrhythmias.
- Include Prototype: verapamil (Calan, Isoptin) and diltiazem (Cardizem).
- Presentation of calcium channel blockers under the heading of antianginals.

Carbapenems

Carbapenems:
- A class of beta-lactam antibacterials that includes: imipenem-cilastatin sodium (Primaxin) and meropenem (Merrem).
- Their antibacterial spectrum of activity is broader than any other antibacterial to date.

Pharmacotherapeutics: Used alone for mixed aerobic and anaerobic infections, as therapy for serious nosocomial infections, or infections in immunocompromised hosts.

Drug interactions: May interact with other drugs.

Adverse reactions – N, V, D.

Valproic acid

Two major drugs are valproate (Depacon) and divalproex (Depakote).

Pharmacotherapeutics: Used for the long-term treatment of: absence seizures, myoclonic seizures, and tonic-clonic seizures.

Drug interactions: Inhibition of phenobarbital metabolism in the liver.

Adverse reactions:
- Must be used cautiously in young children and in patients receiving multiple anticonvulsants.
- May lead to fatal liver toxicity. This risk limits use.

Hydantoins

The two most commonly prescribed anticonvulsants - phenytoin and phenytoin sodium (Dilantin) - belong to this class. Phenytoin is:
- Absorbed slowly both PO and IM
- Distributed rapidly and is highly protein-bound
- Metabolized in the liver
- Excreted in the urine.

Pharmacotherapeutics: Used to treat complex partial seizures and tonic-clonic seizures.

Drug interactions: Interact with a number of drugs.

Adverse reactions: Drowsiness

Fibric acid derivative drugs

Fibric acid derivates:
- Two derivatives of this acid that is produced by fungi are Prototype: clofibrate (Atromid-S), gemfibrozil (Loprid), and fenofibrate (Tricor).
- Reduce high triglyceride and LDL levels.

Pharmacotherapeutics: Used primarily to reduce triglyceride levels and secondarily to reduce blood cholesterol levels.

Drug interactions: May displace acidic drugs such as phenytoin, thyroid derivatives, and digoxin.

Adverse reactions: GI effects.

Adenosine

Adenosine: An injectable antiarrhythmia drug used for the acute treatment of parozxysmal supraventricular tachycardia.

Pharmacotherapeutics: Effective against reentry tachycardias (when an impulse depolarizes an area of heart muscle and returns and repolarizes it) that involve the AV node.

Drug interactions: Caffeine antagonizes the effect requiring larger doses.

Adverse reactions: facial flushing, shortness of breath, dyspnea, chest discomfort.

Antidepressant and antimanic drugs

Anti-depressant and anti-manic drugs:
- Used to treat affective disorders which are disturbances in mood characterized by depression or elation.
- Unipolar disorders (depression) are treated with MAO inhibitors, tricyclic antidepressants, or other antidepressants.
- Bipolar disorders (depression and mania) are treated with lithium.

Tricyclic antidepressants

Pharmacotherapeutics:
- Used to treat episodes of major depression.
- Less effective in patients with hypochondriasis, atypical depression, or depression with delusions.
- Also being investigated for use with migraine headaches, phobias, urinary incontinence, attention deficit disorder, ulcers, and diabetic neuropathy.
- Cimetidine (Tagamet) impairs metabolism.

Adverse reactions: Orthostatic hypotension and sedation

Depolarizing blocking drugs

Depolarizing blocking drugs:
- Succinylcholine is the only therapeutic drug in this class.
- Acts like acetylcholine but isn't inactivated by cholinesterase.
- It is the drug of choice for short-term muscle relaxation.

Pharmacotherapeutics: The drug of choice for short-term muscle relaxation (during intubation and ECT).

Drug interactions: Potentiated by a number of anesthetics and antibiotics.

Adverse reactions: apnea and hypotension

Expectorants

These drugs thin mucous so it's cleared more easily out of airways.

Pharmacotherapeutics:
- Used for the relief of coughs from: colds, minor bronchial irritation, bronchitis, influenza, sinusitis, bronchial asthma, emphysema, and other respiratory disorders.
- May be taken with antitussives, analgesics, antihistamines, or decongestants.

Drug interactions: Administration with anticoagulants may increase the risk of bleeding.

Loop diuretic drugs

Include: bumetanide (Bumex), ethacrynate sodium, ethacrynic acid (Edecrin), and Prototype: furosemide (Lasix).

Pharmacotherapeutics: Used to treat hypertension and edema that is associated with heart failure, and liver and kidney disease.

Drug interactions: a significant number of interactions exist.

Adverse reactions: fluid and electrolyte imbalances.

Central acting skeletal muscle relaxants drugs

Central acting:
- Act on the central nervous system to treat acute spasms caused by: anxiety, inflammation, pain, trauma.
- Baclofen and diazepam (Valium)

Pharmacotherapeutics: Treat acute, painful musculoskeletal conditions along with rest and physical therapy.

Drug interactions: Taken with other CNS depressants increase CNS effects.

Adverse reactions: Dependence

Polyethylene glycol-electrolyte

GoLYTELY (Polyethylene glycol-electrolyte solution):
- Used as bowel prep for colon surgery & GI procedures
- Induces diarrhea, cleanses bowel. Isotonic
- 1 gallon, needs to be reconstituted
- Fast at least 3 hrs prior, no meds< 1 hr prior
- Instruct patient to drink 250 cc/10 minutes until clear watery stools
- Onset 30-60 min, duration 4 hrs

SE: nausea, fullness, bloating

Sulfonamides

Sulfonamides were the first effective systemic antibacterial drugs. Drugs include: (prefix - sulf & suffix - azole).

Pharmacotherapeutics: Frequently used to treat acute UTI's.

Drug interactions:
- Have few significant interactions.
- Increase the hypoglycemic affects of oral diabetic agents.

Adverse reactions – urinary crystals, hypersensitivity.

Epoetin alfa

Epoetin alfa stimulates RBC production.

Pharmacotherapeutics: Used to treat patients with:
- Normocytic anemia caused by chronic renal failure.
- Anemia associated with zidovudine therapy in patients with HIV infection.
- Certain types of anemia decreasing the need for transfusions.

Drug interactions: No known drug interactions.

Adverse reactions: Hypertension

Lactulose

Lactulose:
- Used primarily for prevention of hepatic encephalopathy in liver failure
- Binds to ammonia in the blood
- In acute phase, 30-45cc/hr until diarrhea; then 3-4 times/day
- Dosage adjusted to produce 2-3 soft stools/day

Monitor patient's mental status & level of consciousness, ammonia levels

Side effects: flatulence, abd. bloating, diarrhea

Antimalarial drugs

Antimalarial/protozoal drugs:
- One of the major drugs used to prevent and treat malaria is chloroquine.
- Action results from its incorporation into the DNA of the parasite, rendering it ineffective.
- Antiprotozoal drugs are used for a variety of disorders including pneumocystis carinii infections, giardiasis, trichomoniasis, and toxoplasmosis.

Antitubercular drugs

Antitubercular drugs:
- Used to treat tuberculosis which is caused by mycobacterium tuberculosis.
- These drugs can halt the progression of an infection but are not always curative.
- Because of drug-resistant TB strains, a four-drug regimen is recommended that includes: isoniazid, rifampin, pyrazinamide, and streptomycin or ethambutol.

Anti-Lipemics

Anti-Lipemics:
- Used to lower abnormally high blood levels of lipids such as cholesterol, triglycerides, and phospholipids.
- Include: bile-sequestering drugs (bile acid sequestrants), fibric acid derivatives (fibrates), and cholesterol synthesis inhibitors (HMG-CoA reductase inhibitors – hydroxymethylglutaryl-coenzyme A reductase) or STATINS.

Bulk-forming laxatives

Bulk-forming laxatives:
- Metamucil, Citrucel, etc.
- Swell in water to form gel that increases bulk and softens stool, increases peristalsis
- Similar to the action of dietary fiber
- Useful in chronic constipation, and in irritable bowel syndrome
- Onset: 12-24 hrs
- Powder needs reconstitution in at least 8 oz water or juice

Barbiturates

Pharmacodynamics: Depress the sensory cortex of the brain, decrease motor activity, alter cerebral function, and produce drowsiness, sedation, and hypnosis.

Pharmacotherapeutics: Clinical indications include: daytime sedation; insomnia; preop sedation and anesthesia; anxiety relief; anticonvulsant.

Barbiturates

Barbiturates:
- Reduce overall CNS alertness.
- Phenobarbital is the prototype drug in this class.

Pharmacokinetics:
- Absorbed well from the GI tract
- Distributed rapidly
- Metabolized by the liver
- Excreted in the urine.

Barbiturates

Drug interactions: Interact with many other drugs.

Phenytoin (Dilantin) and valproic acid (Depacon) may increase toxic effects.

Adverse reactions: Tolerance, psychological and physical dependence.

Fluoroquinolones

Fluoroquinolones:
- Structurally similar synthetic antibiotics.
- Used to treat UTI's, URI's, pneumonia, and gonorrhea.
- Drugs include: (suffix - floxacin & oxacin)

Pharmacotherapeutics: Used to treat a variety of UTI's.

Drug interactions: Several interactions may occur.

Adverse reactions: Few but may include N, V, and D.

Carafate

Carafate (sucralfate):
- Forms a protective barrier on the GI mucosa, high affinity for areas of ulceration
- Local acid neutralization

Uses: gastric, duodenal and oral ulcers, GI bleed, stress ulcer prevention

Minimal absorption

Dosing: 1 g qid, 1 hr before meals & HS

Side effects: constipation

NSAIDS and recommended dosages for adults

The following are 5 Key NSAIDS and normal recommended dosages for adults:
- Naproxen,500 to 1,500 mg per day in 2 doses
- Ketoprofen, (Brand) Orudis, 200 to 225 mg per day in 3 or 4 doses
- Indomethacin, (Brand) Indocin, 50 to 200 mg per day in 2 to 4 doses
- Ibuprofen, Motrin- 1,200 to 3,200 mg per day in 3 or 4 doses
- Piroxicam, Feldene- 20 mg per day in 1 or 2 doses

Antianginals

Anti-Anginals work by reducing myocardial oxygen demand, increasing the supply of oxygen to the heart, or both. Three classes include:
- Nitrates - treat acute angina.
- Beta blockers - long-term prevention.
- Calcium channel blockers - used when other drugs fail.

Proton pump inhibitors

Proton pump inhibitors inhibit HCL production in the stomach. Effects may last up to 72 hours. They are used for peptic ulcer and GERD. The side effects include (mild) nausea, headache, diarrhea, constipation, flatulence. They may affect absorption of other drugs.

Omeprazole (Prilosec)
Lansoprazole (Prevacid)

Cytotec

Cytotec (misoprostol):
- Prostaglandin analog
- Reduces gastric acid secretion
- Enhances mucosal resistance to injury

Uses:
- Prevention and treatment of NSAID-related ulcers
- NSAIDs inhibit prostaglandins

Side effects: Nausea, vomiting, abdominal pain

Anti-anxiety drugs

Pharmacotherapeutics: Used to treat generalized anxiety states; not useful in panic attacks.

Drug interactions: Hypertensive reaction may occur when given with MAO inhibitors.

Adverse reactions: Dizziness and lightheadedness.

Antipyretics

The key antipyretics are:
- Salicylates: aspirin (also called acetylsalicylic acid or ASA), choline salicylate, magnesium salicylate, and sodium salicylate;
- Acetaminophen; and Nonsteroidal anti-inflammatory drugs (NSAIDs): ibuprofen, naproxen sodium, and ketoprofen.

Stool softeners

Stool softeners:
- Docusate (Colace, Doss)
- Reduce surface tension in the bowel increasing water absorption into stool
- Onset: 24-48 hrs (up to 3-5 days)

Side effects: (rare) GI pain, cramping, rash

Administer with adequate fluids

Calcium channel blockers

Calcium channel blockers decrease coronary vascular resistance and increase coronary blood flow. They also decrease peripheral resistance via vasodilatation of arterioles. They are without significant effect on venous tone at normal doses. Calcium channel blocking agents affect the movement of calcium into the cells of the heart and blood vessels. As a result, they relax blood vessels and increase the supply of blood and oxygen to the heart while reducing its workload. Some of the calcium channel blocking agents are used to relieve and control angina pectoris (chest pain). Some are also used to treat high blood pressure (hypertension). High blood pressure adds to the workload of the heart and arteries. If it continues for a long time, the heart and arteries may not function properly. This can damage the blood vessels of the brain, heart, and kidneys, resulting in a stroke, heart failure, or kidney failure. High blood pressure may also increase the risk of heart attacks. These problems may be less likely to occur if blood pressure is controlled.

Ten calcium channel blockers are:
- Bepridil
- Diltiazem
- Felodipine
- Flunarizine
- Isradipine
- Nicardipine
- Nifedipine
- Nimodipine
- Verapamil
- Amlodipine

Benzodiazepines

Benzodiazepines

The three types of Benzodiazepines that provide anticonvulsant effects are:
- diazepam (parenteral) - status epilepticus
- clonazepam (Klonopin) - long-term epilepsy
- clorazepate (Tranxene) - adjunct in treating partial seizures

Milk of magnesia

Milk of magnesia:
- Osmotic saline laxative
- Used in simple constipation & postop
- Suspension
- Use cautiously in renal impairment
- Potential for hypermagnesemia due to reduced excretion

Tramadol

The dosage of Tramadol is 50 to 100 mg every 4 to 6 hours as needed. Possible side effects are constipation diarrhea, dizziness, drowsiness, increased sweating, loss of appetite, and nausea.

Gastric acidity

Three types of drugs that are used to control gastric acidity are:
- Histamine (H2) receptor antagonists
- Proton pump inhibitors
- Antacids

Diuretics

Diuretics are used to increase the rate of urine flow. Osmotic diuretics include glycerin, isosorbide, mannitol, and urea. Osmotic diuretics are filtered at the glomerular level and are typically given in large doses. Osmotic diuretics not only cause increased urine excretion, but excretion of sodium, potassium, calcium, chloride and bicarbonate. Loop diuretics include lasix, bumex, torsemide, and azosemide. Loop diuretics increase urine output and the excretion of sodium, potassium, and chloride. Thiazide and thiazide like diuretics act to cause decreased reabsorption within the renal proximal tubule. Common thiazide diuretics used today include naturetin, hydrodiuril, enduron, lozol, and zaroxolyn.

Dyslipidemia and hypercholesterolemia

Hyperlipidemia is a leading cause of atherosclerosis and coronary heart disease as well as ischemic cerebrovascular disease, and peripheral vascular disease. Drug treatment for dyslipidemia includes statin drugs which includes atorvastatin, and simvastatin. Nicotinic acid or Niacin is also used to control dyslipidemia. Niacin has a favorable affect on all aspects of lipids. Niacin lowers the low density lipoproteins, elevates the high density lipoproteins and lowers the triglycerides. Bile acid sequestrants such as cholestyramine and colestipol are also used for the treatment of dyslipidemia. Fibric acid derivatives are also utilized as treatment for dyslipidemia. Fibric acid derivatives include medications such as clofibrate, gemfibrozil, and ciprofibrate.

Pharmacology suffixes

The following are the various suffixes in pharmacology along with their actions:
- Benzodiazepine-azepam
- Phenothiazine-azine
- Anti-fungal-azole
- Penicillin-cillin
- Antibiotic-cycline
- Tricyclic Anti-depressant-ipramine
- Protease Inhibitor-navir
- Beta Antagonist-olol
- Cardiac glycoside-oxin
- Methylxanthine-phylline
- ACE Inhibitor-pril
- Beta 2 Agonist-terol
- H2 Antagonist-tidine
- Pituitary Hormone-trophin
- Alpha 1 Antagonist-zosin

ACE inhibitors

Used to treat heart disease, and are commonly prescribed for CHF patients. They commonly end in "pril". They work to lowers blood pressure by relaxing blood vessels. Nursing interventions include monitor blood pressure frequently.

Important Therapeutic Drug Levels

Digoxin	0.5-2.0 mg/mL
Lithium	0.8-1.5 mEq/L
Dilantin	10-20 mcg/dL
Theophylline	10-20 mcg/dL
Warfarin	2.0-3.0 (afib,MI,DVT,PE)
Warfarin	2.5-3.5 (for mechanical heart valves)

Common Toxicity Reversal Agents

Heparin- protamine sulfate
Coumadin- vitamin K
Ammonia- Lactulose
Acetaminophen- n-Acetylcysteine
Iron- deferoxamine
Digoxin- digibind
Alcohol withdrawal- librium

Total parenteral nutrition

Total Parenteral Nutrition is nutrition that is maintained totally by central intravenous routes, or nongastrointestinal routes. The purpose of total parenteral nutrition is to provide calories, nutrients, lipids, and protein to the body. Total parenteral nutrition maintains a positive nitrogen balance that will allow for healing. Total parenteral nutrition is a mechanism to replace lost electrolytes, vitamins, and minerals to the body. Total parenteral nutrition can be administered via a peripherally inserted catheter (termed a picc line), or a centrally inserted catheter (central line).

Electrolytes, vitamins, and minerals can be added to provide 100% of daily requirements for individuals using the parenteral method of feeding. Parenteral feedings contain no milk products and often are accompanied by infused lipids to provide the required amount of dietary fats. Total Parenteral Nutrition or TPN as it is called requires the monitoring of electrolytes, weight, blood glucose levels, intake and output as well as physical assessment daily. The nurse is responsible to assess the site for possible infections that may occur, tissue damage such as infiltration, and phlebitis or inflammation. Continuous monitoring of the IV insertion site is needed to avoid complications.

Enteral nutrition

Enteral feedings require a tube to be placed into the stomach or jejunum via the abdominal wall; this feeding tube provides liquid nutrition while maintaining the functionality of the gastrointestinal system. Enteral feedings can be temporary or permanent and provide 100% of the daily nutritional requirement of individuals in multiple situations. Feedings are specific to disease process as with the pulmonary, renal and cardiovascular systems, and often contain milk products. It is common to begin enteral feeding at a slow rate and graduate hourly intake to a maintenance goal. Enteral feedings often cause diarrhea upon initial usage, but this does clear with time and gastrointestinal adjustment. Keep in mind feeding tube should be kept patent and placement checked per facility policy at minimum every shift.

Oral tube feedings

Short-term tube feeding can be administered orally via the nose or the mouth. The tube is progressed from either the nose or mouth into the stomach or jejunum. Nutrition is provided by bolus feedings of prescribed formula or can be given continuously over a period of hours or a combination of both may be utilized. One hundred percent of daily nutritional requirements can be maintained short-term using oral (OG/orogastric) or nasogastric (NG) tubes. Formulas are prescribed to enhance the healing process or increase functionality with disease processes. Feeding formulations are dosed per need of the client, weight of the client, and allergies.

J tube and G tube

A J tube feeds directly into the jejunum and a G tube goes directly to the stomach. Note: the J tube allows feeding without involving the stomach.

NG- tube

This is a long thin tube that is inserted through the child's nose, throat and esophagus down into the stomach. A pump or gravity feed may be used to supply the food through the tube. Feeds can be given in bolus or continuous amounts. Bolus meaning large amounts over a short period of time. For example, mealtimes can be mimicked by giving three large meals a day through the tube.

NJ-tube (N-Naso, J-Jejunum)

This is similar to the NG tube except once in the stomach it continues through the pyloric valve, duodenum (first part of the small bowel) and into the jejunum (second part of the small bowel). NJ tubes have the same drawbacks of the NG tube but because the end of the tube is in the jejunum instead of the stomach, NJ tubes can help reduce vomiting associated with reflux.

Reduction of Risk Potential

Cholesterol

HDL, LDL, and triglycerides
High-density lipoprotein (HDL): Normal (Good Cholesterol) HDL is considered the friendly cholesterol and consists of 50% protein and assists with decreasing plaque deposits in blood vessels.
Adult desired level: 29-77 mg/dl. Risk for CHD (coronary heart disease) <35mg/dl. Moderate risk level is 35-45 mg/dl. Low risk level is 46-59 mg/dl. Very low risk is >60mg/dl.

Low-density lipoprotein (LDL): Normal (Bad Cholesterol)
Adult desired level: 60-160mg/dl. Risk for CHD: High risk level is >160mg/dl. Moderate risk level is 130-159 mg/dl. Low risk level is <130 mg/dl.
Desirable level is 100 mg/dl.

Triglyceride level: Normal is 10-190 mg/dl.

These are among the leading contributors to atherosclerosis and coronary artery disease. The nurse should educate the client to remain NPO (have nothing by mouth) the 12 hours prior to testing, consume a regular diet the 72 hours prior to the lab, and consume no alcohol 24 hours prior to the exam.

Cholesterol levels and coronary artery disease risk
Total Cholesterol: Normals
Adult desired level: <200 mg/dl. Moderate risk: 200-240 mg/dl. High risk: >240 mg/dl. Children: Infant normal: 90-130 mg/dl. Children age 2-19 years: 130-170 mg/dl. Moderate risk: 171-184 mg/dl. High risk: >185mg/dl.

Cholesterol is a blood lipid synthesized by the liver and found in red blood cells, cell membranes, and muscles. Serum cholesterol is used as an indicator of atherosclerosis and coronary artery disease. Hypercholesterolemia causes plaque deposits in the coronary arteries which makes elevated cholesterol levels a risk factor for MI (myocardial infarction/heart attack), and atherosclerosis. Elevated cholesterol has familial tendency. When preparing the client for a cholesterol level to be drawn the nurse should educate the client to remain without food for the 12 hours prior to the test. The nurse should also be aware that aspirin and cortisone can alter the cholesterol level causing an increase or decrease. Vented patients or patients with hypoxemia may have elevated cholesterol levels, and hemolysis of the specimen can cause false elevations.

Normal ranges

- Bleeding time (template) Less than 10 minutes
- Erythrocyte count 4.2-5.9 million/cu mm
- Erythrocyte sedimentation rate (Westergren) Male: 0-15 mm/hr; female: 0-20 mm/hr
- Hematocrit, blood Male: 42-50%; female: 40-48%
- Hemoglobin, blood Male: 13-16 g/dL; female: 12-15 g/dL

- Mean corpuscular volume 86-98 fL
- Prothrombin time, plasma 11-13 seconds
- Partial thromboplastin time (activated) 30-40 seconds
- Platelet count 150,000-300,000/cu mm
- Reticulocyte count 0.5-1.5% of red cells

Normative values for PO2, PCO2, Bicarbonate, pH and Bicarbonate-serum

- Arterial studies, blood (patient breathing room air)
- PO2 75-100 mm Hg
- PCO2 38-42 mm Hg
- Bicarbonate 23-26 mEq/L
- pH 7.38-7.44
- Oxygen saturation 95% or greater
- Bicarbonate, serum 23-28 mEq/L

Normative values for glucose, phosphorus, pre-albumin, and BUN

- Glucose, plasma Normal (fasting): 70-115 mg/dL
- Borderline: 115-140 mg/dL
- Abnormal: greater than 140 mg/dL
- Phosphorus, serum 3.0-4.5 mg/dL
- Proteins, serum:
- Pre-Albumin .2 - 0.4 g/dL
- Albumin 3.5-5.5 g/dL
- Urea nitrogen, blood (BUN) 8-20 mg/dL

Normative values for serum sodium, potassium, chloride, and bicarbonate

- Electrolytes, serum:
- Sodium 136-145 mEq/L
- Potassium 3.5-5.0 mEq/L
- Chloride 98-106 mEq/L
- Bicarbonate 23-28 mEq/L

Normative values for serum phosphorus, and triglycerides

- Phosphorus, serum 3.0-4.5 mg/dL
- Triglycerides, serum (fasting) Normal: less than 250 mg/dL
- Borderline: 250-500 mg/dL
- Abnormal: greater than 500 mg/dL

Renal function labs

Albumin

Normal Albumin levels: Adult: 3.5-5.0 g/dl. 52-68% of total protein Children: Newborn normal is 2.9-5.4 g/dl. Infant normal is 4.4-5.4 g/dl. Child normal is 4.0-5.8 g/dl. Albumin levels are used to determine the amount of albumin circulating in the blood or urine.

Elevated levels are associated with liver disease, burns, malnutrition, renal disorders, and dehydration.

BUN (Blood Urea Nitrogen)
Normal BUN of the serum is: Adult: 5-25 mg/dl. Infant: 5-15 mg/dl. Child: 5-20 mg/dl. Elderly are slightly higher than the adult normal. The BUN is utilized to detect disorders of the kidney such as dehydration, liver damage, over hydration, kidney function (renal insufficiency), and sepsis.

Creatinine
Normal Creatinine for adults is 0.5-1.5mg/dl. (Females are slightly lower related to lower muscle mass.). Child Normals: Newborn: 0.8-1.4mg/dl. Infant: 0.7-1.7mg/dl Child: 2-6yrs 0.3-0.6mg/dl. Older Child: 0.4-1.2 mg/dl. Creatinine is a byproduct of muscle catabolism; creatinine production is proportional to muscle mass. Creatinine is filtered by the glomeruli and is excreted in the urine. Creatinine is elevated with acute and chronic renal failure.

Low magnesium and high creatinine signals renal failure.

Liver function labs

Alkaline Phosphatase (ALP)
Normals: Adult: 42-136 U/l. Child: 0-12 yrs. 40-115 U/l.   Child: 13-18 yrs. 50-230 U/l. Elderly normal is slightly higher than that of an adult. Alkaline phosphatase is an enzyme produced mainly in the liver and bone. Alkaline phosphatase is used to assist in diagnosis of liver and bone disease. The nurse should remember that ALP levels may be naturally elevated in children who are experiencing bone growth.

ALT/SGPT
Alanine aminotransferase (ALT)/Serum Glutamic Pyruvic Transaminase (SGPT). Adult Normals: 10-35 U/l. Males may have a slight elevation in these numbers. Child Normals: Infant can be twice as high as an adult, and children are very similar to the adult level. Elderly levels are slightly higher than that of an adult. ALT/SGOT assists in the detection of liver disorders such as viral (acute) hepatitis, necrosis of the liver, and drug or chemical toxicity. Cirrhosis, cancer, and alcohol intoxication are also associated with elevated ALT levels.

AST/SGOT
Aspartate aminotransferase (AST) Normals: Adult Normals: 8-38 U/l. Females may experience slightly lower values than men. Child Normals: Newborns have a level 4 times the normal of an adult. Children's levels are similar to that of an adult. Elderly levels may be slightly higher than that of an adult.

ALT/SGOT
Elevated levels assist in the determination of heart and liver muscle damage. ALT is also uses in conjunction with CK and LDH in diagnosing an acute MI. Bilirubin: The normal adult bilirubin is 0.1-1.0 mg/dl.

Pancreatic function labs

Amylase
Normal Amylase levels for the Adult are 60-160. Elderly levels are slightly higher than that of an adult. Amylase is an enzyme that originates within the pancreas, the salivary glands and the liver. The function of amylase is to change starch into sugar. The individual who is experiencing acute pancreatitis will have amylase levels that are double the normal range. (Other signs and symptoms of acute pancreatitis include inflammation, severe pain, and necrosis caused by tissue death.) The nurse should be aware that glucose in an IV may cause a false negative amylase.

Lipase
Normal lipase levels: Adult 20-180 IU/l (the nurse should keep in mind values of labs often times vary between laboratories); Normal lipase for children is Infant: 6-105 IU/l, and Child 20-136 IU/l. Lipase is secreted by the pancreas and digests fat. Acute pancreatitis is the most common cause of an elevated lipase level. Decreased levels may indicate late cancer, or hepatitis.

Electrolytes (K, Na, Cl)

K-Potassium normal for Adults is 3.5-5.3 mEq/l. Potassium normal for children is 3.5-5.5 mEq/l. Infant potassium normal is 3.6-5.8 mEq/l.
The most frequent cause of hyperkalemia or elevated potassium level >5.5 mEq/l is renal insufficiency.

MURDER is a helpful mnemonic to assist you to remember the symptoms of hyperkalemia.

Muscle cramps
Urine abnormalities
Respiratory distress
Decreased cardiac contractility
EKG changes
Reflexes

MACHINE is a helpful mnemonic to assist you to remember the causes of hyperkalemia.
Meds: ACE inhibitors, NSAIDS, Diuretics (potassium sparing)
Acidosis: metabolic and respiratory
Cellular destruction: burns, traumatic injury
Hypoaldosteronism and hemolysis
Intake: excessive dietary (eg: salt replacements that contain potassium)
Nephrons: renal failure
Excretion: impaired

Hyperkalemia Treatment: C BIG K DROP is a mnemonic to assist you to remember the treatment for hyperkalemia. The acronym sounds like "see big K+ drop".
Calcium
Bicarbonate
Insulin
Glucose
Kayexalate

D(rop)iuretics and dialysis

6 L's is a helpful mnemonic to assist you to remember the symptoms of Hypokalemia.
Lethargy
Leg cramps
Limp muscles
Low, shallow respirations
Lethal cardiac dysrhythmias
Lots of urine (polyuria)

Na-Sodium normal for Adults and children is 135-145 mEq/l. Sodium normal for infants is 135-150mEq/l.
Hypernatremia is elevated sodium levels (>145 mEq/l.) might be caused by anuria or no urine production, and acute renal failure.
Hyponatremia is characterized by a sodium level <135mEq/l. Hyponatremia can result from tubular disorders associated with the inability to reabsorb sodium.

Ample Salt is a helpful mnemonic to assist you to remember the symptoms of Hypernatremia.
Ascites, Edema
Mouth that is dry
Personality/mental status changes (irritable, confused, restless, anxious)
Low urine output
Elevated blood pressure and fluid retention

Skin flushed
Agitation
Low-grade fever
Thirst

Chloride (Cl): Normal Chloride levels for the Adult are 95-105 mEq/l.
Normal Chloride levels for Children: Newborn 94-112 mEq/l. Infant 95-110 mEq/l. Child 98-115 mEq/l.

Chloride provides information on acid/base balance as it relates to potassium and sodium.

CATS is a helpful mnemonic to assist you to remember the symptoms of hypocalcemia.
Convulsions
Arrhythmias
Tetany
Stridor and Spasms

Calcium and Phosphorus relationship
Calcium decrease = phosphorus increase
Phosphorus decrease – calcium increase
Serum calcium: 9.0-11.0 mg/dL
Phophorus: 3.0-4.5 mg/dL

- 168 -

TSH

The normal TSH (Thyroid stimulating hormone) values are: Adult 0.35-5.5 uIU/ml. Newborn: <25 uIU/ml. Thyroid stimulating hormone is secreted by the anterior pituitary gland (anterior hypophysis) in response to thyroid releasing hormone (TRH) from the hypothalamus. Thyroid stimulating hormone (TSH) is a catalyst (stimulates) the production of T4 (thyroxine) from the thyroid gland. TSH is dependent upon the negative feedback mechanism of the body; decreased levels of T4 cause the release of TRH and in turn stimulate the production of TSH. Thyroid stimulating hormone (TSH), and T4 (thyroxine) measurements are utilized to differentiate thyroid and pituitary functions among individuals with hormonal irregularities, and suspect disease states. Thyroid stimulating hormone is often utilized to determine hypothyroidism caused by the pituitary. Decreased levels of TSH may indicate secondary hypothyroidism related to pituitary problems. The nurse should keep in mind that ASA (aspirin), steroids, dopamine and heparin will alter the results of TSH and may cause false readings.

Thyroid function labs

Calcitonin: Normal calcitonin levels are: Adult Male: <40ng/l Adult Female: < 25 pg/ml. Normal Child Values: Newborn: Normally higher than the adult levels. Child: <70 pg/ml. Calcitonin is a hormone secreted by C cells of the thyroid gland, and aids in the maintenance of serum calcium and phosphorus levels. Calcitonin is secreted in reaction to elevated serum calcium levels. Calcitonin is elevated with carcinoma of the thyroid, and hyperplasia of the adenoma. Free thyroxine (Free T 4): Normal ranges for T-4 are: Adult 4.5-11.5 ug/dl. Normal ranges for the Child are: Newborn: 11-23 ug/dl. Children age 1-4 months 7.5-16.5, children 4-12 months old 5.5-14.5 ug/dl, children 1-6 years old 5.5-13.5, children 6-10 years old 5-12.5 ug/dl. Thyroxine (T4) is the major hormone derived and secreted by the thyroid gland; T4 is commonly used to identify function of the thyroid gland. T4 is used in the diagnosis of hypo and hyperthyroidism. Decreased levels of T4 indicate hypothyroidism, and elevated levels of T4 indicate hyperthyroidism. T4 is also used as a comparison of labs to determine thyroid function. T4 is often done with various other thyroid labs to determine and diagnose disease of the thyroid. Triiodothyronine (T3): Normal ranges for T3 are: Adult 80-200 ng/dl. Child: Newborn 40-215 ng/dl. Children ages 5-10 years 95-240 ng/dl. Children ages 10-15 years 80-210 ng/dl. Triiodothyronine is a thyroid hormone that is always present in small amounts. Serum T3 is secreted in reaction to TSH.

Ketones

Ketones are found in both the serum and the urine. Normal adult serum ketone level is 0.5-4 mg/dl. Normal levels of ketones for children are the same; a newborn will have a slightly higher level of ketones. Serum ketones of the blood or acetone ketone bodies are composed of acetone, acetoacetic acid, and betahydroxybutric acids that are a product of fat metabolism, and fatty acids. Ketone bodies are present in abundance with uncontrolled diabetes. Starvation also produces excessive ketones. During periods of diabetic ketoacidosis the client will have a ketone level of >50 mg/dl. Ketones are excreted in the urine also, but first elevation and notice of rise occurs within the blood. Serum ketones can be utilized to monitor acidosis of the diabetic, and determine effectiveness of treatment. Urine Ketones levels are negative in both the adult and child. Ketones are produced and utilized for energy when the body does not have enough carbohydrates or the carbohydrates cannot be utilized for energy. Diabetic acidosis and starvation are two usual causes of urine ketone production. Urine ketones assist in the diagnosis of an acidotic state within the body.

HbGA1c and diabetes

HbGA1c is the major determinant for glycosylated hemoglobin. Normal for the non diabetic adult is 2-5% of glycosylated hemoglobin. HbGA1c normal for the diabetic adult who is controlled well with insulin or oral diabetic agents is 2.5-6.0% (it is best to always discuss this lab and the normal as <7%). The average is 6.1-5.5%. Uncontrolled diabetes is >8%. Hemoglobin A1C is a representation of blood glucose levels over the past 1-4 months (health care providers typically say over the last 90 days). HbGA1c is used to determine effectiveness of diabetic therapy. The nurse should be aware that false levels of HbGA1c occur with decreased levels of hemoglobin. HbGA1c is also used as a diagnostic tool for diagnosis of diabetes.

BNP and B-ANP

B-natriuretic peptide (BNP) is a peptide that is released into the blood stream (circulation) of individuals with heart failure. B-ANP (atrial natriuretic peptide/atrial natriuretic factor /hormone) is present the plasma of heart failure patients. ANP promotes renal salt and water excretion, increases capillary function, and decreases atrial pressure and secretion of renin, angiotensin, aldosterone, and antidiuretic hormone. ANA or ANF/H acts as an antagonist to renin and aldosterone. ANA is released during atrial expansion causing vasodilatation and an increased glomerular filtration rate. ANH causes a reduction of renal absorption of sodium, blocks renin release by the kidney, and aldosterone secretion from adrenal glands that promote an antihypertensive effect that cause a reduced pre and afterload as well as decreased blood volume. Elevated ANH is an indicator of cardiovascular disease, early indicator of left ventricular disorders, and congestive failure. In individuals with chronic congestive failure the ANH may be low.

Glucose and diabetes

Fasting Blood Glucose (sugar) FBG normals: Adult 70-110 mg/dl., Panic level is < 40 mg/dl or > 700 mg/dl. Normal glucose for the newborn is 30-80 mg/dl. And normal for the child is 60-100 mg/dl. Normal glucose for an elderly individual is 70-120 mg/dl. Glucose is formed from carbohydrates taken in with food and stored in the liver and skeletal muscles. Glucose levels are maintained by insulin production in the pancreas. Elevated glucose (hyperglycemia) indicates not enough insulin production to utilize carbohydrates for energy and glucose remains in the blood in whole form. Decreased levels of glucose (hypoglycemia) indicate inadequate food consumption. Postprandial glucose is a glucose level done two hours (2hrs.) after consuming a meal; this is also termed feasting glucose. The normal two hour postprandial (PPBS) glucose levels are: Adult <140 mg/dl/2h in the serum or plasma, and <120 mg/dl/2h in the blood. Elderly PPBS is <160 mg/dl/2h in the serum and <140 mg/dl/2h in the blood. Self-monitoring glucose is done with capillary blood or finger stick method. Normal capillary blood values are 60-110 mg/dl for an adult, and 50-85 mg/dl, for a child. Self-monitoring is done to control glucose levels on an hourly or daily basis and is utilized when frequent glucose readings are needed.

WBC

The white blood count (WBC) is used to assist in the determination of infectious disease and infectious processes. The white blood count is part of a complete blood count (CBC). White blood cells are also called leukocytes. White blood counts are also used to diagnose health problems. The white blood cells have two groups; the poly (multi)morphonuclear group which consist of neutrophils, eosinophils, and basophils, and mononuclear leukocytes which consist of monocytes and lymphocytes. Leukocytes are part of the body's own natural defense system. White blood cells immediately respond to invasion of organisms by going directly to the affected site. Leukocytosis is an elevated white blood cell count, and leucopenia is a decreased white blood cell count. The normal white blood cell levels are: Adult: Total white cell count is 4500-10,000 ul. Child: Newborn 9000-30,000 ul., 2yrs old 6000-17000 ul., 10 yrs old 4500-13500 ul.

Troponin

Troponin is a form of globular protein in muscle with an increased affinity to calcium ions. Calcium ions are a regulatory protein for muscle contractions. C, 1 and 2 are found is cardiac skeletal muscle, and cardiac muscle. The cardiac forms of Troponin 1 and Troponin T are specific enough to assist in the diagnosis of cardiac conditions. Troponin is released with injury or necrosis of the myocardium. There are 2 cycles of Troponin release that allow early detection of damage; within 4-6 hours of cardiac injury the Troponin will elevate. The Troponin will also rise seven to ten days following a cardiac injury. Peak activity of Troponin is Troponin I 18-20 hours, Troponin T 10-24 hours. Elevation during injury occurs for Troponin I within 4-6 hours and for Troponin T within 3-4 hours following injury.

Normal levels typical for an MI:
Troponin T >0.1 ng/ml
Troponin 1 >2.5 ng/ml

Urinalysis and culture and sensitivity

Urinalysis may be performed to assist in detecting problems with renal function, disease processes, urinary tract infections, diabetes, prenatal examinations, and routine examinations. The nurse should remember that drugs and foods can alter the color of urine. Normal results:
- Color: Straw (Cloudiness may be due to phosphates and urates and are considered normal)
- Turbidity: Clear
- Sp.Gr. 1.001-1.020 (low may indicate tubular defects such as sickle cell anemia, diabetes, and diabetes insipidus)
- Dipstick: ph 4.5-7.5
- Protein: Negative (protein often indicates disease processes such as nephritic syndrome, renal tubular disease, pyelonephritis, and polycystic kidney disease)
- Sugar: Negative (glucose in the urine may indicate diabetes or other endocrine disease)
- Acetone/ketones: Negative (ketones may indicate non-controlled diabetes, alcoholism, starvation)
- Bile: Negative

- Hemoglobin: Negative
- Nitrite: Negative (indicates bacteria)
- Leukocyte Esterase: Negative
- Urobilinogen: Positive

CBC

A complete blood count (CBC) is a combination of red blood cells, white blood cells, erythrocytes indices, hematocrit, differential blood cells count, and may include the platelet count. Complete blood counts are used as diagnostic exams to assist in determination of anemia, blood loss, blood values, hydration status as well as routine exams, and current physical blood status during hospitalization, exam or pre-procedural exams. Normal CBC Values: RBC: Adult Male 4.5-6.0, Female 4.0-5.0 ul. Children 3.8-5.5, and Elderly Male is 3.7-6.0 decreased levels of RBC may indicate hemorrhage, anemia, or overhydration; elevated levels may indicate dehydration, and polycythemia vera.
Hb: Adult Male is 13.5-18.0 g/dl. Female is 12.0-16.0 g/dl. Children 11.0-16.0 and infant normal is 10.0-15.0. Elderly normal is 11.0-17.0 dl/g in males, and 11.5-16.0 g/dl in females. Elevated Hb levels may indicate hemoconcentration/dehydration, and polycythemia vera. Decreased level may indicate anemia, acute blood loss, and hemodilution. Hct: Adult Male is 40-54%, Female is 36-46%, Elderly 38-42%, Children ranges are 29-40%. Decreased Hct levels indicate anemia, and folic acid deficiency. Elevated levels may indicate dehydration, and polycythemia vera. WBC: Adult 5,000 to 10,000 ul, Children 6,000-17,000, and elderly normals are 4200-1600 for the male, and 3100-10,000 for the female.

CBC components

The complete blood count (CBC) has six components. The six components of the blood count include RBC (red blood cell count), the hemoglobin (Hb/Hgb), the hematocrit (Hct), the RBC erythrocyte indices, the MCV (mean corpuscular volume), the MCHC or mean corpuscular hemoglobin, and the RBC distribution width (RDW). The white blood count and differential white blood cell count are also part of the complete blood count. The complete blood count is utilized to determine hematologic conditions, and diagnose anemia such as iron deficiency (microcytic), and aplastic, hemolytic, and pernicious or macrocytic anemia. The Complete blood count is utilized for determination of bleeding disorders, and blood cell changes.

Electrocardiography

An electrocardiogram is utilized to identify heart size, structure, function, and valvular disease; electrocardiography is a non-invasive procedure. The normal findings for an electrocardiography are: Normal heart size, normal heart structure, normal valve mechanisms, and normal chambers of the heart. Various types of electrocardiography are performed including:
- M-Mode which is used to determine motion of the heart.
- Two-dimensional echocardiography which records motion and gives a cross-sectional view of the heart.
- Spectral doppler measures amount, speed and direction of blood as it flows thru the heart.

- Color doppler determines direction of blood flow thru the heart as well as regurgitation, stenosis, holes, and abnormal prosthetic valve function.
- Transesophageal echocardiography (TEE) is utilized to obtain visual images of structures closely associated with the heart; mitral or aortic valve disorders, esophageal problems, thrombus, and dissection of the aorta.
- Contrast echocardiography assists in determining perfusion problems, ischemia and intracardiac communication.

CPK / CK

Normal values: CPK for the Adult Male: 5-35 ug/ml. Adult female: 5-25 ug/ml. CPK (creatine phosphokinase) for the child Male: 0-70 IU/l, Female: 0-50 IU/l,
Normal values for the CPK Isoenzymes:
- CPK-MM (muscle) is 94-96% (Elevated levels indicate muscular dystrophy (MD), delirium tremens (DTs), crush injury, trauma, surgery, post-surgical states, IM injections (this may indicate false positives when trying to rule out an MI, it is best to use IV meds prior to this lab), hemophilia, hypokalemia, and hypothyroidism.)
- CPK-MB (heart) is 0-6% (Elevated levels indicate acute MI/heart attack, severe angina pectoris, cardiac surgical procedures, cardiac ischemia, myocarditis, and hypokalemia.)
- CPK-BB (brain) is 0% (Elevated levels indicate CVA (stroke), subarachnoid damage, brain cancer (CA), acute brain injury, Reye's syndrome, pulmonary embolism and infarction, as well as seizures.)

Creatine kinase also termed creatine phosphokinase is an enzyme found in high levels within the heart and skeletal muscles, and in low levels within the brain. CPK becomes elevated with muscle disease, myocardial infarction (MI/heart attack), and cerebrovascular disease as well as intramuscular injections, and vigorous exercise.

Angiography and arteriography

Angiography is a term for an examination of the blood vessels. Arteriography is a term used for examination of arteries. Angiography and arteriography are used interchangeably. Angiographies assist in determination of patency of blood vessels and assist with identification of tumors and normal vascularization. The nurse needs to be aware of potential life-threatening air embolisms, and clot emboli that can occur with angiography. The angiography is used to assist with diagnosis of aneurysms, thrombosis, emboli, lesions, stenosis, plaque, and for the evaluation of renal, pulmonary and cerebral blood flow. The normal findings of an angiography are normal structure and potency (function) of blood vessels. There are various types of angiography:
- Cerebral angiography: Cerebral angiography is utilized for visualization of the carotid artery, vertebral artery, vessels of the circle of Willis and cerebral arterial branches.
- Pulmonary angiography: Pulmonary angiography is utilized to visualize the pulmonary vessels.
- Renal angiography: Renal angiography offers visualization of the renal vessels, and parenchyma.

CT scans

The computed tomography (CT) scan offers imaging of sections of the body from various angles. Computed tomography will assist in early diagnosis of disease and disease processes. The CT is approximately 100 times more sensitive than the normal x-ray. Computed tomography can be performed with or without contrast dye (media). Contrast offers enhanced views of the organs and structures being examined; an example is increased visibility of small tumors or abnormalities. The computed tomography is utilized for viewing the brain, head, chest, abdomen, pelvis, spine, and bones of the body. Computed tomography (CT) is utilized most often in determining coronary artery disease, lesions of the head, liver, and kidney. CT also assists in the diagnosis of tumors, edema, abscesses, infection, metastatic diseases, vascular disorders, stroke, and bone destruction and deformity. CT is also used to locate and identify foreign object within soft tissue.

Barium enema

A barium enema is a fluoroscopic study of the lower intestinal tract using a contrast medium. Barium sulfate suspension is the normal contrast used. A barium enema uses x-ray to examine the large intestine for detection of polyps, masses within the intestines, diverticulitis, intestinal stricture or obstruction and ulcerations within the colon. The nurse should be aware of the prep needed for a barium enema and educate the client on pre-examination preparations. Normal findings of the barium enema are normal filling of the large intestine (colon), and normal structure of the large intestine (colon).

Arthrography and arthroscopy

Arthrography is an x-ray used to examine a joint. Arthrography can be done with air, contrast media, or both; these are used to fill joint spaces for visualization of abnormalities. Arthrography will assist in detection of abnormal cartilage or ligaments. The most common joints examined using arthrographies are the knee and shoulder. Normal findings include: Normal medial meniscus, and normal bicipital sheath, joint capsule, and intact bursa. Arthroscopy is an endoscopic examination of the interior of a joint; fiberoptic examination of the interior of a joint is done with arthroscopy. Normal findings: Normal lining of the synovial membrane, membrane intact, ligaments and tendons intact with smooth, white cartilage.

Cystography

A cystography is a visualization of the bladder with use of radiopaque media. Cystography allows for visualization of not only the bladder, but the urethra, prostatic urethra, and orifices (openings) of the urethra. Cystography is a diagnostic exam used to determine renal calculi, obtain tissue biopsy of the bladder, bladder wall, urethra, or renal pelvis. A cystography will assist in determination of ruptured bladder, neurogenic bladder, fistulas or tumors. Cystography is used to remove renal stones and assist in determining causation of hematuria, and urinary tract infections (UTI). Normal findings of the cystoscopy are: normal structure of the urethra, normal structure of the bladder, normal prostatic urethra and normal urethral orifices.

Bronchoscopy

A bronchoscopy is an inspection of the interior of the tracheobronchial tree for either diagnosis, biopsy, or foreign body removal. A bronchoscopy can be used to visualize the larynx, trachea, and bronchi. With utilization of a bronchoscopy the patient may have examinations of tissue, secretion removal, or specimen collection done. Normal findings of a bronchoscopy include normal structure and normal lining of the larynx, trachea, and bronchi. The nurse is responsible for educating the client on the procedure she/he may be responsible for witnessing the consent, removal of dentures, glasses, jewelry, and contact lenses. The nurse will obtain vital signs prior to the examination/procedure. The nurse should educate the client on relaxation techniques prior to the procedure, and the mechanisms and actions of the anesthetic to be used.

Electromyography

The electromyogram is an examination of the electrical currents associated with muscle action. Electromyogram is presented in the form of a graph. Electromyography is a measurement of skeletal muscles while they are at rest and during voluntary muscle contraction. Electromyograms are used to diagnose neuromuscular disorders such as muscular dystrophy, peripheral neuropathy, and diabetic neuropathy, neuropathy related to alcoholism, myasthenia gravis, and central neuronal degeneration. The nurse should be aware of medications that have the potential to alter test results and should consult the physician related to withholding these medications. The nurse should also be aware that increased age may alter the outcome of the test. The normal findings of an electromyography are:
* At rest: Minimal electrical activity
* Voluntary Muscle Contraction: Markedly increased electrical activity.

Electroencephalography

The electroencephalography is a reading of the electropotentials within the brain. The electroencephalogram measures electrical impulses of brain cells. The electroencephalography is an assistive tool for diagnosing seizure disorders, neoplasm of the brain, cerebral vascular accident/strokes, trauma of the brain, and infectious processes of the brain and nervous system. Electroencephalogram is also used to determine brain death. Electroencephalography is also useful in diagnosis of intracranial hemorrhage, and intracranial abscess. The normal findings of an EEG are the same for the adult or child. Normal tracing and regular short waves are the expected findings of the EEG. The nurse should be aware of the potential for drugs such as sedatives, and stimulants to alter the outcome of the EEG. Alcohol will decrease the response of the EEG and the use of hairspray and normal oils within the hair can also alter responses.

Biopsy, cholecystogram, ultrasonography, and cholangiography

A biopsy is a sampling of tissue by tissue removal. Biopsy can be performed by needle aspiration, surgical procedure (excision or incision), brushing, or scraping of tissue for cells or any other mechanism of cell removal for inspection. Cholecystogram is a visualization of the gallbladder that allows for a radiographic recording of structure and function. The nurse should prepare the client by giving nothing by mouth (especially if contrast media is utilized) and administer preparatory procedures prior to the procedure. If the

- 175 -

cholecystogram is done on an outpatient basis the nurse should educate the client on preparation that should be done at home. Ultrasonography is the location and measurement or delineation of deep structures by measuring reflected high frequency ultrasonic waves to provide a two dimensional image. Cholangiography is a radiographic examination of the bile ducts. Dye is injected directly into the biliary tree to give a clear picture of the hepatic duct, cystic duct, and gallbladder.

Gastrointestinal series

A gastrointestinal series is an examination using x-ray. The gastrointestinal series uses fluoroscopy to visualize the esophagus, stomach, and small intestine. The individual will be asked to ingest oral contrast such as barium meal or meglumine diatrizoate. The contrast media is observed under fluoroscopy while it passes thru the digestive tract. The gastrointestinal series is used to determine and diagnose inflammation, ulcerations, and tumors. The gastrointestinal series is also used to detect and diagnose hiatal hernias, pyloric stenosis, gastroenteritis, gastric polyps, foreign bodies, and malabsorption of the gastrointestinal system. Esophageal varices, obstructions, and strictures are also visible using a gastrointestinal series. The normal findings of a GI (gastrointestinal) series is; Normal structure of the esophagus, stomach, small intestine, and normal peristalsis.

Pharmacological agents in a GI Series

A gastrointestinal series is an examination using x-ray. The gastrointestinal series uses fluoroscopy to visualize the esophagus, stomach, and small intestine. The individual will be asked to ingest oral contrast such as barium meal or meglumine diatrizoate. The contrast media is observed under fluoroscopy while it passes thru the digestive tract. The gastrointestinal series is used to determine and diagnose inflammation, ulcerations, and tumors. The gastrointestinal series is also used to detect and diagnose hiatal hernias, pyloric stenosis, gastroenteritis, gastric polyps, foreign bodies, and malabsorption of the gastrointestinal system. Esophageal varices, obstructions, and strictures are also visible using a gastrointestinal series. The normal findings of a GI (gastrointestinal) series is; Normal structure of the esophagus, stomach, small intestine, and normal peristalsis.

Labs for bone disease and disorders

The following are labs associated with bone disease and disorders:
- Phosphorus (P): Phosphorus is the main intracellular anion; phosphorus is combined with calcium in the body (80-85%). Phosphorus metabolizes carbohydrates, fats and maintains acid-base balance, use of vitamin B-12, and promotes muscle and nerve activity.
  Normals:
  Adult 1.7-2.6 mEq/l   Newborn 3.5-8.6 mEq/l
  Infant 4.5-6.7 mEq/l   Child 4.5-5.5 mg/dl
- Total protein: Total protein consists of albumin and globulin; total protein is significant with diseases such as collagen disorders, cancer, and infection, and water intoxication.
  Normals:
  Adult 6.0-8.0 g/dl   Newborn 4.6-7.4 g/dl
  Infant 6.0-6.7g/dl   Child 6.2-8.0g/dl

- Uric acid (serum): Uric acid is produced from purine metabolism. Elevated levels may indicate alteration in liver function, and Uric acid levels are the main diagnostic of gout (hyperuricemia)
  Normals:
  Adult Male 3.5-8.0 mg/dl   Adult Female 2.8-6.8 mg/dl

  Panic Values: >12 mg/dl
  Child: 2.5-5.5 mg/dl   Elderly: 3.5-8.5 mg/dl

Bone disorder labs

Three labs associated with bone disorders are:
- Albumin: Albumin makes up more than half of the plasma protein, and is synthesized by the liver. Albumin increases osmotic pressure resulting in edema with low levels. Decreased levels may indicate liver disease, renal disorders, severe burns and malnutrition, prolonged immobilization as with bone fractures, and protein-losing enteropathies. Elevated levels of albumin indicate dehydration, severe vomiting, and severe diarrhea. Normals for the adult are 3.5 to 5.0 g/dl; 52% to 68% of total protein. Children-- Newborn: 2.9-5.4 g/dl; Infant: 4.4-5.4 g/dl. Child: 4.0-5.8 g/dl.
- Alkaline Phosphatase (ALP): Alkaline phosphatase is produced mainly by the liver and bone; alkaline phosphatase also can come from the liver, intestine and kidney. ALP is a diagnostic tool used for the indication and diagnosis of liver and bone diseases. Cancer of the bone can be determined with use of the ALP. The ALP also indicates Paget's disease, healing fractures, osteitis deformans, multiple myeloma, and osteomalacia. Normals: Adult 42---136 U/l Child age 0-12 yrs. --- 40-115 U/l Child 13-18 yrs. --- 50-230 U/l Elderly is slightly higher than that of the adult.
- Calcium: Calcium is found most often in bones and teeth. Approximately 50% of calcium is ionized; only the ionized calcium is utilized by the body. Calcium is responsible for nerve impulses and contractility of the myocardium and skeletal muscles.

Arthritis labs

The following are labs associated with Arthritis:
- ASO (Antistreptolysin): Streptolysin is secreted by beta-hemolytic streptococcus and is capable of lysing red blood cells (RBC's). Streptolysin has the same action as antigens to stimulate the antibodies of the immune system. ASO levels that are elevated can indicate Rheumatic fever, acute glomerulonephritis and recent streptococcal infections. Adult: <100; Toddlers <160 IU/ml; Newborn similar to mother.
- ANA (Antinuclear antibodies): The ANA is a diagnostic tool for screening systemic lupus erythematosus (SLE) as well as other collagen disorders such as rheumatoid arthritis, scleroderma, leukemia, and infectious mononucleosis. Elevated---- Positive is >1:20.
- ESR (Erythrocyte sedimentation rate): ESR is the rate in which red blood cells settle in unclotted blood in millimeters per hour. Adult: Male <50 yrs. 0-15mm/hr, Female <50 yrs. 0-20mm/hr, Males >50 yrs. 0-20mm/hr, Female >50 yrs. 0-30mm/hr

- Children: Newborn 0-2mm/hr, 4-14 yrs. 0-10mm/hr
- CRP (C-reactive protein): CRP is apparent in the bloodstream within 10 hours after the onset of an inflammatory process in which tissue destruction is involved. CRP is used to monitor acute inflammatory phases of rheumatoid arthritis and rheumatic fever. *CRP will only elevate during bacterial infections and does not rise during viral infections. Adult: Not usually present   Children: Not usually present
- Rheumatoid factor (RF): Rheumatoid factor is a test utilized to measure antibodies IgM, IgG, and IgA found with rheumatoid arthritis.

Cardiac evaluation labs

AST: AST is found in heart muscle and in the liver. AST will be elevated following an MI (heart attack). With heart muscle damage the AST will peak within 24 to 48 hours and return to normal in 4 to 6 days following initial damage.
(AST: Aspartate aminotransferase)
Normal:

Adult: 8-38 U/l	Newborn: 4 times the normal adult level
Child: similar to adults	Elderly: slightly higher than adult levels

CPK: (Creatinine phosphokinase)/ CK: Creatine kinase: CPK is found in high concentration in heart and skeletal muscle and in low concentration in brain tissue. Elevated CPK is an indicator of an MI (heart attack/myocardial infarction). CK will indicate damage to the specific area of concern and will provide documentation to support or rule out disease processes.
Normals:

Adult Male 5-35 ug/ml	Adult Female 5-25 ug/ml
Newborn 65-580	
Child Male 0-70 IU/l	Child Female 0-5 IU/l

Lipid profile labs

Total Cholesterol: Total cholesterol is utilized to determine the amount of cholesterol found in the red blood cells, cell membranes, and muscles. Serum cholesterol is used to determine and detect atherosclerosis and coronary artery disease. Hypercholesterolemia causes plaque deposits in the coronary arteries and this contributes to myocardial infarction (MI).
Normal Values: Adult <200 mg/dl.
Moderate risk levels: 200-240 mg/dl.
High risk levels: >240 mg/dl

Triglycerides: Triglycerides are blood lipids formed by esterification of glycerol. Triglycerides function to provide energy for heart and skeletal muscle.
Normal Values: Adult 12-29 years; 10-140 mg/dl
30-39 years; 20-150 mg/dl
40-49 years 30-160 mg/dl
>50 years 40-190 mg/dl
Infants 5-40mg/dl
Children 5-11 years 10-135 mg/dl

Triglycerides are a major contributing factor in arterial diseases.

Coagulation studies

APTT (Activated partial thromboplastin time): APTT will reveal clotting deficiencies. APTT is more sensitive than the PT alone.
Normal Values: Adult PTT 60-70 seconds. APTT 20-35 seconds: Child is greater than that of an adult.
PT (Prothrombin Time): Normal Values: Adult 10-13 seconds. Prothrombin time measures the clotting ability of factors I, II, V, VII, and X.
INR (International Normalized Ratio): Normal Value is 2.0-3.0. INR is utilized to monitor clotting time among individuals who are taking warfarin (coumadin) therapy.
Platelet count: The platelet count is used to determine basic elements of the blood that promote coagulation (clotting). Platelets are small, and clump and stick to rough surfaces and injured sites when coagulation is needed. A decreased platelet count of <50% of the normal value will cause bleeding; this decreased platelet count places the individual at risk for hemorrhage.
Normal Values: Adult: 150,000-400,000 ul.   Child: 200,000-475,000 ul.
Factor assay: Factor assays are ordered to detect deficiencies of blood coagulation components. There are 12 factor assays and are equally important for blood clotting.

Pyelogram

Most people are familiar with x-ray images, which produce a still picture of the body's interior by passing small, highly controlled amounts of radiation through the body, and capturing the resulting shadows and reflections on film. An IVP study uses a contrast material to enhance the x-ray images. The contrast material is injected into the patient's system, and its progress through the urinary tract is then recorded on a series of quickly captured images. The exam enables the radiologist to review the anatomy and the function of the kidneys and urinary tract.

Common uses of IVP Studies
A radiologist can use an IVP study to find the cause of a wide variety of disorders, including frequent urination, blood in the urine, or pain in the side or lower back. The IVP exam can enable the radiologist to detect problems within your urinary tract resulting from kidney stones; enlarged prostate; tumors in the kidney, ureters, or urinary bladder; and other changes.

Lithotripsy

Lithotripsy is a technique used to break up stones that form in the kidney, bladder, ureters, or gallbladder. There are several ways of doing this, although the most common is extracorporeal shock wave lithotripsy. The shock waves are focused on the kidney stone and break the stone into tiny pieces, which are passed out of the body naturally during urination. While most kidney stones are treated with this type of lithotripsy, not all stones can be treated this way. Sometimes a laser is used to pulverize the stone, but when a laser is used, the doctor must use an endoscope, which is a tube introduced into the body, via the urinary tract, to get close to the stone. Extracorporeal shock wave lithotripsy is a very safe procedure with few complications.

TB testing and therapeutic management

TB Testing
Recommended procedure is Mantoux test
Uses purified protein derivative (PPD), Standard dose and administration technique
Positive reaction
>5-mm induration
>10-mm induration
>15-mm induration

Therapeutic management of TB
INH- isoniazid
Rifampin, PZA- pyrazinamide, 6 month regimen
Multi-drug resistant—streptomycin IM, Prophylaxis for high-risk pt: INH 9-12 mos

Prognosis-serious if HIV, less than 2 or adolescent

Prevention- avoid contact, BCG vaccine

Nursing considerations- contagious airborne precautions and neg pressure room, follow up.

Mental exam

This part of the examination tests the level of consciousness (alert to comatose); the degree of orientation (notation x 4: knowledge of (1) time, (2) place, (3) person and (4) purpose of visit); the use of language (fluency of spontaneous speech; naming objects such as a pen or watch; repetition of rhymes, e.g., "Mary had a little lamb"; comprehension of verbal commands); and short term memory (ask the patient to recall three items, such as, rose, umbrella, truck, minutes after hearing the words). Abnormalities in mental state indicate damage above the level of the foramen magnum, i.e., in the brain.

Level of consciousness

Level of consciousness is the most important aspect of the neurologic exam. Deterioration of LOC is usually the first neurologic change to be noted. One component of mental status and is usually only component that is assessed in serial assessments done in ICU.

Components of consciousness:
- Arousal: (Alertness) The lowest level of consciousness and centers on the patient's ability to respond to verbal or noxious stimuli in an appropriate manner.
- Awareness: (Awareness) Higher level function and addresses the patient's orientation to person place and time.

Categories of consciousness:
- Alert
- Lethargic
- Obtunded
- Stuporous
- Comatose

Glasgow Coma Scale

Eye opening:
- Spontaneous 4
- To voice 3
- To pain 2
- None 1

Verbal response:
- Oriented 5
- Confused 4
- Inappropriate words 3
- Incomprehensible words 2
- None 1

Motor response:
- Obeys commands 6
- Localizes pain 5
- Withdraws from pain 4
- Flexion (decorticate) 3
- Extension (decerebrate) 2
- None 1

Scoring guide:
- Minimum score 3
- Maximum score 15
- Mild brain injury 13 or higher
- Moderate brain injury 9 to 12
- Severe brain injury 8 or lower

Brudzinski's Sign and Kernig's Sign

Brudzinski's Sign: When the neck is flexed, flexion of the knees also occurs (present in meningeal irritation). Flexion of the neck is passive.

Kernig's Sign: Flexion of the knee with the lower extremity in a "raised position" that causes pain Note: In cases of a herniated lumbosacral disk, straight leg raising with flexion of the hip may be limited on the affected side.

Decorticate and decerebrate positioning

Decorticate (flexion) posturing
The patient will have the following: flexion of the head and trunk, adduction and internal rotation of the arms, pronation and flexion of the forearm, flexion of the wrists and fingers, flexion of the hips, knees, ankles, and toes, internal rotation of the legs, and inversion of the feet.

Decerebrate (extension) posturing

The patient will have the following: extension and internal rotation of all four extremities and may also show extension of the body and head (opisthotonus).
Decerebrate posturing indicates a lesion of the midbrain or lower. It is also associated with a mortality rate of 70%.

Deep tendon reflexes

Reflexes are graded 0 to 4, where 0 is absent, 1 is reduced, 2 is normal, 3 is increased, and 4 is clonus. Reflexes are tested over the biceps, triceps, brachioradialis, quadriceps, and Achilles tendons. Reflexes graded 0 and 1 indicate lower motor neuron damage (i.e., damage to anterior horn cell, anterior nerve root, peripheral nerve, or neuromuscular junction of muscle). Reflexes graded 3 and 4 indicate an upper motor neuron damage (i.e., in the cerebrum, brain stem or spinal cord).

Romberg's test

Romberg's test is a simple bedside sensitive clinical test that pinpoints to sensory ataxia as the cause in a patient presenting with postural imbalance. It must be carried out in all patients presenting with dizziness, imbalance, and falls. Romberg's test is a commonly performed test during the neurological examination to evaluate the integrity of dorsal columns of the spinal cord. Early detection of reversible causes is desirable as they may be remediable and their treatment can prevent permanent dysfunction and disability. Cerebella damage is indicated by a + Romberg exam.

Secondary prevention and nutrition

With secondary prevention the individual is attempting to identify disease processes in the earliest stages; with early detection of disease or illness the outcome will be improved as opposed to identification of the disease or illness in the later stages. Early indications of dietary deficiencies may prevent disease, illness, long-term or chronic illness, as well as assist in the determination of treatments, and with modifications to promote health. With early identification of dietary insufficiencies severity of disease may be reduced with diet modifications. An example of secondary prevention with regard to nutritional intake would be the reduction of dietary sodium to decrease blood pressure therefore reducing the risk of coronary artery disease and cerebral vascular accidents.

Amniocentesis

Removal of some fluid surrounding the fetus for analysis. Fetus location is identified by US prior to the procedure. Results may take a month. Used to check for:
- Spina bifida
- Rh compatibility
- Immature lungs
- Down syndrome

Surgical wound infections

Surgical wound infections typically occur approximately the fifth postoperative day. There may be initial symptoms present during the first thirty-six to forty-eight hours following a surgical procedure. Causative agents of surgical wound infections include, but are not limited to Staphylococcus aureus, Escherichia coli, Pseudomonas aeruginosa, Proteus vulgaris, and Aerobacter aerogenes. Assessment of wound infections includes temperature, pulse, respirations, and blood pressure. Observe the wound for edema, erythema, drainage (document color, amount and odor), tenderness, pain (document pain level), and appearance of wound site. Wound cultures should be taken prior to antibiotic therapy to ensure proper treatment is given. Administer antibiotics and antipyretics as ordered. Monitor for systemic effects. Apply and change dressings as ordered (always document amount, color and odor of drainage on dressing).

TURP procedure

Transurethral resection of the prostate (TURP) is the most common operation for BPH. A long thin instrument called a resectoscope is passed into the urethra. With a light source and lens on the end it acts as a telescope, allowing the surgeon to view the prostate either directly or on a video monitor. A precisely controlled electric current, applied by a loop of wire at the end of the resectoscope, is used to shave off sections of the enlarged prostate. TURP is an effective procedure with over 90% of men reporting an improvement after the operation. However, as with any surgical procedure there is a risk of side-effects and complications. A common side-effect of this procedure is retrograde ejaculation.

Important terms

- Emergency - Must be done immediately to save the client's life. Ex: appendectomy, repair of traumatic amputation, internal bleeding.
- Diagnostic - Surgical exploration, Ex: Lap, biopsy.
- Ablative - Excision or removal of diseased body part, ex: amputation, appendectomy, debridement of necrotic tissue, cholecystectomy, colostomy.
- Palliative - Relieves or reduces symptoms, pain, will not cure: Ex: colostomy, ca, debridement.
- Reconstructive - Restores function or appearance of tissue. Ex: scar revision, ORIF.
- Transplant - Replaces failing organs. Ex: kidney, heart, lung, liver, cornea.
- Constructive - Restores function lost or reduced from congenital deformities. Ex: cleft palate and lip, Atrial septal defects repair.
- Cosmetic/plastic - Improves appearance of client. Ex: facelift, Rhinoplasty, Blepharoplasty
- Inpatient surgery - After surgery pt. stays in hospital for at least 24hrs.
- Outpatient surgery - (Ambulatory/same day surgery) After procedure client is released following recovery from anesthesia.
- Major - Organs are altered, higher risk surgery, extensive reconstruction. Ex: CAB, colon resection, lung resection.
- Minor - Minimal alterations of organs, minimal risks. Ex: cataract, tooth, skin graft.
- Elective - Client's choice, not always necessary, palliative in nature. Ex: bunionectomy, hernia repair, plastic surgery.
- Urgent - Necessary for client's health, may prevent additional problems. Ex: CABG, tumor removal, cholecystectomy for stones.
- Tympanic percussion - Lung is hyperexpanded with air as in asthma, emphysema, chronic bronchitis and cystic fibrosis
- Dull percussion - Lung filled with fluid , pus, pleural effusion

- Decreased breath sounds - Over obstructed areas (cancer), or decreased lung tissues (emphysema) or increased air
- Increased breath sounds - Lung tissues density increased (pneumonia)
- Wheezes - Found where bronchi are narrowed (asthma, chronic bronchitis, cystic fibrosis, localized tumor)

Physiological Adaptation

Pathophysiology

Patho is a Greek term that means to suffer. Pathophysiology is the study of suffering caused by abnormalities and disease. Pathophysiology is a mechanism to learn and understand categorization of disease, and disease recognition. Pathophysiology is learning the different diseases, disease processes, and causative factors for disease. Pathology explains in detail the clinical manifestations of disease, disease interactions, and signs and symptoms of disease. Pathology teaches the interactive mechanisms of organisms as they affect the body and cause disease. Pathophysiology teaches the cellular level changes of disease, and disease processes from time of organism invasion to presenting signs and symptoms.

Phagocytosis

Phagocytosis is carried out by polymorphonuclear leucocytes (mainly on pyogenic bacteria) and macrophages (mainly on bacteria, viruses and protozoa capable of intracellular life). There are many different forms of macrophages which carry out phagocytosis – Kupffer cells in the liver, alveolar macrophages, brain microglia, osteoclasts, mesangial glomerular cells, etc. Complement facilitates phagocytosis as adherence reactions activate phagocytic cells to engulf and destroy microbes. Microbes bind to the phagocyte receptors, a process that can be aided by opsonins – factors that bind to both the microbes and the phagocytic cells to facilitate uptake. Membrane protrusions called pseudopodia form around the microbes, which are ingested to form a phagosome. The phagosome fuses with lysosomes containing enzymes and granules which kill and digest the microbe. The degradation products are then released from the phagocyte.

Cytokines

IL-1 Primarily stimulate of fever response. Helps activate B and T cells. Produced by macrophages.
IL-2 Aids in the development of Cytotoxic T cells and helper cells. Produced by helper T cells.
IL-3 Aids in the development of bone marrow stem cells. Produced by T-cells.
IL-4 Aids in the growth of B cells. Produced by helper T-cells. Aids in the production of IgG and IgE
IL-5 Promotes the growth of eosinophils. Produced by helper T-cells. Also promotes IgA production.
IL-8 Neutrophil factor
TNF-a Promotes the activation of neutrophils and is produced by macrophages.
TNF-b Produced by T lymphocytes and encourages the activation of neutrophils
g-interferon (Activates macrophages and is produced by helper T cells.)

Defense against bacterial infection

The first line of defense is part of the innate (primary) immune response, which is a non-specific form of defense against infection. The skin provides a barrier to entry of bacteria. Fatty acids, lactic acids of sweat and sebaceous secretions also contribute to the first line of defense. The mucous lining of the respiratory and GI tracts traps bacteria and the trapped particles are removed by coughing and sneezing, aided by ciliated epithelial cells. Tears, saliva and urine contain enzymes and acids that kill bacteria. Normal bacterial flora in humans defend against infectious bacteria by competitive inhibition – competing for nutrients, space to grow, etc.

Chickenpox

Chickenpox is caused by a virus called varicella zoster. Incubation 11-21 days. The blisters are small and sit on an area of red skin that can be anywhere from the size of a pencil eraser to the size of a dime. Fever may be noted. Patient must be kept in isolation. If the patient scratches the lesions they will spread. Chickenpox may start out seeming like a cold: You might have a runny or stuffy nose, sneezing, and a cough. But 1 to 2 days later, the rash begins, often in bunches of spots on the chest and face. From there it can spread out quickly over the entire body - sometimes the rash is even in a person's ears and mouth. Chickenpox is very contagious.

Innate and acquired immunity

Innate immunity is also called natural immunity. Innate immunity consists of all the immune defenses that lack immunologic memory. Innate immunity is acquired at birth and all humans have a resistance to certain types of organisms. Acquired immunity includes active acquired immunity and passive acquired immunity. Acquired immunity is gained post birth as a result of an immune response. Active or passive immunity occurs related to the stimulation process and whether the response is activated by a donor or by the host. Active acquired immunity is produced by a host after exposure either from an antigen or immunization. Passive acquired immunity is produced when preformed antibodies or T lymphocytes are transferred to the individual.

Humoral and cell mediated immunity

Humoral immunity is associated with circulating antibodies, and B-cells are the primary source of humoral immunity. The primary immunocyte of the immune response is the lymphocyte. The process of humoral immunity involves the lymphocyte migration through lymphatic system and blood vessels. As lymphocytes make their way through the lymph they become B-cells. B-cells that encounter antigens are stimulated to mature into plasma cells that produce antibodies by the process of referred clonal selection.

Immunoglobulins

Immunoglobulins are antibodies that are produced from serum glycoprotein in plasma cells in response to an immunogen. Immunoglobulins are receptors on the surfaces of mature B cells. Immunoglobulins have specific sensitivity to antigens. There are five molecular classes of immunoglobulin. The five classes of immunoglobulin are IgG, IgA, IgM, IgE, and IgD:
- IgG is responsible for most antibody functions such as precipitation, agglutination, and complement activation.
- IgA is primarily responsible for normal body secretions. The IgA antibodies protect the body from infectious enzymes and secretions.
- IgM is the largest immunoglobulin with ten antigenic binding sites; only 5 of which are functional. IgM is the first antibody produced during the initial primary response to an antigen.

- IgD is found in low concentrations in the blood, and the function is unknown.
- IgE is the least concentrated immunoglobulin in circulation. IgE is the primary antibody with allergic reactions.

Antigens and immunogens

Antigens are molecules or molecular complexes that react with preformed components of the immune system such as lymphocytes and antibodies. Antigenicity is the molecules innate capacity to react with those preformed components. Self-antigens are produced within the body and nonself antigens are foreign to the body or not formed by the body. Immunogen is an antigen that has the capacity to initiate an immune response. Immunogens and antigens result in stimulation of an immune response by the body. The body responds with antibodies or immune cells when activated to protect the body from invasion of bacteria, viruses and/or any other inflammatory process, illness or injury.

Hypomagnesemia

Secreting too much aldosterone (the hormone that regulates the body's salt-fluid balance), ADH (a hormone that inhibits urine production), or thyroid hormone can cause hypomagnesemia. Severe magnesium deficiency can cause seizures, especially in children. People who have hypomagnesemia usually experience loss of weight and appetite, bloating, and muscle pain, and they pass stools that have a high fat content. Also, they may be listless, disoriented, confused, and very irritable. Other symptoms of hypomagnesemia are: Nausea, Vomiting, Muscle weakness, Tremor, Irregular heartbeat, Delusions and hallucinations, Leg and foot cramps. Hypermagnesemia is most common in patients whose kidneys cannot excrete the magnesium they derive from food or take as medication. Patients may feel flushed and drowsy, perspire heavily, and have diarrhea. Breathing becomes shallow, reflexes diminish, and the patient becomes unresponsive. Muscle weakness and hallucinations are common. The patient's heart beat slows dramatically and blood pressure plummets. Oral magnesium supplements or injections are usually prescribed to correct mild magnesium deficiency. Intravenous furosemide (Lasix) or ethacrynic acid (Edecrin) can increase magnesium excretion in patients who get enough fluids and whose kidneys are functioning properly.

Babinski's reflex

Common causes of Babinski's reflex are:
- Generalized tonic-clonic seizure (there may be a temporary Babinski's reflex for a short time after a seizure)
- Amyotrophic lateral sclerosis, Brain tumor (if it occurs in the corticospinal tract or the cerebellum), Familial periodic paralysis, Friedreich's ataxia, Head injury, Hepatic encephalopathy, Meningitis, Multiple sclerosis, Pernicious anemia
- Poliomyelitis (some forms), Rabies, Spinal cord injury, Spinal cord tumor, Stroke, Syringomyelia, Tuberculosis (when it affects the spine)

Coma, persistent vegetative state, and brain death

Coma is a state of unconsciousness in which both wakefulness and awareness or absent. The patient cannot be aroused and does not display any purposeful reactions to noxious stimuli. The coma state is really a continuum from light to deep and patients can fall anywhere on the continuum regarding their level of reactions. In a persistent vegetative state, wakefulness is present but awareness is absent. Sleep wake cycles and hypothalamic and brain stem functions are present but they are not aware of self or environment due to lack of cerebral function. Brain death is the complete, irreversible cessation of function of the entire brain and brain stem. Spinal reflexes may or may not be present. When brain death occurs the patient is dead regardless of the presence of a heartbeat, or mechanical ventilator assisted respirations.

Hyperkalemia and hypokalemia

At resting membrane, concentration of K in the cell is very high, and in the extra-cellular fluid it is slow. There is a passive flow of K out of the cell.
Hyperkalemia, extracellular K is high - prevent the passive flow - more K in the cell – depolarization
Arrhythmias, Muscle Weakness, Cramps
Hypokalemia, extracellular is slow - stimulate passive flow - more K goes out of cell - hyperpolarization
Decreased reflexes, Muscle Weakness, CNS depression

Risk factors for developing phantom pain

The following have been associated with an increased risk of developing phantom pain:
- Poorly controlled pre-amputation pain
- Persisting stump pain afterwards
- Bilateral amputations (both legs)
- Lower limb more than upper limb amputations
- Chronic Sciatica - There is a weak suggestion that phantom pain may occur more commonly in those who have had chronic sciatica in the leg prior to amputation. In some patients MRI scanning of the lumbar spine reveals a disc prolapse large enough to be causing lower lumbar nerve root irritation and referred pain to the leg.

5 P's of compartment syndrome

Compartment syndrome is excessively high pressure in a compartment of the body (most often the legs, arm, or abdomen) that usually results from blood or edema filling the area and then impeding blood flow. It is a medical emergency. There are the 5 P's associated with the development of compartment syndrome:
- Paraesthesia
- Pain
- Paralysis
- Pallor
- Pulselessness.

Arterial occlusions

Acute arterial occlusions happen when blood flow to an extremity (most often the leg) is suddenly stopped. It occurs most often in patients with a history of peripheral artery disease or in the post-operative period after many cardiovascular surgeries. It is an emergent condition that needs to be recognized immediately. The 4 P's are helpful to remember the signs of arterial occlusion.

- Pain
- Pulselessness or absent pulse
- Pallor
- Paresthesia

Common gastrointestinal (GI) problems

(GERD) is a common term utilized today to describe the return of gastric (stomach) content into the esophagus. GERD is characterized by a cough, burning sensation in the stomach, chest, red, sore throat, and pain in the gastric region. Often patients with GERD will experience the presence of gastric content returning into the oral cavity (mouth) upon lying down at night. Common causes of GERD include caffeine, consuming large meals before bed, over eating, spicy or fatty foods, binding clothing, acidic drinks, lack of mastication with meal consumption, and constipation. Emesis (vomiting) is another common GI problem as well as a protective mechanism of the body. Emesis is the opposite action of normal peristalsis; food is not moved downward in the GI tract, instead it is propelled upward via the esophagus into the oral cavity and exits the mouth. The most common causes of emesis production include altered equilibrium, gluttony, viral or bacterial illness, and purposeful production for weight control as with bulimia or anorexia nervosa. Flatulence (intestinal gas) or flatus is a natural occurrence in the gastrointestinal tract. Intestinal gas is formed by bacteria and/or carbohydrates that have been ingested without proper mastication and have fermented in the GI tract. Individuals who are unable to tolerate or alter the mechanical structure of lactose have an increased production of gas in the intestinal tract as well.

Acute respiratory failure

Acute respiratory failure is characterized by an altered level of consciousness which may present as altered cognition or the individual may be totally unresponsive. Other signs and symptoms include, but are not limited to nasal flaring, sweating, wheezing, visualization of the intercostal spaces retracting, and use of accessory muscles for respiration. Acute respiratory failure occurs suddenly (acute) with a sharp decrease or cease in respirations. With acute respiratory failure there is little or no air to gas exchange related to constricted bronchi or impediment within the lungs. Clients who suffer acute respiratory failure require a diet plan that limits the amount of carbon dioxide production. Respiratory diets often contain high kilocalories, high protein, moderate or high fats along with increased amounts of carbohydrates. This diet will allow for energy production to aid with healing and assist with the malnutrition that almost always accompanies acute respiratory failure.

Endometriosis

Endometriosis: abnormal tissue growth outside the uterus.

Symptoms:
- Spotting
- Infertility
- LBP
- Periods (painful)
- Sexual intercourse painful

Tests:
- Pelvic US
- Laparoscopy
- Pelvic exam

Treatment:
- Progesterone treatment
- Pain management
- Surgery
- Hormone treatment
- Synarel treatment

Endometriosis is the occurrence of endometrial tissue in areas other than the uterine cavity (ectopic/out of place or out of proper position). Endometriosis may be diagnosed with endometrial tissue growth on the peritoneal surfaces, fallopian tubes, lymph nodes, ovaries or bowels. Endometriosis may also be characterized by an ectopic growth of endometrial tissue in more than one of these sites as well. Signs and symptoms associated with endometriosis include dyspareunia (painful intercourse), dysmenorrhea, dyschezia (difficult production of stool), pelvic pain (acute or chronic), premenstrual spotting, and spontaneous abortion. Endometriosis can occur in a woman at any age.

Hirsutism

Hirsutism: development of dark areas of hair in women that are uncommon.

Causes:
- Cushing's syndrome
- Congenital adrenal hyperplasia
- Hyperthecosis
- PCOS
- High Androgen levels
- Certain medications

Treatment:
- Laser treatment
- Birth control medications
- Electrolysis
- Bleaching

Cervicitis

Cervicitis: infection, foreign bodies of chemicals that cause inflammation of the cervix.

Symptoms:
- Pain with intercourse
- Vaginal discharge
- Pelvic pain
- Vaginal pain

Tests:
- Pelvic examination
- STD tests
- Pap smear

Treatment:
- Laser therapy
- Antibiotics/antifungals
- Cryosurgery

Sheehan's syndrome

Sheehan's syndrome: hypopituitarism caused by uterine hemorrhage during childbirth. The pituitary gland is unable to function due to blood loss.

Symptoms:
- Amenorrhea
- Fatigue
- Unable to breast-feed baby
- Anxiety
- Decreased BP
- Hair loss

Tests:
- CT scan of Pituitary gland
- Check pituitary hormone levels

Treatment: Hormone therapy

Pelvic inflammatory disease

Pelvic inflammatory disease: infection of the fallopian tubes, uterus or ovaries caused by STD's in the majority of cases.

Symptoms:
- Vaginal discharge
- Fever
- Pain with intercourse

- Fever
- Nausea
- Urination painful
- LBP
- No menstruation

Tests:
- Pelvic exam
- Laparoscopy
- ESR
- WBC count
- Pregnancy test
- Cultures for infection

Treatment:
- Antibiotics
- Surgery

Toxic shock syndrome

Toxic shock syndrome: infection of (S. aureus) that causes organ disorders and shock.

Symptoms:
- Seizures
- Headaches
- Hypotension
- Fatigue
- Multiple organ involvement
- Fever
- Nausea
- Vomiting

Tests:
- Check BP
- Multiple organ involvement

Treatment:
- Dialysis- if kidneys fail
- BP medications
- IV fluids
- Antibiotics

Monitor the patient for:
- Kidney failure
- Liver failure
- Extreme shock
- Heart failure

Diabetes

The National Institutes of Health (NIH) recognizes the following as classifications of diabetes:

- Diabetes Mellitus (DM): Diabetes Mellitus is an umbrella term that includes Type I diabetes or Insulin Dependent Diabetes, Type II or Non-Insulin Dependent Diabetes, nonobese is a non-insulin dependent form of diabetes, and obese non-insulin dependent diabetes.
- Impaired Glucose Tolerance (IGT): Impaired glucose tolerance occurs when there is an increased amount of circulating blood glucose after consuming an increased amount of carbohydrates.
- Gestational Diabetes Mellitus (GD): Gestational diabetes is a form of diabetes mellitus that occurs during pregnancy characterized by the pregnant women's intolerance of carbohydrates.

Diabetes mellitus (DM)

Diabetes Mellitus (DM) results from the lack of insulin production by the pancreas; with DM insulin can be produced in decreased amounts or is not produced at all. Carbohydrate use is impaired, while lipid and protein use is enhanced. Diabetes is diagnosed when blood glucose levels are equal to or greater than 126 mg/dl on two separate occasions, with glucose tolerance testing, or with a glycosylated hemoglobin/HgbA1c levels. Clinical note: HgbA1c levels are drawn only every 90 days as the red blood cells replenish themselves. HgbA1c is a measurement of the blood glucose levels over the past 3 month period. Diabetes Mellitus is a chronic condition that can be controlled with diet, exercise, education, and medication.

Type I diabetes mellitus

Diabetes Mellitus - literally this means the overproduction of a sweet urine. Type I, a.k.a. Insulin Dependent Diabetes Mellitus, IDDM. (Formerly called childhood onset diabetes because typically it surfaces early in life, before the age of 30). In these individuals the beta cells of the Islets of Langerhans have suffered damage, usually due to autoimmunity, childhood disease, exposure to toxins, or congenital damage. As a result the pancreas produces inadequate amounts of insulin, sometimes none. Because of this the individual is unable to maintain normal plasma glucose concentration, and is unable to uptake and use glucose in metabolism. Treatment is by means of insulin administration, either by injection or orally depending on the individual.

Complications include:

- Hypoglycemia from overdose of insulin - this results in weakness, sometimes fainting, and, in the extreme, coma, all reversible with administration of glucose.
- Ketoacidosis from fat metabolism when insulin is under-administered. This complication can be life threatening.
- Hyperglycemia when insulin administration is imprecise. Hyperglycemia damages cells and tissues.

Diabetes type 1 is also known as juvenile diabetes and characteristically occurs at an early age (normally diagnosed prior to age 25) with abrupt onset of symptoms. The pancreas has ceased to produce insulin in type 1 diabetes. Beta cells are destroyed in the type one diabetic patient as the result of autoimmune dysfunction. The actual cause of Type I diabetes is unknown, although it has been linked to genetic predisposition, environment, and viral organisms. Type I diabetic patients are at a high risk of developing atherosclerosis at an accelerated rate, neuropathy, retinopathy, and nephropathy. Symptoms of Type I diabetes include polyuria, polyphagia, polydipsia, anorexia may be present, weight loss, fatigue, lethargy, muscle cramps, irritability, and vision changes. Other symptoms of type 1 diabetes include emotional lability, altered thought processes that affect performance, headache, and anxiety, and chest pain, shortness of breath (SOB), nausea, diarrhea, and constipation.

Type II diabetes mellitus

Type II - Non Insulin Dependent Diabetes Mellitus, NIDDM. (Formerly adult onset diabetes because it tends to show up after the age of 30, usually around middle age). This type is caused by insulin-resistant receptors on the target cells. Insulin resistance can be the result of:

- Abnormal insulin - this might result from mutation to the beta cells.
- Insulin antagonists - this can be the result of adaptation to hypersecretion of insulin.
- Receptor defect - this can be:
  - The result of an inherited mutation.
  - Due to abnormal or deficient receptor proteins. This is the result of adaptation to hypersecretion of insulin.

Diabetes type II is characterized by insulin resistance in the peripheral tissues along with a decreased production of insulin by the beta cells of the pancreas. When insulin in the pancreas is not performing to regulate carbohydrate metabolism the normal rise in insulin production does not occur allowing blood glucose levels to concentrate in the blood stream causing elevated blood glucose (sugar) levels. NIDDM usually occurs in those ages 40 and over and those who suffer from obesity and who are overweight. Diabetes mellitus type II causes the same systemic effects as type I diabetes, neuropathy, nephropathy, retinopathy and increased rates of atherosclerosis leading to cardiovascular disease. Symptoms of NIDDM include polyuria, polydipsia, polyphagia, weight loss, weakness, fatigue, increased rates of infection, and increased healing time.

Treatment

Gain control of the blood glucose is the first goal of treatment; desired range is 70-110 mg/dl. Routine follow-up visits. Home glucose monitoring should be done before every meal and at bedtime and at any time the individual feels they have an elevated or decreased blood glucose level. Diet education should be given that includes following a diet that consists of 10-20% of the calories coming from protein; < 10% of the caloric intake coming from saturated and non-saturated fats, with the remainder of the diet consisting of calories from monounsaturated fat and carbohydrates. Sugar is not prohibited but should be limited and monitored for the effects on the blood glucose post-prandially.

The following phrases can help you quickly identify hyper and hypoglycemia:
Hot and dry: sugar high/hyperglycermia
Cold and clammy: need some candy/hypoglycemia

Diabetic Ketoacidosis

Diabetic Ketoacidosis can be fatal and should be dealt with in a rapid and responsible manner. With diabetic ketoacidosis the body does not have an adequate supply of insulin to meet the demand for the amount on nutrient intake that is present. Ketones are present with diabetic ketoacidosis; the body is utilizing fatty acids for energy thus producing an abnormal amount of ketones (ketosis). With ketoacidosis the glucose level is elevated and the patient is suffering life-threatening hyperglycemia. Symptoms include Kussmaul' respirations; this is a respiratory rate that is deep and shallow. The individual with DKA will have fruity odor to the breath, dry mucous membranes related to the dehydration occurring within the cells, anorexia or polyphagia, polydipsia, hypotension, hypothermia, confusion, tachycardia, tachypnea, hypothermia, weakness, malaise, lethargy, nausea, and/or vomiting. Patients suffering DKA will need immediate fluids (1000ml the first hour is standard) and intravenous insulin, blood glucose monitoring.

PIG FUME is a helpful mnemonic to assist you to remember the treatment for Diabetic Ketoacidosis (DKA).

Potassium
Insulin
Glucose: once serum level drops
Fluids (Crystalloids)
Urea (Continue to monitor)
Monitor creatinine and cath as needed
Evaluate for NGT or OGT

Hypoglycemia

Hypoglycemia is a blood glucose level that falls below the established normal for the client; frequently noted as <70 mg/dl. Hypoglycemic symptoms include headache, visual disturbances, confusion, personality changes, emotional instability, convulsions, and if left untreated coma will proceed. Other symptoms of hypoglycemia include diaphoresis, tremors, and nervousness. Reactive hypoglycemia takes place 2-3 hours post prandially (after food consumption) and may be caused by drugs or specific nutrients. Spontaneous hypoglycemia occurs with conditions of the pituitary and adrenal glands. Hypoglycemia is a hormonal reaction of the endocrine and metabolic systems. Causes of hypoglycemia include the intake of increased amounts of carbohydrate and then dumping syndrome occurring, hyperinsulinemia, exercise, illness, pregnancy, malnutrition, and sepsis.

Pathology of HIV and AIDS

H - Human: because this virus can only infect human beings.
I - Immuno-deficiency: because the effect of the virus is to create a deficiency, a failure to work properly, within the body's immune system.
V - Virus: because this organism is a virus, which means one of its characteristics is that it is incapable of reproducing by itself. It reproduces by taking over the machinery of the human cell.

Some people newly infected with HIV will experience some "flu-like" symptoms. These symptoms, which usually last no more than a few days, might include fevers, chills, night sweats and rashes (not cold-like symptoms). Other people either do not experience "acute infection," or have symptoms so mild that they may not notice them. When immune system damage is more severe, people may experience opportunistic infections (called opportunistic because they are caused by organisms which cannot induce disease in people with normal immune systems, but take the "opportunity" to flourish in people with HIV).

CHF

CHF:
- Inability of heart to pump adequate amt of blood to systemic circulation at nl filling pressure to meet metabolic demands
- Volume overload, pressure overload, decreased contractility, high cardiac output demands

Generally results from cardiac defects that cause increased volume or increased pressure on ventricles (coarctation of aorta, myocardial failure, disease of organs especially lungs) Eventually R side has trouble pumping blood forward to lungs, dilates, hypertrophies, and signs of R sided failure are seen.

Cor pulmonale=CHF from obstructive lung disease (CF or bronchopulmonary dysplasia)

Compensatory Mechanisms (Cardiac reserve)- Hypertrophy and dilation of cardiac muscle and stimulation of SNS

Multiple sclerosis

An unpredictable disease of the central nervous system, multiple sclerosis (MS) can range from relatively benign to somewhat disabling to devastating, as communication between the brain and other parts of the body is disrupted. In the case of MS, it is the nerve-insulating myelin that comes under assault. Such assaults may be linked to an unknown environmental trigger, perhaps a virus. Most people experience their first symptoms of MS between the ages of 20 and 40; the initial symptom of MS is often blurred or double vision, red-green color distortion, or even blindness in one eye. Most people with MS also exhibit paresthesias, transitory abnormal sensory feelings such as numbness, prickling, or "pins and needles" sensations. Some may also experience pain. Speech impediments, tremors, and dizziness are other frequent complaints. Occasionally, people with MS have hearing loss. Approximately half of all people with MS experience cognitive impairments such as difficulties with concentration, attention, memory, and poor judgment, but such symptoms are usually mild and are frequently overlooked. Depression is another common feature of MS.

Bell's palsy

Bell's palsy is a form of temporary facial paralysis resulting from damage or trauma to one of the two facial nerves. Symptoms of Bell's palsy usually begin suddenly and reach their peak within 48 hours. Symptoms range in severity from mild weakness to total paralysis and may include twitching, weakness, or paralysis, drooping eyelid or corner of the mouth, drooling, dry eye or mouth, impairment of taste, and excessive tearing in the eye. There is no cure or standard course of treatment for Bell's palsy. The most important factor in treatment is to eliminate the source of the nerve damage. The prognosis for individuals with Bell's palsy is generally very good. The extent of nerve damage determines the extent of recovery. With or without treatment, most individuals begin to get better within 2 weeks after the initial onset of symptoms and recover completely within 3 to 6 months.

Hyperthermia

Regardless of extreme weather conditions, the healthy human body keeps a steady temperature of 98.6 F (37 C). In hot weather, or during vigorous activity, the body perspires. As this perspiration evaporates from the skin, the body is cooled. If challenged by long periods of intense heat, the body may lose its ability to respond efficiently. When this occurs, a person can experience hyperthermia.

Hyperthermia prevention:
- Drink plenty of liquids, even if not thirsty.
- Dress in light-weight, light-colored, loose-fitting clothing.
- Avoid the mid-day heat and do not engage in vigorous activity during the hottest part of the day (noon - 4 p.m.).
- Wear a hat or use an umbrella for shade.
- If possible, use air conditioners liberally or try to visit air-conditioned places such as libraries, shopping malls, and theaters. For an air conditioner to be beneficial it should be set below 80 F.
- If not used to the heat, get accustomed to it slowly by exposing yourself to it briefly at first and increasing the time little by little.
- Avoid hot, heavy meals. Do a minimum of cooking and use an oven only when absolutely necessary.

Delirium tremens

Delirium tremens (DT) is a potentially fatal form of ethanol (alcohol) withdrawal. Symptoms may begin a few hours after the cessation of ethanol, but may not peak until 48-72 hours. Emergency physicians must recognize that the presenting symptoms may not be severe and identify those at risk for developing DT. DT is caused by the direct effect that ethanol has on the benzodiazepine-GABAa-chloride receptor complex. Persistent effects of ethanol lead to the down-regulation of the receptor complex. When ethanol is withdrawn, a functional decrease in the inhibitory neurotransmitter GABA is seen. This results in an unopposed increase in sympathetic activity with a resultant increase in plasma and urinary catecholamines. Ethanol withdrawal seizures typically occur 6-48 hours after the last drink. DT usually begins 24-72 hours after cessation or reduction of ethanol use.

Symptoms may include the following:
Tremors, Irritability, Insomnia, Nausea/vomiting (frequently secondary to gastritis or pancreatitis), Hallucinations (auditory, visual, or olfactory), Confusion, Delusions, Severe agitation, Seizures - Begin 6-48 hours after the last drink.

MODS

Multiple organ dysfunction syndrome (MODS) results from SIRS and is the failure of several interdependent organ systems. MODS is the major cause of death of patients in the critical care units. The progressive physiologic failure of two or more separate organ systems. Approximately 7 to 15% of critically ill patients experience dysfunction of at least two organ systems. Outcome is directly related to the number of organs that failure. The failure of three or more organs is associated with a 90 to 95 % mortality rate.

Clinical Course of Secondary MODS: Organ failure may occur in a progressive pattern or they may fail simultaneously.
The lungs are generally the first organ and the most common organ to be affected. Persistent hypermetabolism occurs after the initial insult and may last 14-21 days and is the result of sustained systemic inflammation.
The persistent hypermetabolism causes autocatabolism. Decrease in lean body mass, severe weight loss, increased CO and VO2, alterations in nutrient metabolism. GI, hepatic, and immunologic dysfunction may occur concurrently. Cardiovascular instability and central nervous system dysfunction may be present.

Heat cramps, heat exhaustion, and heat stroke

Heat cramps are painful muscle spasms in the abdomen, arms, or legs following strenuous activity. The skin is usually moist and cool and the pulse is normal or slightly raised. Body temperature is mostly normal. Heat cramps often are caused by a lack of salt in the body, but salt replacement should not be considered without advice from a physician. Heat exhaustion is a warning that the body is getting too hot. The person may be thirsty, giddy, weak, uncoordinated, nauseous, and sweating profusely. The body temperature is usually normal and the pulse is normal or raised. The skin is cold and clammy. Although heat exhaustion often is caused by the body's loss of water and salt, salt supplements should only be taken with advice from a doctor. Heat stroke can be LIFE-THREATENING! Victims of heat stroke almost always die so immediate medical attention is essential when problems first begin. A person with heat stroke has a body temperature above 104 F. Other symptoms may include confusion, combativeness, bizarre behavior, faintness, staggering, strong rapid pulse, dry flushed skin, lack of sweating, possible delirium or coma.

Paget's disease

The cause of Paget's disease (Osteitis Deformans) is unknown. Early viral infection and genetic causes have been theorized. The disease is characterized by excessive breakdown of bone tissue, followed by abnormal bone formation. The new bone is structurally enlarged, but weakened and filled with new blood vessels. The disease may localize to one or two areas within the skeleton, or become widespread. Frequently, the pelvis, femur, tibia, vertebrae, clavicle, or humerus are involved. The skull may enlarge head size and cause hearing loss, if the cranial nerves are damaged by the bone growth.

Symptoms/Signs:
- Bone pain (may be severe and persistent)
- Joint pain or joint stiffness
- Headache
- Bowing of the legs
- Warmth of skin overlying affected bone fracture
- Neck pain
- Reduced height
- Hearing loss

Note: Most patients have no symptoms

Cardiomyopathies

Cardiomyopathies: Dilated, Hypertrophic, or Restrictive:
- Dilated: enlarged four-chamber dilatation, but wall of normal thickness --> myocardial fibrosis --> ventricular thrombi, valve regurgitation. Can be associated with alcohol abuse, infectious myocarditis, nutritional deficiencies, toxins, idiopathic
- Hypertrophic: IHSS (Idiopathic Hypertrophic Subaortic Stenosis) - stenosis of the outflow tract in the left ventricle due to septal hypertrophy, with myofiber disarray. Associated with limited ventricular filling (diastolic dysfunction), as well as obstruction to left ventricular outflow (systolic dysfunction). Can lead to sudden death, or heart failure. Familial
- Restrictive: ventricular wall is stiffened due to infiltrative process (diastolic dysfunction). Causes: Amyloidosis, hemochromatosis, carcinoid, sarcoidosis, metastases to the heart, etc.

Lobar vs. Bronchopneumonia and Community vs. Nosocomial vs. Immunocompromised

Lobar vs. Bronchopneumonia:
- Lobar - large confluent areas involved, virulent organism, 4 stages.
- Bronchopneumonia - patchy consolidation of multiple areas, lower virulent organisms - usually host resistance is decreased

Community vs. Nosocomial vs. Immunocompromised:
- Community Acquired-
  - Typical, Abrupt onset, high fever, rigor, chest pain, productive cough. Organisms: strep pneumonia, H. flu. Klebsiella, anaerobes, S. aureus., GNB, (Legionella).
  - Atypical - Slow onset, fever, nonproductive cough, headache, myalgias. Organisms: mycoplasm, chlamydia, viruses. Risk factors: age, tobacco, ETOH, chronic diseases
- Nosocomial-Risk factors: intubation, in hospital > 48 hrs, post sx, elderly, obese, malnutrition. Organisms: gram neg, anaerobes (aspiration), Staph aureus
- Immunocompromised - anything! (bacteria, TB, fungi, CMV, PCP)

Myelomeningocele

Myelomeningocele is one of the most common birth defects of the central nervous system. It is a neural tube defect in which the bones of the spine do not completely form, and the spinal canal is incomplete. This allows the spinal cord and meninges (the membranes covering the spinal cord) to protrude out of the child's back. Spina bifida includes any congenital defect involving insufficient closure of the spine. Myelomeningocele accounts for about 75% of all cases of spina bifida and may affect as many as 1 out of every 800 infants. The rest of the cases are most commonly spina bifida occulta (where the bones of the spine do not close, the spinal cord and meninges remain in place, and skin usually covers the defect) and meningoceles (where the meninges protrude through the vertebral defect but the spinal cord remains in place).

Autonomic Dysreflexia

Autonomic dysreflexia is a potentially life threatening emergency that involves over reaction of the autonomic nervouse system to a stimulus. It occurs most often in patients with T6 or higher spinal cord injuries, but it can occur in those with lower spinal cord injuries as well. The patient will present with a sudden onset of hypertension, flushing, sweating, and bradycardia, due to stimuli below the level of spinal injury, with the stimuli often being fecal impaction, urinary retention, pain, or another disease process.
Interventions:
Elevate head of bed to 90 degrees
Looser restrictive clothing
Asses for bladder distention and bowel impaction
Administer antihypertentive meds
Can cause stroke, MI, seizure

Pleural effusion and empyema

Pleural effusion: are common in pneumonia and result because of irritation of the pleural space resulting in capillary leak and decreased lymphatic clearance in the pleural space. When these effusions consist only of this fluid, the effusion is considered uncomplicated and will resolve spontaneously as the pneumonia resolves.

Empyema: when infection enters the usually sterile pleural space then the effusion is said to be complicated or an empyema (pus in the pleural space). This complication requires open tube drainage of the pleural space in addition to antimicrobial therapy. It is impossible to differentiate a simple from a complicated effusion radiologically and requires obtaining a sample via a procedure termed a thoracentesis.

Treatment for Myasthenia Gravis

Myasthenia gravis can be controlled. Some medications improve neuromuscular transmission and increase muscle strength, and some suppress the production of abnormal antibodies. These medications must be used with careful medical follow-up because they may cause major side effects. Thymectomy, the surgical removal of the thymus gland (which often is abnormal in myasthenia gravis patients), improves symptoms in certain patients and may cure some individuals, possibly by re-balancing the immune system. Other therapies include plasmapheresis, a procedure in which abnormal antibodies are removed from the blood, and high-dose intravenous immune globulin, which temporarily modifies the immune system and provides the body with normal antibodies from donated blood.

SIRS

Systemic Inflammatory Response Syndrome (SIRS) is a generalized systemic inflammation in organs remote from an initial insult. The advances in medicine in the last several years have increased survival rates.

Clinical conditions associated with SIRS:
- Infection, Infection of vascular structures (heart and lung)
- Pancreatitis, Ischemia
- Multiple trauma with massive tissue injury

- Hemorrhagic shock, Immune-mediated organ injury
- Exogenous administration of tumor necrosis factor
- Aspiration of gastric contents, Massive transfusion
- Host defense abnormalities

Clinical manifestations:
- Temperature < 38 degrees C, Heart rate > 90 beats/min
- Respiratory rate > 20 breaths/min or PaCO2 < 32 torr
- WBC > 12,000 or < 4000 or > 10% immature (bands) forms

Fe deficiency

Microcytic (decreased MCV)
Hypochromic (decreased MCH)
There is a defect in heme synthesis in Fe deficiency. Absorption occurs in the duodenum and upper jejunum. The amount of Fe absorbed is increased with Fe deficiency.

Causes of iron deficiency:
- Blood loss
- Decreased absorption in the duodenum and proximal jejunum
- Decreased intake (especially in children)
- Increased requirements (menstruating women, pregnant women)

Clinical features:
- Angular stomatitis and glossitis
- Pica
- Koilonychia
- Fatigue and weakness

Abnormalities:
- Decreased serum Fe
- Decreased ferritin (storage form)
- Increased TIBC
- Low reticulocyte count
- If becomes chronic laboratory findings: low Fe, low TIBC (not making adequate proteins)

GERD

GERD (gastroesophageal reflux disease) - an esophagitis.
Pathology: Decreased tone with smoking, alcohol, fatty meals. Reflux worse with obesity, pregnancy, impaired gastric emptying, Prone positioning and peristaltic dysfunction

Clinical: heartburn typical, cough or hoarseness (irritation larynx) less common. Often asymptomatic, dissociation between symptoms and degree of reflux, prolonged exposure (especially nocturnal) -> mucosal damage

Damage can include ulceration, erosion and Barrett's metaplasia (intestinal metaplasia)

Histology: squamous epith replaced by columnar cell glandular mucosa

Diagnosis: pH monitoring, Treatment: decrease acid, alter diet, raise head of bed, surgery

Infections associated with AIDS

The following are 10 opportunistic infections associated with AIDS:
- Salmonellosis, Syphilis and Neurosyphilis
- Tuberculosis (TB), Bacillary angiomatosis (cat scratch disease)
- Aspergillosis, Candidiasis (thrush, yeast infection)
- Coccidioidomycosis, Cryptococcal Meningitis
- Histoplasmosis, Kaposi's Sarcoma
- Lymphoma, Systemic Non-Hodgkin's Lymphoma (NHL)
- Primary CNS Lymphoma, Cryptosporidiosis
- Isosporiasis, Microsporidiosis
- Pneumocystis Carinii Pneumonia (PCP, Toxoplasmosis)
- Cytomegalovirus (CMV), Hepatitis
- Herpes Simplex (HSV, genital herpes), Herpes Zoster (HZV, shingles)
- Human Papilloma Virus (HPV, genital warts, cervical cancer)
- AIDS Dementia Complex (ADC)

Hypothermia

When more heat is lost than your body can generate, hypothermia can result. The key sign of hypothermia is an internal body temperature that drops to less than 95 F.

Signs/Symptoms:
- Shivering
- Slurred speech
- Abnormally slow breathing
- Cold, pale skin
- Loss of coordination
- Fatigue, lethargy or apathy

Symptoms usually develop slowly. Someone with hypothermia typically experiences gradual loss of mental acuity and physical ability and so may be unaware of the need for emergency medical treatment. Older adults, infants and young children, and people who are very lean are at particular risk.

Seborrheic keratosis and actinic keratosis

Seborrheic keratosis: The development of skin "tags" or the barnacles of old age. Usually found in people over 30 years old. Appear to be tabs growing in groups or individually on your skin. Can be treated with Scrapping, Freezing or Electrosurgery.

Actinic keratosis: A site that can become cancerous, usually small and rough on the skin that has been exposed to the sun a lot. Usually treated with cryosurgery and photodynamic therapy.

Congestive heart failure

Class I describes a patient who is not limited with normal physical activity by symptoms. Class II occurs when ordinary physical activity results in fatigue, dyspnea, or other symptoms. Class III is characterized by a marked limitation in normal physical activity. Class IV is defined by symptoms at rest or with any physical activity.

Causes:
- CAD
- Valvular heart disease
- Cardiomyopathies
- Endocarditis
- Extracardiac infection
- Pulmonary embolus

Symptoms:
- Skin cold or cyanotic
- Wheezing
- Mitral valvular deficits
- Lower extremity edema
- Pulsus alternans
- Hypertension
- Tachypnea

UNLOAD FAST is a helpful mnemonic to assist you to remember the management of Congestive Heart Failure.
Upright Position
Nitrates
Lasix
Oxygen
Ace Inhibitors
Digoxin

Fluids (decrease)
Afterload (decrease)
Sodium Restriction
Test (digoxin level, ABGs, K level)

Ventricular Tachyarrhythmias

Ventricular Tachycardia- Presence of 3 or greater PVC's (150-200bpm), possible abrupt onset. Possibly due to an ischemic ventricle. No P waves present.

LAMB is a helpful mnemonic to assist you to remember the treatment of Ventricular Tachycardia.
Lidocaine
Amiodarone
Magnesium/Mexiletine
Beta Blocker

(PVC)- Premature Ventricular Contraction- In many cases no P wave followed by a large QRS complex that is premature, followed by a compensatory pause.

Ventricular fibrillation- Completely abnormal ventricular rate and rhythm requiring emergency intervention. No effective cardiac output.

Hypothyroidism

Hypothyroidism: Poor production of thyroid hormone:
Primary- Thyroid cannot meet the demands of the pituitary gland.
Secondary- No stimulation of the thyroid by the pituitary gland.

Causes:
- Surgical thyroid removal
- Irradiation
- Congenital defects
- Hashimoto's thyroiditis (key)

Symptoms:
- Constipation
- Weight gain
- Fatigue
- Hoarse vocal sounds
- Joint pain
- Depression
- Muscle weakness
- Poor speech
- Color changes

Tests:
- Decreased BP and HR
- Chest X-ray
- Elevated liver enzymes, prolactin, and cholesterol
- Decreased T4 levels and serum sodium levels
- Presence of anemia
- Low temperature
- Poor reflexes

Treatment:
- Increase thyroid hormone levels
- Levothyroxine

Monitor the patient for:
- Hyperthyroidism symptoms following treatment
- Heart disease
- Miscarriage
- Myxedema coma if untreated

Bradyarrhythmias

AV block (primary, secondary (I,II) Tertiary
Primary- >.02 PR interval
Secondary (Mobitz I) – PR interval Increase
Secondary (Mobitz II) – PR interval (no change)
Tertiary- most severe, No signal between ventricles and atria noted on ECG. Probable use of Atrophine indicated. Pacemaker required.
Right Bundle Branch Block (RBBB)/Left Bundle Branch Block (LBBB)
Sinus Bradycardia- <60 bpm, with presence of a standard P wave.

Atopic dermatitis and contact dermatitis

Atopic Dermatitis: Scaling, Itching, Redness and Excoriation. Possible lichenification in chronic cases. Most common in young children around the elbow and knees. Adults are more common in neck and knees. May be associated with an allergic disorder, hay fever, or asthma.

Contact Dermatitis: Itchy, weepy reaction with a foreign substance (Poison Ivy) or lotions. Skin becomes red.

Legg-Calve-Perthes disease

Legg-Calve-Perthes disease: poor blood supply to the superior aspect of the femur. Most common in boys ages 4-10. The femur ball flattens out and deteriorates. 4x higher incidence in boys + Bony crescent sign.

Symptoms:
- Hip and knee pain
- Limited AROM and PROM
- Pain with gait and unequal leg length.

Tests:
- X-ray Hip
- Test ROM of hip

Treatment:
- Surgery
- Physical therapy
- Brace
- Bed rest

Klinefelter's Syndrome

A congenital male chromosomal abnormality resulting in an XXY configuration rather than the typical XY. The addition of the X sex chromosome produces the following female characteristics: tendency to grow less body hair, small testicular (testes) size, long arms and legs, narrow shoulders, poor beard growth, female pubic hair pattern, and narrow shoulders.

Middle Cerebral Artery CVA

Symptoms and Signs:
- Dysphasia (if Left hemisphere involvement)
- Dyslexia
- Dysgraphia
- Contralateral Hemiparesis or Hemiplegia
- Contralateral hemisensory disturbance
- Rapid progression in Decreased Level of Consciousness
- Vomiting
- Homonymous Hemianopia
- Denial or lack of recognition of paralyzed extremity
- Eyes look toward lesion
- Inability to turn eyes toward the affected side

Differences in lung volumes between restrictive and obstructive conditions

Restrictive/Obstructive
decreased TLC - normal or increased TLC
increased elastic recoil/decreased compliance - visa versa
decreased FEV1, FVC - decreased FEV1FVC
increased FEV1% - decreased FEV1%
decreased pO2 - decreased pO2

Conjunctivitis

Inflammation of the conjunctiva that can be caused by viruses or bacteria. Also known as pink eye. If viral source can be highly contagious.

Antibiotic eye drops and warm cloths to the eye helpful treatment.

Conjunctivitis can also be caused by chemicals or allergic reactions. Re-occurring conjunctivitis can indicate a larger underlying disease process.

Hyperthyroidism

Hyperthyroidism: excessive production of thyroid hormone.

Causes:
- Iodine overdose
- Thyroid hormone overdose
- Graves' disease (key)
- Tumors affecting the reproductive system

Symptoms:
- Skin color changes
- Weight loss
- Possible goiter

- Nausea
- Exophthalmos
- Diarrhea
- Elevated BP
- Sweating

Tests:
- Elevated Systolic pressure noted
- T3/T4 (free) levels increased
- TSH levels reduced

Treatment:
- Radioactive iodine
- Surgery
- Beta-blockers
- Antithyroid drugs

Glaucoma

An increase in fluid pressure in the eye leading to possible optic nerve damage. More common in African-Americans. Minimal onset symptoms, often picked up too late. Certain drugs may decrease the amount of fluid entering the eye. Two major types of glaucoma are open-angle glaucoma and \angle-closure glaucoma.

Slipped capital femoral epiphysis

Slipped capital femoral epiphysis: 2x greater incidence in males, most common hip disorder in adolescents. The ball of the femur separates from the femur along the epiphysis.

Symptoms:
- Hip pain
- Gait dysfunction
- Knee pain
- Abnormal Hip AROM

Tests:
- X-ray
- Palpation of the hips

Treatment: Surgery

Wilson's disease

High levels of copper in various tissues throughout the body. (Genetically linked- Autosomal recessive).

Key organs affected are:
- Eyes
- Brain
- Liver
- Kidneys

Symptoms:
- Gait disturbances
- Jaundice
- Tremors
- Abdominal pain/distention
- Dementia
- Speech problems
- Muscle weakness
- Splenomegaly
- Confusion

Various lab tests:
- Bilirubin/PT/ SGOT increased
- Albumin/Uric acid production decreased
- MRI
- Genetic testing
- Low levels of serum copper
- Copper is found in the tissues
- Kayser-Fleisher Rings in the eye

Treatment:
- Pyridoxine
- Low copper diet
- Corticosteroids
- Penicillamine

Monitor the patient for:
- Cirrhosis
- Muscle weakness
- Joint pain/stiffness
- Anemia
- Fever
- Hepatitis

Cushing's syndrome

Abnormal production of ACTH which in turn causes elevated cortisol levels.

Causes:
- Corticosteroids prolonged use
- Tumors

Symptoms:
- Muscle weakness
- Central obesity distribution
- Back pain
- Thirst
- Skin color changes
- Bone and joint pain
- Htn
- Headaches
- Frequent urination,
- Moon face
- Weight gain
- Acne

Tests:
- Dexamethasone suppression test
- Cortisol level check
- MRI-check for tumors

Treatment:
- Surgery to remove tumor
- Monitor corticosteroid levels

Monitor the patient for:
- Kidney stones
- Htn
- Bone fractures
- DM
- Infections

Systemic lupus erythematosus

Systemic lupus erythematosus: autoimmune disorder that affects joints, skin and various organ systems. Chronic and inflammatory. 9x more common in females.

Symptoms:
- Butterfly rash
- Weight loss
- Fever
- Hair loss
- Abdominal pain
- Mouth sores
- Fatigue
- Seizures
- Arthritis
- Nausea
- Joint pain
- Psychosis

Tests:
- CBC
- Chest X-ray
- ANA test
- Skin rash observation
- Coombs' test
- Urine analysis
- Test for various antibodies

Treatment:
- NSAIDS
- Protective clothing
- Cytotoxic drugs
- Hydroxychloroquine

Monitor the patient for:
- Seizures
- Infection
- Hemolytic anemia
- Myocarditis
- Infection
- Renal failure

Pneumonia

Types of pneumonia: Viral pneumonia, Walking pneumonia, Legionella pneumonia, CMV pneumonia, Aspiration pneumonia, Atypical pneumonia

Symptoms:
- Fever
- Headache
- SOB
- Cough
- Chest pain

Tests:
- Chest X-ray
- Pulmonary perfusion scan
- CBC
- Cultures of sputum
- Presence of crackles

Treatment:
- Antibiotics if caused by a bacterial infection
- Respiratory treatments
- Steroids
- IV fluids
- Vaccine treatments

Rheumatoid arthritis

Rheumatoid arthritis: inflammatory autoimmune disease that affects various tissues and joints.

Symptoms:
- Fever
- Fatigue
- Joint pain and swelling
- ROM decreased
- Hand/Feet deformities
- Numbness
- Skin color changes

Tests:
- Rheumatoid factor tests
- C-reactive protein
- Synovial fluid exam
- X-rays of involved joints
- ESR increased

Treatment:
- Physical therapy
- Moist heat
- Anti-inflammatory drugs
- Corticosteroids
- Anti-malarial drugs
- Cox-2 inhibitors
- Splinting

Scleroderma

Scleroderma: connective tissue disease that is diffuse.

Symptoms:
- Wheezing
- Heartburn
- Raynaud's phenomenon
- Skin thickness changes
- Weight loss
- Joint pain

- SOB
- Hair loss
- Bloating

Tests:
- Monitor skin changes
- Chest X-ray
- Antinuclear antibody test
- ESR increased

Monitor the patient for:
- Renal failure
- Heart failure
- Pulmonary fibrosis

Diverticulitis

Abnormal pouch formation that becomes inflamed in the intestinal wall.

Symptoms:
- Fever
- Diarrhea
- Nausea
- Vomiting
- Constipation

Tests:
- Barium enema
- WBC count
- Colonoscopy
- CT Scan
- Sigmoidoscopy

Must be on a low residue diet. No nuts, seeds, peas. Pain is LL Quadrant.

Pulmonary actinomycosis

Bacterial infection of the lungs caused by (propionibacteria or actinomyces)
Causes: Microorganisms

Symptoms:
- Pleural effusions
- Facial lesions
- Chest pain
- Cough
- Weight loss
- Fever

Tests:
- CBC
- Lung biopsy
- Thoracentesis
- CT scan
- Bronchoscopy

Monitor patient for:
- Emphysema
- Meningitis
- Osteomyelitis

Heart valve infection

Endocarditis (inflammation), probable valvular heart disease. Can be caused by fungi or bacteria.

Symptoms:
- Weakness
- Fever
- Murmur
- SOB
- Night sweats
- Janeway lesions
- Joint pain

Tests:
- CBC
- ESR
- ECG
- Blood cultures
- Enlarged spleen
- Presence of splinter hemorrhages

Treatment:
- IV antibiotics
- Surgery may be indicated

Monitor the patient for:
- Jaundice
- Arrhythmias
- CHF
- Glomerulonephritis
- Emboli

Pulmonary hypertension

Causes: May be genetically linked, more common in women

Symptoms:
- Fainting
- Fatigue
- Chest Pain
- SOB with activity
- LE edema
- Weakness

Tests:
- Pulmonary arteriogram
- Chest X-ray
- ECG
- Pulmonary function tests
- CT scan
- Cardiac catheterization

Treatment:
- Manage symptoms
- Diuretics
- Calcium channel blockers
- Heart/Lung Transplant if necessary

Ulcerative colitis

Chronic inflammation of the rectum and large intestine.

Symptoms:
- Weight loss
- Jaundice
- Diarrhea
- Abdominal pain
- Fever
- Joint pain
- GI bleeding

Tests:
- Barium enema
- ESR
- CRP
- Colonoscopy

Treatment:
- Corticosteroids
- Mesalamine

- Surgery
- Ostomy
- Azathioprine

Monitor the patient for:
- Ankylosing spondylitis
- Liver disease
- Carcinoma
- Pyoderma gangrenosum
- Hemorrhage
- Perforated colon

ARDS

Causes: Trauma, Chemical inhalation, Pneumonia, Septic shock

Symptoms:
- Low BP
- Rapid breathing
- SOB

Tests:
- ABG
- CBC
- Cultures

Treatment:
- Echocardiogram
- Auscultation
- Cyanosis
- Chest X-ray
- Mechanical Ventilation
- Treat the underlying condition

Monitor the patient for:
- Pulmonary fibrosis
- Multiple system organ failure
- Ventilator associated pneumonia
- Acidosis
- Respiratory failure

Pulmonary valve stenosis

Causes: Congenital, Endocarditis, Rheumatic Fever

Symptoms:
- Fainting
- SOB

- Palpitations
- Cyanosis
- Poor weight gain

Tests:
- Cardiac catheterization
- ECG
- Chest-X-ray
- Echocardiogram

Treatment:
- Prostaglandins
- Diuretics
- Anti-arrhythmics
- Blood thinners

Respiratory Alkalosis

Causes: Anxiety, Fever, Hyperventilation

Symptoms:
- Dizziness
- Numbness

Tests:
- ABG
- Chest X-ray
- Pulmonary function tests

Treatment:
- Paper bag technique
- Increase carbon dioxide levels

ROME is a helpful mnemonic to assist you to remember the Acid-Base Balance rules.
Respiratory
Opposite
Metabolic
Equal

RSV (Respiratory syncytial virus)

Symptoms:
- Fever
- SOB
- Cyanosis
- Wheezing
- Nasal congestion
- Croupy cough

Tests:
- ABG
- Chest X-ray

Treatment:
- Ribavirin
- Ventilator in severe cases
- IV fluids
- Bronchodilators

Monitor the patient for:
- Pneumonia
- Respiratory failure
- Otitis Media

Neoplastic disorders

Neoplastic disorders are cancers or the uncontrolled or uncontrollable proliferation of abnormal cells. Cancer cells typically tend to be immature and abnormal. Cancer cells are encapsulated and this allows for easy invasion of surrounding cells. Cancer cells metastasize at a rapid rate, invade multiple other tissues, cells and organs and if not controlled prove to be fatal. Causative factors associated with cancers include, but are not limited to viruses, sunlight exposure to skin, chronic irritation of skin or other tissues, chemicals such as tobacco smoke, high fat diets, and diets with low fiber tend to be precursors for cancer. Other factors associated with cancer include increased carbohydrate intake, animal proteins, air and industrial pollutants, chemicals, drugs and genetic weaknesses or traits.

CAUTION UP is a helpful mnemonic to assist you to remember the early warning signs of cancer.
Change in bowel or bladder
A lesion that does not heal
Unusual bleeding or discharge
Thickening or lump in breast or elsewhere
Indigestion or difficulty swallowing
Obvious changes in wart or mole
Nagging cough or persistent hoarseness
Unexplained weight loss
Pernicious Anemia

Infectious endocarditis

Infectious endocarditis and inflammatory process of the endocardium or internal layers of the heart muscle. The endocardium includes the subendothelial connective tissue, the atrial wall, and smooth muscle of the heart. Infectious endocarditis is a disorder or disease that encompasses the valves of the heart and the endothelial surface of the heart. Infectious endocarditis is typically caused by a viral or bacterial infection that produces abnormalities in the valves of the heart. Acute endocarditis may be caused by bacteria, fungi, and the rickettsia virus. Sub-acute endocarditis is typically caused by streptococcus viridans. Factors that may contribute to infectious endocarditis include history of valvular disease, surgical procedures, immunosuppressive drug therapy such as steroids, and heroin addiction. Infectious endocarditis also may be caused by extensive indwelling catheters, and prolonged IV antibiotics.

Cancer and neoplasms

Carcinomas
Originate from the epithelial tissue of the skin, lung, gastrointestinal tract, breast and uterine lining. Carcinomas traditionally begin to spread via the lymph system, followed by the blood stream. Carcinomas are named according to the type of cells involved. Examples include carcinoma of the prostate, breast, and/or lung. The two major types of carcinoma are the glandular (adenocarcinoma), and squamous cell carcinoma. Squamous cell carcinoma is the most frequently diagnosed type of cancer.

Sarcoma
A neoplasm of the connective tissue. Sarcomas have an increased risk of malignancy, and originate from an excessive proliferation of mesodermal cells. Sarcomas are common among the soft tissue such as bone, and muscle. Sarcomas are generally characterized by large masses that may or may not metastasize to other areas of the body.

Lymphoma
Neoplasms of the lymph or reticuloendothelial tissue. Lymphomas are typically solid tumors that traditionally appear in the lymph nodes, spleen, or any other organ tissue. Hodgkin's disease is an example of lymphoma. Lymphomas are categorized according to cell involvement (B or T cells).

Leukemia
Both acute and chronic and encompasses the blood producing organs. Leukemia is a progressive proliferation of abnormal leukocytes. Categorized by cell type and duration from initial onset to time of demise.

Aplastic anemia

Aplastic anemia is characterized by a decreased production of red blood cells within the bone marrow, causing a decreased amount of circulating erythrocytes in the circulating blood. Aplastic anemia may also include low levels of circulating leukocytes and platelets. Causes of aplastic anemia include, but are not limited to erythrocyte destruction caused by drugs and/or chemicals, anti-tumor agents, 6-mercaptopurine, antimicrobials, heavy metals, and damage due to radiation. Signs and symptoms of aplastic anemia include dyspnea, ecchymoses, petechiae, fatigue, and fever, hemorrhage, menorrhagia, occult blood, epistaxis, pallor, palpitations, weakness, retinal hemorrhage, and weight loss.

Thromboangiitis obliterans (Buerger's disease)

Thromboangiitis obliterans is an inflammatory process of the arteries and veins. Thromboangiitis obliterans occurs most often in young and middle-aged men, especially those who smoke. Thromboangiitis obliterans is characterized by occlusions of the extremities (both upper and lower), that are caused by thrombus formations that occlude the vessels. Thromboangiitis obliterans traditionally was the cause of gangrene infections. Signs and symptoms of thromboangiitis obliterans include ulcerations of the extremities especially the digits, coolness and pallor in the hands and feet, increased sensitivity to cold. Paresthesias such as numbness, tingling, burning often occur as the result of thromboangiitis obliterans. Intermittent claudication (traditionally caused by ischemia, characterized by pain) often occurs in the arch of the foot or legs; it is rare to have claudication in the forearm or hands. Buerger color is often noted in the hands and feet. Buerger color is characterized by cyanotic hands and feet.

Crohn's disease (regional enteritis)

Crohn's disease is a chronic inflammatory disorder of the intestinal tract. The causative agent associated with Crohn's disease is unknown. Characteristics associated with Crohn's disease include deep ulcerations, fistula formation, narrow, thick bowels, and lymphocytic infiltration. The terminal ileum is the major area affected by Crohn's disease. Those with Crohn's disease experience frequent exacerbations and remissions. Crohn's disease does have a familial tendency, with no preference to sexual orientation. Crohn's disease most often occurs during the 20's and 30's. Signs and symptoms of Crohn's disease include, but are not limited to diarrhea, abdominal pain and discomfort, and weight loss ranging from 5 to 20 pounds. Other signs and symptoms of Crohn's disease include potential for abdominal masses, perirectal, bladder, vaginal, and skin fistulas. Hemorrhage is often associated with Crohn's disease. Fever, emesis, and cachexia are also signs and symptoms associated with Crohn's disease.

Hodgkin's disease

Hodgkin's disease is a malignant neoplasm characterized by enlarged lymph tissue. Hodgkin's disease origination is unknown, but it is thought that the Epstein Barr virus is associated with the development of Hodgkin's disease. It is thought that Hodgkin's disease mainly encompasses the B-cells, with some potential alteration in T-cells. Hodgkin's disease produces an excessive proliferation of Reed-Sternberg cells. Signs and symptoms include lymphadenopathy (traditionally cervical or supraclavicular), fever may accompany Hodgkin's disease, night sweats, weight loss, fatigue, and anorexia are also associated symptoms of Hodgkin's disease. Other signs and symptoms of Hodgkin's disease include unexplained itching and pain that is induced by alcohol intake. Stages that accompany Hodgkin's disease are:
- Stage I: single lymph node group
- Stage II: two or more groups of lymph nodes on the same side of the body
- Stage III: involved lymph nodes on both sides of the body
- Stage IV: dissemination of the disease that includes organ involvement

Ulcerative colitis

Ulcerative colitis is an inflammatory disorder of the colon and rectal areas. Ulcerative colitis is characterized by ulcerations of the colon and rectum, rectal bleeding, mucosal crypt abscesses, and polyps. Often mega colon and peritonitis occur as a result of ulcerative colitis. The client with ulcerative colitis will experience episodes of exacerbation and remission. Ulcerative colitis does have a familial history. Those ages 15 to 35 are at highest risk for the disease as well as those over age 70. The cause of ulcerative colitis is unknown, but is assumed to be related to diet allergies, or abnormal immune responses. Signs and symptoms of ulcerative colitis include abdominal pain, bloody diarrhea, anemia, hypoproteinemia, electrolyte imbalances, fever, weight loss, arthralgias, and arthritis.

Treatments include sulfasalazine or other antibiotics, steroid enemas, mesalamine aminosalicylic acid enemas, and oral steroids are used for severe inflammation. Educate the client on the importance of maintaining routine appointments for disease evaluation.

Crohn's disease

Crohn's disease or regional enteritis will include mechanisms of treatment such as weight maintenance, and maintaining nutritional balance. The nurse will need to educate the client on monitoring for fat malabsorption. Fat malabsorption is noted with fatty stools. The client should be taught to report these as well as to decrease the amount of fat in the diet. Sitz baths and excellent, careful peri-care will assist with comfort and healing. Treatment may include surgical procedures such as draining of abscesses, and fistula repair. Folate supplements might be utilized. Prevention mechanisms for bone destruction and bone loss may be considered. Diet is traditionally as tolerated. Increase fiber in diet with diarrhea stools.

Dysphagia and medical nutritional therapy

Dysphagia is difficulty swallowing. Dysphagia can result from multiple disease processes. The most frequent of those being cerebral vascular accident (CVA) or commonly known as stroke. Oral Candida (thrush), Alzheimer's disease, any disorder that causes decreased or altered muscle functioning such as multiple sclerosis (MS), trauma, Parkinson's, stricture or cancers. Nutrition is provided to these patients with altered diets such as pureed or mechanical soft, and feedings such as Enteral or Parenteral. Medical nutritional therapy is a form of providing adequate nutritional intake to individuals who cannot perform acts of normal swallowing. Swallowing occurs in a sequence of oral intake, chewing and salivation, followed by progressive movement into the oropharyngeal cavity, and down the esophagus into the stomach.

Appendicitis

Appendicitis is an acute inflammation of the vermiform appendix. A cardinal sign is maximum tenderness at McBurney's point. Males seem to be afflicted by appendicitis more commonly than females. Signs and symptoms include abdominal pain, right lower quadrant pain that is decreased with flexion of the right thigh. The patient will guard the area of pain and tenderness. Other signs and symptoms include anorexia, nausea and vomiting, constipation or mild diarrhea, elevated temperature, rapid heart rate, positive Rovsing's sign, and positive Psoas sign (pain with right thigh extension). Treatment will include fluids for correction of any fluid or electrolyte imbalances, broad-spectrum antibiotics, and surgical procedures to remove the appendix or drain any abscess that may have occurred. The nurse should assist with immediate mobility following surgery, and educate the client that full activity should return within six weeks post-surgical procedure. Resume diet as bowel function resumes (typically 24 to 48 hours post-op). Educate the client that activity should be restricted following surgery, and notify the physician for nausea, vomiting, pain, fever and chills.

Hiatal hernia

Hiatal hernia describes an area of the stomach that has protruded upward into the chest via the esophageal hiatus. Hiatal hernias may occur due to weakness in the diaphragm, eructation (belching) on a routine basis, pregnancy, reduced motility of the esophagus (scleroderma), and gastric emptying delays. Disease processes such as Zollinger-Ellison syndrome, and Heller's myotomy are also known causes of hiatal hernia. Treatment consists of refraining from lying flat in bed, not going to bed on a full stomach or directly after consuming a meal, avoiding restrictive clothing, weight loss (as the pressure of additional abdominal weight pushes the abdominal contents upward), dietary modifications such as avoiding caffeine and spicy foods, the use of antacids, and histamine receptor 2 antagonists such as Zantac (ranitidine), Pepcid (famotidine) or Tagamet (cimetidine). Proton pump inhibitors (PPIs) such as Nexium (esomeprazole), Prevacid (lansoprazole) are also utilized. Clinical note: the H2 receptor agonists all have the suffix -ine, and PPIs all end in -azole.

Esophagitis

Esophagitis is an inflammation of the esophagus. (Clinical note: -itis as a suffix always refers to inflammation) Esophagitis can be caused by bacteria or viral organisms. Other forms of esophagitis include inflammation caused by reflux of gastric content, and taking medications such as daily pill ingestion. Esophagitis is a self-limiting disorder in the individual who is not immune compromised. Esophagitis is treated with antimicrobial agents depending on the organism. Fungal, bacterial or viral agents are all utilized as necessary. Viscous lidocaine is often used as a method of controlling the pain that is associated with esophagitis. Clear liquid or bland diets are utilized to decrease irritation and maximize nutrition.

Dumping syndrome

Dumping syndrome is a term used to describe a rapid cycle of gastric emptying. Symptoms associated with dumping syndrome include flushing, diaphoresis, weakness, dizziness, nausea, abdominal cramping, diarrhea, and potential vasomotor failure (tachycardia, orthostatic or positional hypertension). When large volumes of food are placed into the small intestine too quickly, fluid is pulled from within the cells to accommodate digestion and hypovolemia occurs causing the symptoms associated with dumping syndrome. Dumping syndrome occurs most often after ingestion of a large meal (post-prandially). It is not uncommon for a client to experience both intestinal and vascular symptoms together or have a mono reaction of the intestinal symptoms or the vascular symptoms.

Peptic ulcer disease

Peptic ulcer disease designates an area of altered integrity of the gastric mucosal protective layer. Gastric content irritates the ulcerated areas causing pain and discomfort. A leading cause of PUD is Helicobacter pylori infection (H. Pylori). Inadequate bicarbonate a base used to neutralize stomach acid is also a leading cause of peptic ulcer disease. Treatments consist of diet alterations, symptom relief including antacids and PPIs, healing the mucosal lining, and prevention mechanisms to decrease further incidence. Peptic ulcers occur as chronic erosions greater than 5 mm in diameter. Factors associated with PUD include the use of aspirin, NSAIDs, corticosteroids, smoking, familial tendency, and history of ulcers.

Inflammatory bowel disease

Chronic Ulcerative Colitis (CUC) along with Crohn's disease is designated as inflammatory bowel disease. Inflammatory bowel disease is a chronic disorder of the large or small intestine with an unknown cause. Symptoms include abdominal pain, weight loss, occasional mass of the abdomen, perirectal area, bladder, skin or vaginal fistula formations, possible production of blood in the urine or stool, enlarged colon (Mega colon), and obstruction of the bowel. Treatment consists of weight management, balanced diet, hygiene, and surgical repair of fistulas or abscesses. Inflammatory bowel disease occurs most often between the ages of 15 and 30 and/or between the ages of 60 and 80. Inflammatory bowel disease is most often caused by NSAIDs, stress and may occur upon cessation of smoking.

Celiac disease

Celiac Disease occurs when the microvilli of the small intestine are damaged by gliadin. Gliadin is the protein of gluten found in wheat, rye, oats and barley. Symptoms include loose stools, often diarrhea (clinical note: diarrhea is only diarrhea when 2,000 ml of liquid stool is produced daily), fatty stools (steatorrhea), flatus, bloating, weakness and reduction of weight. Atrophy and inflammatory processes in the small intestine are the result of Celiac disease. Celiac disease often impairs the absorption of vitamins and minerals causing malnutrition, anemia, and clotting disorders. Treatment consists of removing products that contain gluten from the diet. Celiac disease is most often associated with children, but does occur in adults.

Celiac disease is a metabolic alteration causing reactions to gluten. With celiac disease there is damage to the gastrointestinal mucosa causing a malabsorption of nutrients. Celiac disease is characterized by inflammation and atrophy of the upper portion of the small intestine. Signs and symptoms include diarrhea, malabsorption, fatty stools (steatorrhea), vitamin and nutrient deficiencies, anemia, and failure to thrive. The nursing assessment should include observation of stool, abdominal distention, abdominal pain, emesis, anorexia. The nurse should monitor for changes in personality such as lethargy or irritability. The nurse should ensure the client maintains the ordered diet that is traditionally free of wheat, rye, oat, and barley gluten. The nurse should monitor weight on a routine basis, document diet consumption, monitor growth patterns, and educate the family and client regarding the disease process.

Fatty liver

Fatty liver is also referred to as hepatic steatosis and is characterized by greater than 30% of liver cells having fat deposits. The condition of fatty liver occurs as the result of alcohol intake, increased amounts of kilocalories in the diet, obesity, the use of corticosteroids, elevated triglycerides are also linked to fatty liver. The majority of patients remain asymptomatic while some develop localized pain over the area of the liver, hepatomegaly, splenomegaly, fatigue, ascites, and edema. Treatments include weight reduction, maintenance of triglyceride levels, control diabetes if this is a factor, discontinue use of alcohol, and daily physical exercise.

Ileostomy and colostomy

An Ileostomy occurs as the result of total removal of the colon and the rectum, the anus is sutured closed and an opening in the lower abdominal wall in the area of the ileum is formed to allow for fecal evacuation. A colostomy is formed when the colon is routed to an opening in the abdominal wall forming an artificial opening for feces to be removed and collected. The anus is also sutured with a colostomy. The colon is no longer attached to the natural anal structure for emptying. Both serve as mechanisms for waste collection related to disease processes occurring either in the colon, rectal or anal areas. Clinical note: keep in mind this is often a traumatic event in the lives of your patients, please be professional and sensitive with the care given to these individuals.

Iron-deficiency anemia

Iron-deficiency anemia is caused by a decreased supply of or inadequate absorption of iron. With iron-deficiency anemia hemoglobin synthesis is diminished along with a decreased amount of oxygen in the blood due to lack of oxygen carrying cells. Characteristics of iron deficiency anemia include low serum iron, an increase in the serum iron binding capacity, a decreased serum ferritin level, and decreased iron stores in the bone marrow. Iron deficiency may occur as an acute illness from a rapid loss of blood or may be a chronic condition that has developed related to a slow steady blood loss or a constant poor diet. Iron-deficiency is traditionally asymptomatic, but may present as respiratory difficulty (especially on exertion), fatigue, elevated heart rate (tachycardia), heart palpitations, and orthostatic hypotension or other vasomotor disturbances. Individuals with iron-deficiency anemia often complain of headaches, inability to concentrate, and irritability. Those with iron-deficiency anemia may display spoon shaped, brittle nails, and have an increased risk of infection. Hemoglobin in those with iron-deficiency anemia is normally below 12g/dl. Nursing considerations include monitoring stools for blood (occult/hidden), monitoring diet, providing education, and monitor and decrease the amount of milk in the diet, and perform an in-depth patient history upon initial assessment.

Atopic dermatitis

Atopic dermatitis is an inflammatory reaction to the skin that is traditionally caused by allergens that come in contact with the skin. With atopic dermatitis the individual will experience itching (pruritus), and erythema to the affected areas. Lesions may appear on the face, trunk, limbs, or head. The nurse will need to assess for secondary infection related to scratching. Characteristics of atopic dermatitis include erythema, papules, and macules that may or may not produce exudates. Vesicles may also be present with atopic dermatitis. At the time of initial exam the nurse should assess for exposure to chemicals, take a complete history that includes current allergies and any history of skin infections, determine emotional status and current level of stress, determine climate exposure that includes excessive heat and cold as well as determination of any changes currently taking place within the household. The nurse should educate the individual to limit or avoid stress as possible, minimize over exposure to heat or cold, take tepid baths, use oatmeal in the bath to assist with pruritus, decrease or limit the use of perfumed soaps, decrease sun exposure, and avoid lotions that contain alcohol. Do stress the use of emollient creams.

Thalassemia

Thalassemia is an autosomal, inherited recessive trait that occurs primarily in the Asian, Middle Eastern, and Mediterranean populations. Thalassemia is characterized by the abnormal formation, and decreased life span of red blood cells. There are two types of thalassemia, alpha and beta. The specific type will be associated with the altered synthesis of alpha or beta globin. Individuals with thalassemia may present with pallor, jaundice, anorexia, hepatomegaly, splenomegaly, fatigue, decreased appetite and poor diet, altered growth patterns, dyspnea, gall-stones (cholelithiasis), and pathologic (unexplained) fractures. Thalassemia may cause mongoloid faces in older children. Treatment will include blood transfusions in which the nurse will need to monitor for transfusion complications, and anaphylactic reactions. Desired hemoglobin will be 9.3 g/dl at minimum. Folate may be given and iron chelation (a mechanism of treatment to remove specific particles from the blood) therapy may be utilized. Daily penicillin may be used as a prophylaxis mechanism. The nurse should counsel the patient to avoid strenuous exercise, and strenuous activity, and also to avoid iron rich foods.

Wilm's Tumor

Wilm's tumor is traditionally malignant and is a tumor of the kidney. Wilm's tumor is characteristically diagnosed in childhood prior to the fifth year of life, and has traits of an inherited autosomal dominant disorder. Wilm's tumor is a renal neoplasm in which blastema (a cellular mass), stromal, and/or epithelial cells are present. Wilm's tumor is normally asymptomatic, palpable upon inspection, and produces abdominal pain with exam. Signs and symptoms of Wilm's tumor include fever, anemia, cardiac murmur, hepatomegaly, splenomegaly, abdominal ascites, well defined abdominal wall veins, and metastases to the gonadal area. Treatment consists of chemotherapy, and radiation. The nurse should educate the family and client on the disease, assist with mechanisms to control pain, and anxiety, and mechanisms of care for the child with Wilm's tumor.

Symptoms:
- Fever
- Vomiting
- Fatigue
- Irregular urine coloration
- Abdominal pain
- Constipation
- Abdominal mass
- Increased BP

Tests:
- BUN
- Creatinine
- Analysis of the urine
- X-ray
- CT Scan
- Family history of cancer
- CBC

Treatment:
- Surgery
- Chemotherapy
- Radiation

Intussusception

Intussusception is the inversion of one portion of the intestine into another resulting in intestinal obstruction. Signs and symptoms include severe abdominal pain with drawing up of the lower extremities. Diarrhea, or jelly type stools that have the presence of blood and/or mucous may be noted. Abdominal pain may be intermittent or constant. The individual may appear lethargic and experience lethargy that progresses with disease progression. Abdominal masses may be palpable with the individual who is experiencing intussusception. Fever and pallor also may accompany intussusception. Bile containing emesis and abdominal distention are traditionally present. Treatment may consist of barium enema or surgical repair. The nurse will need to monitor for signs of dehydration, and infection while maintaining a constant level of pain control.

Otitis media

Otitis media is a bacterial infection of the inner (middle) ear or tympanum. Otitis media is a common disorder among young children related to the short, wide eustachian tube. Otitis media is often associated or accompanied by upper respiratory infections. Characteristics of otitis media include fluid, and/or inflammation of the middle ear. With otitis media the tympanic membrane will be erythematous, bulging, and have no bony land marks or light reflex. Signs and symptoms of otitis media include ear pain, fever, altered or decreased hearing, and otorrhea with perforation of the tympanic membrane. Other symptoms of otitis media include irritability in children, sleeping difficulty, pulling or tugging at the ear in children, vertigo, and/or loss of balance.

Pneumonia

Pneumonia treatment consists of antibiotic therapy (sputum culture will assist in determining the exact causative agent), oxygen if the patient is experiencing hypoxia or cyanosis, increased fluids, rest, and analgesics for pain and discomfort often felt with pneumonia. The client should be placed on bed-rest, and consume a diet that is tolerable. Corticosteroids in short duration will assist with the respiratory inflammation and assist with healing time. Antipyretics are often given to assist in the reduction of temperature. Bronchodilators may be used to open airways and facilitate appropriate, effective gas exchange. The client should be educated on causes of pneumonia and discuss preventive mechanisms as well.

Cerebral palsy

Cerebral palsy is present at birth or noted early in childhood. Cerebral palsy is generally diagnoses within the first 3 years of life. Cerebral palsy can be acquired or inherited. Cerebral palsy is a non-progressive disorder of the nervous system in which the individual is unable to control voluntary muscles. Males are typically affected by cerebral palsy more often than females. There are 3 types of cerebral palsy; spastic, dyskinetic, and ataxic. Spastic cerebral palsy is characterized by increased muscle tone. Dyskinetic cerebral palsy is characterized by involuntary athetoid (constant slow) movements. Ataxic cerebral palsy is characterized by poor posture and decreased muscle control and coordination. The nursing assessment will include assessment of muscle tone, coordination, posture, reflexes, motor development, and sensory deficits. An in-depth history should be taken to determine any seizure activity. The patient and/or family should be educated on how to maintain the highest level of functioning.

Acute glomerulonephritis

Acute glomerulonephritis is characterized by inflammation of the glomeruli. Acute glomerulonephritis is most often caused by an antigen-antibody response to group A beta hemolytic streptococcus. Signs and symptoms of acute glomerulonephritis include blood in the urine (hematuria), oliguria (small or scant amounts of urine production), anuria (no urine production), edema, hypertension, and occasional fever, but the person who is experiencing acute glomerulonephritis is traditionally afebrile. Protein and nitrates are often found in the urine, along with white blood cells, epithelial cells, and casts. The blood, urea, and nitrogen are elevated (elevated BUN), and the individual will most likely have an elevated sedimentation rate.

Urinary tract infection

Urinary tract infections are characteristically bacterial infections that cause inflammation in one or more areas of the urinary tract. Escherichia coli are the most common organisms seen with urinary tract infection. Signs and symptoms of urinary tract infection include abnormally high fever, polyuria, and urgency with urination, dysuria, urinary retention, and enuresis (episodes of incontinence). Pain often is associated with urinary tract infections and may occur in the low back, flank area, and lower abdominal area. Urinary tract infection is an umbrella term used to describe cystitis (bladder infection), pyelonephritis (kidney infection), and urethritis.

Staging of pressure ulcers

Stage one pressure ulcers have intact skin that may be cool to touch, feel firm or boggy, may not blanch, and may be accompanied by pruritus and tenderness. Stage one ulcers may have a constant appearance of discoloration that may present as dark pink, pink, bluish, or red. Stage two pressure ulcers have a partial loss of skin thickness. The epidermis or dermis is involved with stage two pressure ulcers. Stage two pressure ulcers have the appearance of bullae, erythema, or superficial skin loss. Stage three pressure ulcers appear as skin damage or loss that encompasses the subcutaneous tissue as well as the epidermis and dermis. Stage three pressure ulcers may involve necrosis. Stage three pressure ulcers do not include the fascia. Stage four pressure ulcers may include the muscle and/or bone. Stage four pressure ulcers have widespread loss of tissue and broad tissue necrosis.

Infectious mononucleosis

Infectious mononucleosis is a viral infection caused by the Epstein-Barr virus. Infectious mononucleosis characteristically occurs in young adults and most often is transmitted via saliva. Infectious mononucleosis causes generalized lymphadenopathy. Signs and symptoms of infectious mononucleosis include sore throat, dysphagia, fever, and swollen lymph nodes. Inflammation of the pharynx is also associated with infectious mononucleosis. Other signs and symptoms include, but are not limited to malaise, splenomegaly, headache, anorexia, chills, nausea and vomiting, and generalized malaise. Those at risk for infectious mononucleosis include students (both high school and college), those who engage in kissing, and individuals who have been exposed to infection, particularly strep infection.

Osteosarcoma and Ewing's sarcoma

Both Osteosarcoma and Ewing's sarcoma are bone tumors. Osteosarcoma is the most common and malignant bone tumor known today. Osteosarcoma characteristically affects the ends of long bones of the lower extremities. Osteosarcoma is a tumor of the osteoblasts. Osteosarcoma is a cellular lesion formed from cartilaginous tissue. There is historically a genetic alteration in the individual with osteosarcoma. The individual will have experienced a loss in suppressor retinoblastoma and p53 genes. Ewing's sarcoma is characterized by a small, blue round cell neoplasm that forms from bone marrow cells. Ewing's sarcoma occurs most often in the shaft of the femur, tibia or humerus. Ewing's sarcoma is noted to have chromosomal dislocation, and fusion proteins. Signs and symptoms: Bone pain with weight bearing and at rest, swelling, tenderness, traumatic fracture, and injury to the area.

Viral hepatitis A

Hepatitis A is a systemic viral infection or short incubation type hepatitis that involves the liver. Hepatitis A is extremely contagious and caused by an RNA enterovirus. Hepatitis A is transmitted via the fecal-oral route or paternally. Hepatitis A is traditionally acquired when the individual ingests contaminated food, milk or other milk products that are contaminated. Hepatitis A can be transmitted via contaminated water, and seafood from contaminated waters. Hepatitis A is characterized by an inflammation of the liver. Signs and symptoms of hepatitis A include, but are not limited to fever, malaise, nausea and vomiting, anorexia, jaundice, enlarged liver (hepatomegaly), dark urine, transient pale stools, upper right abdominal quadrant pain, and fatigue. Patient education should include education on the disease and disease process, education on hygiene, handwashing, vaccinations to prevent hepatitis A, and educate the individual to cover broken or open skin. To confirm the diagnosis of hepatitis A the individual is tested for hepatitis A antibodies.

Shock

Shock is characterized by inadequate cellular metabolism due to poor tissue perfusion. Signs/Symptoms include hypertension, weak, rapid pulse, cool, clammy skin, altered level of consciousness, decreased urine output, less than 20cc an hour. Rapid breathing and thirst are also signs and symptoms of shock. The types of shock are:
- Hypovolemic shock: Due to decreased amounts of fluid in the body, this can be intra or extracellular. Causes include blood-loss (hemorrhage). Classifications of Hypovolemic shock include: Mild: up to 20% of blood volume loss; Moderate: 20 to 40% of blood volume loss; Severe: 40% or more of blood volume loss
- Cardiogenic shock: A decreased ability of the heart to pump blood related to poor perfusion of the coronary vessels. Causes include myocardial infarction (MI or heart attack), congestive heart failure, and arrhythmias.
- Neurogenic shock: An increase in the size of the vascular bed that results in pooling of venous blood, decreased venous return, and decreased cardiac output. Causes include general anesthesia (deep sedation), injuries to the central nervous system, barbiturate intoxication, spinal anesthesia, and fainting.
- Septic shock: Occurs as a result of toxic substances that act to disrupt the normal mechanism of blood vessels. Causes of septic shock include gram-positive organisms such as pneumococci, staphylococci, and streptococci.

Systemic Lupus Erythematous (SLE)

Systemic Lupus Erythematous (SLE) is an inflammatory process of the connective tissue. There are two types of SLE, discoid lupus erythematous that only affects the skin and is characterized by circular or disc shaped lesions, and systemic lupus erythematous that affects not only the skin, but multiple organ systems as well. Systemic lupus erythematous can be fatal. Characteristics of SLE include fever, weakness, fatigue, joint pain and arthritis, dispersed skin lesions on the upper body, a red or pink rash spread across the nose and cheeks called the butterfly rash, and lymphadenopathy. Exacerbations and remissions are part of the disease process of systemic lupus erythematous. Possible factors contributing to SLE include immunology, environmental factors, hormone abnormalities, and genetics. Treatment includes routine office visits to monitor condition. The nurse should educate the client to avoid sunlight, wear sunscreen, and a hat while outside. The nurse should educate the individual to contact their health care provider if they become ill or suspect infection. The individual should be counseled to conserve energy, and avoid stress as much as possible.

Atelectasis

Atelectasis is a condition characterized by an area of lung tissue that has a decreased amount of or loss of air in part of or throughout the entire lung. Atelectasis is also termed pulmonary collapse (collapsed lung). Causes of atelectasis include, but are not limited to bronchial obstruction, pleural effusion or pneumothorax, cardiac hypertrophy. The nursing assessment should include painful respirations, anxiety, and cyanosis. Weakness, asymmetrical movement, reduced or absent breath sounds and dullness with percussion are also signs of atelectasis. Temperature, blood pressure, pulse and respiratory rate should also be assessed. Hypoxia is often present with atelectasis related to the decreased blood flow to lung tissue caused by collapse and obstruction. Additional causes include infectious processes, surfactant deficiency, and pulmonary edema.

Pneumothorax

A pneumothorax is a collapsed lung. It is caused by air escaping the lung and entering into the space between the lung and the chest wall, most often causing only a part of the lung to collapse. At times they occur spontaneously, with no cause noted, from trauma, or from an underlying disease. P-THORAX is a helpful mnemonic to assist you to remember the signs of a pneumothorax.
Pleuritic pain
Trachea deviation
Hyperresonance
Onset sudden
Reduced breath sounds (& dyspnea)
Absent fremitus
X-ray shows collapsed lung

Thrombophlebitis

Thrombophlebitis is the formation of clots within the veins. Inflammation of the vessel walls is also evident during episodes of thrombophlebitis. Thrombophlebitis may occur in superficial veins of the upper and lower extremities. Veins most often affected with thrombophlebitis include the saphenous vein of the lower leg, and the soleal veins of the calves. Thrombophlebitis is a major occurrence among individuals with limited mobility, or individuals who have remained in the same position for an extended period of time (example: long/extensive car or plane ride where the body remains in one position).

Valvular diseases

- Mitral Stenosis: A thickening and contracture of the mitral valve cusps of the heart. This thickening and constriction causes narrowing of the opening of the mitral valve. Produces a resistance to diastolic filling of the left ventricle. The most common cause of mitral stenosis is Rheumatic fever.
- Mitral Insufficiency: An incompetent deformity of the mitral valve. Also termed valvular regurgitation and is characterized by valves that do not close tight enough to hinder blood flow back up into the atrium from the ventricles.
- Aortic Valve Stenosis: A narrowing of the opening between the left ventricle and the aorta. It is the most commonly caused by a genetic disorder, rheumatic fever or atherosclerosis.
- Aortic Insufficiency: Characterized by deformed flaps of the heart valves which prevent proper closure. Without proper closure the blood flows back from the aorta into the left ventricle.
- Tricuspid Stenosis: A restriction of the tricuspid valve.
- Tricuspid Insufficiency: A regurgitation of the blood from the right ventricle to the right atrium which occurs during ventricular systole.

Hiatus hernia

Hiatus hernia is an opening in the diaphragm that becomes enlarged allowing part of the stomach to descend upward into the esophagus. Hiatus hernia causes a reflux of gastric content into the lung, esophagus, and or larynx. A hiatus hernia may or may-not have inflammation. Signs and symptoms of hiatus hernia include but are not limited to heartburn (pyrosis), regurgitation, dysphagia (difficulty swallowing), angina like chest discomfort and pain, bronchospasms, exacerbations of asthma, laryngitis, and chronic cough due to gastric juices entering the oral cavity, and pharynx causing irritation.

Pernicious Anemia

Pernicious Anemia is characterized by a deficiency of vitamin B 12 that results from lack of intrinsic factor in the stomach. Pernicious anemia is a chronic disease that has a slow progression and occurs most often in older adults age fifty and older. Signs and symptoms of pernicious anemia include, but are not limited to numbness and tingling, weakness, sore smooth tongue, dyspnea with exertion, faintness and pallor. Pallor occurs not only in the skin, but the mucous membranes as well. Other symptoms of pernicious anemia include faintness, anorexia, diarrhea, weight loss, and fatigue. Other causes of pernicious anemia include atrophic gastritis, and histamine fast achlorhydria.

Hepatitis Cirrhosis/Portal Hypertension

Portal hypertension or hepatitis cirrhosis is a disruption in the normal configuration of hepatic lobules leading to cell death. Portal hypertension also occurs as obstruction of the portal vein takes place. Portal hypertension is characterized by an increased portal venous pressure greater than 10 mm/Hg that is associated with collateral formation and hyperdynamic circulation. Systems involved with portal hypertension include the gastrointestinal, cardiovascular, and nervous systems. Signs and symptoms include splenomegaly, caput medusa (varicose veins that radiate from the umbilicus), umbilical bruit, hemorrhoids, spider angiomata, gynomastia, testicular atrophy, and digital clubbing. Portal hypertension occurs predominantly in older adult males. Risk factors for portal hypertension include cirrhosis, alcohol use, and abuse, viral hepatitis B, hepatitis C, and hemochromatosis. Treatment includes treating the underlying disease or causative agent. Nutritional and metabolic support is also treatment for portal hypertension. The nurse should monitor for level of consciousness changes as this is the first sign of hepatic encephalopathy.

Cushing's syndrome

Cushing's syndrome is a hyper-function of the adrenal cortex that results in excessive production of glucocorticoids, mineralocorticoids, and androgenic steroids. Systems involved with Cushing's syndrome include the metabolic, endocrine, musculoskeletal, skin, exocrine and cardiovascular. Signs and symptoms of Cushing's syndrome include moon face, increased amounts of adipose (fat) tissue on the neck and trunk, central weight gain, emotional lability, hypertension, osteoporosis, stretch marks (striae), diabetes or glucose intolerance, muscle weakness, easy bruising, and hirsutism (presence of excessive body hair). The nurse should be aware that the diet will include potassium supplements, and high protein.

Acute pancreatitis

Acute pancreatitis is an inflammatory process of the pancreas caused by auto digestion of trypsin. Signs and symptoms of acute pancreatitis include, but are not limited to pain, nausea, and vomiting, intestinal ileus. Other symptoms include epigastric pain that radiates to the back. Nausea and vomiting, fever, shock, hypotension, jaundice, and plural effusions may also be present with acute pancreatitis. Flank discoloration or Grey Turner Sign may be present with acute pancreatitis, and Cullen's sign or umbilical discoloration may also be present. Causes of pancreatitis include gallstones (microlithiasis), alcohol, and trauma, treatment for AIDs, antibiotics, diuretics, and treatments for inflammatory bowel disorders. The nurse should be aware that insulin and steroids have the potential to alter lab results in patients with acute pancreatitis.

The acronym PANCREAS is used to assist with memorization of treatment for acute pancreatitis:

- P: pain control: traditionally Demerol (meperidine) was used, now morphine may be utilized.
- A: arrest and shock will require intravenous (IV) fluids.
- N: nasogastric tube utilization to assist with emesis production and prevent aspiration and irritation
- C: calcium monitoring
- R: renal function evaluation
- E: ensure proper and adequate pulmonary function
- A: antimicrobial therapy
- S: surgical or other procedures to assist with treatment

Bed rest is also recommended for the treatment of acute pancreatitis. Teach mechanisms of positioning with pillows for comfort. Clear liquid diet or NPO may be utilized to treat pancreatitis. TPN may be utilized if unable to consume foods. High protein diets are recommended. Education will need to be done for the disease and the disease process.

Parkinson's disease

Parkinson's disease is a neurological disorder characterized by a lack of dopamine (a neurotransmitter). The deficiency of dopamine may occur related to degeneration, vascular disorders or inflammatory changes. Parkinson's is characterized by rhythmic muscle tremors, rigidity with movement, festination (gait in which the trunk, legs, knees, and hips are flexed, but remain stiff), droopy posture, tremors of the hands, pill rolling may also be present. Other signs and symptoms may include a mask like facial expression, and weight loss. The individual with Parkinson's disease may be unable to enunciate words properly. Treatment for Parkinson's consists of medications, treatment of associated depression, and therapies that will include physical, occupational and speech. Education should be given to the patient related to disease, and disease process. The nurse should explain the benefits of small frequent meals, increased amounts of liquid in the diet and increased fiber in the diet. The nurse should also educate the client on support systems available.

Chronic or wide angle/open angle glaucoma

Chronic open angle glaucoma is characterized by impaired vision that can be related to intraocular tension caused by obstruction of the aqueous humor. Chronic open angle glaucoma is thought to be the second most often cause of blindness in the United States. Signs and symptoms of open angle glaucoma include rapid onset of severe eye pain, blurred vision, seeing rainbows in artificial light, halos around lights, nausea, vomiting, and dilated pupils. Gradual loss of peripheral vision is associated with open angle glaucoma. Tonometry, Gonioscopy and visual field examination are the current diagnostic mechanisms for chronic wide/open angle glaucoma.

Chronic bronchitis

Chronic Bronchitis is an inflammation characterized by an increased amount of bronchial secretions. Chronic bronchitis suffers often present with a chronic productive cough that has lasted a minimum of three months a year for at least two years. Large amounts of respiratory exudates obstruct the bronchioles causing a chronic persistent cough, and shortness of breath. With bronchitis there is hypertrophy of the mucus secreting glands and increased mucous production. Increased mucous production is caused by constant irritation. This chronic irritation causes the death of cilia which in-turn causes the ineffective removal of bacteria leading to respiratory infection. Signs and symptoms of bronchitis include cough, sputum production, and frequent recurring infections of the respiratory tract. Dyspnea, hemoptysis, morning headache, pedal edema, cyanosis, wheezing, weight gain, decreased breath sounds and distant or muffled heart sounds are also signs and symptoms of chronic bronchitis.

COPD

Chronic obstructive pulmonary disease (COPD) is an umbrella term for diseases of the bronchi that cause narrowing, and forced expiration is decreased. Diseases often seen as COPD include bronchitis, asthma, cystic fibrosis, bronchiectasis, and emphysema. The airflow obstruction associated with chronic obstructive pulmonary disease is not reversible. The nurse should include assessments of respiratory status and gas exchange. The nurse should educate the client on proper amounts of rest, energy conservation, and pursed lip breathing. Low rate supplemental oxygen may be utilized, stopping smoking, and avoidance of respiratory irritants should be taught by the nurse.

Emphysema

Emphysema is characterized by destruction of lung tissue related to the continuous overfilling of the alveolar sacs. The cause of emphysema is unknown, but can be associated with smoking, asthma, toxins, air pollutants, and allergens. There is thought to be a familial tendency with emphysema. Signs and symptoms of emphysema include minimal coughing, scant production of sputum, difficult respirations, weight loss that may be significant, occasional or infrequent respiratory infections, barrel chest, slight or minimal wheezing, accessory muscle use with respirations, cyanosis, and diminished breath sounds. The individual with emphysema will need to be educated on the disease the disease process and pursed lipped breathing. Diets with increased amounts of protein and decreased amounts of carbohydrates are often prescribed to assist in maintaining the hypercarbia that often accompanies emphysema.

Prostatectomy and causes of prostate disease

Prostate disease is most often attributed to prosthetic hyperplasia and malignancy of the prostate. Several procedures are done to treat prostate problems; these include:
- Suprapubic prostatectomy: Suprapubic prostatectomy is the removal of the prostate gland via an incision in the bladder. With suprapubic prostatectomy the rate of incontinence is decreased.
- Perineal prostatectomy: Perineal prostatectomy is removal of the prostate gland via an incision in the perineum.
- Transurethral resection: A transurethral resection of the prostate occurs with removal of the gland via the urethra. Incontinence and impotence are often the result of transurethral resection.
- Total prostatectomy: A total prostatectomy is the removal of the prostate gland, and the seminal vesicles. Total prostatectomy will often result in impotence, incontinence and rectal injury.

Gout

Gout is a disorder of altered purine metabolism. Gout occurs most often in men and is characterized by elevated uric acid levels that cause inflammation. Gout accompanies severe arthritis as well. Gout has a sudden onset of crystal deposits and sodium urate in the connective tissues and articular cartilage. Gout has a familial tendency. Systems involved with gout include the musculoskeletal, endocrine, metabolic, and renal. Signs and symptoms of gout include, but are not limited to acute onset of swelling, pain, erythema, to one or more joints. Gout is characterized by soft tissue redness, swelling, and warmth. Tenderness and pain often accompany gout. Gout is a recurring disorder. The nurse should teach the patient to rest the area until the acute phase of the disease subsides. The diet of an individual with gout will be characterized by low fat, low or no alcohol, no sardines, anchovies, liver or sweetbread.

Acute coronary syndromes

Acute coronary syndromes include unstable angina, and myocardial infarction. Acute coronary syndromes develop from a gradual progression of atherosclerotic plaque building up within the vessels. Atherosclerotic plaque buildup may either line the walls of the vessels to cause occlusion of the vessel decreasing or stopping blood flow to certain areas of the heart causing muscle death and damage. Atherosclerotic plaque also causes thrombus development that will occlude vessels and arteries causing ischemia and heart muscle loss and damage. Unstable angina that occurs as a result of occlusion is reversible ischemia. Irreversible ischemia causes myocardial infarction and muscle death and damage. Myocardial infarctions are often fatal.

4Es are a helpful mnemonic to remember common precipitating factors for angina.
Exertion
Eating
Emotional Distress
Extreme Temperature

BOOMAR is a helpful mnemonic to assist you to remember nursing interventions for Myocardial Infarction.
Bed rest
Oxygen therapy
Opioids: morphine
Monitoring: vitals, arterial blood gases, cardiac enzymes, and other blood work
Anticoagulation therapy
Reduce clot size

MONA is a helpful mnemonic to assist you to remember the treatment for Myocardial Infarction (or **ON AM** if you want to remember the correct *order*).
Morphine
Oxygen
Nitroglycerin
Aspirin
The correct order of MONA can be remembered by: ON AM (I am ON fire in the AM as I am a morning person)

Rheumatoid arthritis

Rheumatoid arthritis is characterized by cartilage damage that results from one of three processes:

- Neutrophils, T-Cells (particularly CD4 T cells), and other cells in the synovial fluid become activated, degrading the surface layer of the articular cartilage.
- Cytokines (particularly interleukin-1 (IL-1) and tumor necrosis factor-alpha (TNF-a) cause the chondrocytes to attack the cartilage.
- The synovium digests nearby cartilage, releasing inflammatory molecules containing TNF and IL-l.

These leukocytes may be attracted out of the cell into the synovial fluid of the joints causing inflammation, cartilage and bone deformities, and decreased mobility. The phagocytes of inflammation or the neutrophils and macrophages ingest the immune complexes that are normally part of the protective mechanism of the area and form enzymes that degrade synovial tissue and articular cartilage. This inflammatory process can result in hemorrhage, coagulation, and fibrin deposits within the synovial fluid.

Acute respiratory syndrome

The hallmark of acute respiratory distress syndrome (ARDS) is inflammation of the lungs. Early in acute respiratory distress syndrome the pulmonary neutrophils gather in great amounts at the site of inflammation, intraluminal fibrin and platelets also aggregate at the site of inflammation. Injuries from inflammation lead to edema from capillary leaks. This fluid contains plasma proteins that can inactivate the surfactant of the alveoli and cause lack of elasticity with respiration and lead to alveolar collapse. Fibrin clotting then causes obstructed airspaces. The result is decreased respiratory compliance, decreased function, decreased residual volumes, and dead airspace. The end result for the client is ventilation perfusion mismatching, intrapulmonary shunting, and hypoxemia, thrombus, and hypertension, and death.

Peptic ulcers

A peptic ulcer is a mucosal break, 3 mm or greater in size with depth, that can involve the stomach or duodenum. The most important contributing factors are H pylori, NSAIDs, acid, and pepsin. Additional aggressive factors include smoking, ethanol, bile acids, aspirin, steroids, and stress. Important protective or defensive factors are mucus, bicarbonate, mucosal blood flow, prostaglandins, alkaline tide, hydrophobic layer, restitution, and epithelial renewal. When an imbalance occurs, PUD might develop.

Effects of CHF in children

Impaired myocardial function, tachycardia, fatigue, weakness, restless, pale, cool extremities, decreased BP, decreased urine output, Pulmonary congestion, Tachypnea, dyspnea, respiratory distress, exercise intolerance, cyanosis, Systemic venous congestion, Peripheral and periorbital edema, weight gain, ascites, hepatomegaly, neck vein distention

Management:

- Improve cardiac function (Drugs), Digitalis glycosides improve contractility by increasing force and decreasing rate (indirectly increasing diuresis by improving renal flow), SAFETY-Apical pulse, dosage, signs of toxicity.
- Angiotensin converting enzyme (ACE) inhibitors reduced after load-side effects of hypotension, renal problems, cough, hyperkalemia.
- Monitor BP after, Remove excess fluid and sodium, Diuretics (early in day) Sodium restriction- less often in kids than adults, Possible fluid restriction- rare in infants.
- May decrease potassium, which will enhance digoxin

Iron deficiency anemia

Caused by inadequate supply of dietary iron, Generally preventable
Iron-fortified cereals and formulas for infants, Special needs of premature infants. Adolescents at risk due to rapid growth and poor eating habits. Vegetarian diets must be monitored closely; unrefined cereals modify absorption of minerals and are at risk of rickets and iron def. anemia.

Causes: Inadequate supply of iron-rapid growth, excess milk and delayed solids, poor eating habits, exclusively breast fed after 6 months of age. Impaired absorption-presence of iron inhibitors, malabsorptive disorders, chronic diarrhea, Blood loss-hemorrhage, parasite infection
Excessive demand for iron for growth-prematurity, adolescence, pregnancy

Signs: under weight infants, over weight if too much cow's milk, pale. Poor muscle development, prone to infection, edema, growth retardation, decreased serum pro/gamma globulin/ transferrin, irritability, tachycardia, fatigue, glossitis, koilonychia (spoon fingernails)

Hemolytic-Uremic Syndrome (HUS) in children

During dehydrating, acidosis, hypoxia, temp changes sickling occurs (normally a reversible process until repeated cycles); greater viscosity
Normally trait is asymptomatic but can have gross hematuria, Spleen enlarges (repeated insults can cause a splenic infarction) and nl cells replaced with fibrotic cells unable to fight infection
Liver failure and necrosis from impairment of blood flow; moderate hepatomegaly common by 1y/o; rapid RBC destruction increased gallstones
Kidney-from congestion deg ischemia, hematuria, inability to concentrate urine, enuresis
Bone-hyperplasia and congestion of marrow cause osteoporosis, lordosis, kyphosis, osteomyelitis
CNS-occlusion=CVA (peaks btw 4-6y/o), loss of vision, cognitive impairment
Heart-chronic anemia=cardiomegaly, murmur, Other-exercise intolerance, anorexia, joint pain, jaundice, leg ulcers, growth retardation

Beta Thalassemia

Signs: Anemia, chronic hypoxia (HA, bone pain, decreased exercise tolerance, listlessness, anorexia), small stature, delayed sexual maturation, bronzed/freckled complexion, bone changes as older children if untreated (enlarged head, prominent frontal and parietal bosses and malar eminences, flat or depressed nose bridge, enlarge maxilla, protrusion of lips, oriental appearance of eyes), Anemia, splenic enlargement, hemosiderosis (excess iron storage in organs without tissue injury-prophylactically treat with Desferal), growth retardation and delayed sexual maturation

Nursing management:
- Observe for complications of transfusion
- Emotional support to family
- Encourage genetic counseling
- Parent and patient teaching for self-care

Prognosis:
- Retarded growth
- Delayed or absent secondary sex characteristics
- Expect to live well into adulthood with proper clinical management
- Bone marrow transplant is potential cure

Jaundice

Jaundice is the yellowing of the skin, sclera and mucous membranes when plasma bilirubin levels are elevated above normal.
- Type I - Obstructive Jaundice - This occurs when bile made in the liver fails to reach the intestine due to obstruction of the bile ducts (e.g. by gallstone) or cholestasis. It causes increased levels of conjugated bilirubin and increased urinary bilirubin.
- Type II – Hepatocellular Jaundice - This occurs due to disease of the liver cells such as hepatitis where the liver is unable to utilize the bilirubin, which accumulates in the blood. It results in increased levels of unconjugated bilirubin, which being bound to albumin cannot be excreted in the urine. (since albumin is not filtered at the glomerulus)
- Type III – Hemolytic Jaundice (prehepatic jaundice) - This occurs when there is excessive destruction of RBCs in the blood. This can be due to intrinsic red cell defects or an abnormal red cell environment (e.g. antibodies to red cells). This results in increased bilirubin levels, which is bound to albumin and not excreted in urine.

Thalassemia

Thalassemia:
- Inherited blood disorders of hemoglobin synthesis
- Classified by Hgb chain affected and by amount of effect
- Autosomal recessive with varying expressivity

Pathophysiology:
- Anemia results from defective synthesis of Hgb, structurally impaired RBCs, and shortened life of RBCs
- Chronic hypoxia
- Headache, irritability, precordial and bone pain, exercise intolerance, anorexia, epistaxis

- Detected in infancy or toddlerhood
- Pallor, FTT, hepatosplenomegaly, severe anemia (Hgb <6)

Four types:
- Thalassemia minor—asymptomatic silent carrier
- Thalassemia trait—mild microcytic anemia
- Thalassemia intermediate—moderate to severe anemia + splenomegaly
- Thalassemia major "Cooley's anemia"—severe anemia requiring transfusions to survive

Urine and UTI in children

Normal characteristics of urine:
- Color range - Clear
- Newborn production - approx 1-2 mL/kg/hr
- Child production - approx 1 mL/kg/hr

Classification of UTI:
- Upper tract: involves renal parenchyma, pelvis, and ureters, Typically causes fever, chills, flank pain
- Lower tract: involves lower urinary tract, Usually no systemic manifestations

Types of UTIs:
- Recurrent—repeated episodes
- Persistent—bacteriuria despite antibiotics
- Febrile—typically indicates pyelonephritis
- Urosepsis—bacterial illness; urinary pathogens in blood

Pediatric manifestations:
- Frequency
- Fever in some cases
- Odiferous urine
- Blood or blood-tinged urine
- Sometimes NO symptoms except generalized sepsis

Sickle cell anemia crisis

Precipitating factors:
- Anything that increases body's need for oxygen or alters transport of oxygen. Trauma, Infection, fever, Physical and emotional stress
- Increased blood viscosity due to dehydration, Hypoxia
- From high altitude, poorly pressurized airplanes, hypoventilation, vasoconstriction due to hypothermia

Medical management:
- Diagnosis-sear, sickle-turbidity test, hgb electrophoresis, newborn screening
- Prevent sickling, O2 therapy, Blood transfusions- routine; need chelation therapy to prevent iron overload

- Splenectomy if recurrent splenic sequestration, Bed rest to maximize energy and improve oxygenation
- Analgesics-not Demerol, Blood replacement, Antibiotics, Hydration, Heat to painful areas

Nursing management:
- Monitor child's growth—watch for failure to thrive
- Careful multi-system assessment. Assess pain, Observe for presence of inflammation or possible infection.

Epiglottitis

Epiglottitis is a very dangerous infection of the epiglottis (the flap of tissue that closes off the larynx when one swallows - sometimes visible sticking up behind the tongue as a rounded shape) and the area around the voicebox (larynx) with a bacterial germ. Classically, it was almost always caused by Haemophilus influenzae type B, an aggressive bacterium that used to be responsible for many serious infections in children under the age of five.

Signs/Symptoms:
- Drooling, Sore throat, Difficulty swallowing
- Difficulty breathing (patient may need to sit upright leaning slightly forward to breathe adequately) (Tripod position)
- Stridor (noisy breathing, "crowing" sound when inhaling)
- Hoarseness, Chills, Shaking, Fever, Cyanosis (blue skin coloring)

Hemophilia A and B

Types of Hemophilia:
- Hemophilia A
  - "Classic hemophilia"
  - Deficiency of factor VIII
  - Accounts for 80% of cases of hemophilia
  - Occurrence: 1 in 5000 males
- Hemophilia B
  - Also known as Christmas disease
  - Caused by deficiency of factor IX
  - Accounts for 15% of cases of hemophilia

Manifestations of Hemophilia:
- Bleeding tendencies range from mild to severe
- Symptoms may not occur until 6 months of age
- Mobility leads to injuries from falls and accidents

Necrotizing Enterocolitis

Definition: acute inflammatory disease of the bowel in preterm and high-risk infants.

Factors in development of NEC:
- Prematurity
- Intestinal ischemia
- Colonization of pathogenic bacteria
- Substrate in the intestinal lumen

Diagnostic evaluation:
- X-ray appearance
- Lab studies
- DIC

Therapeutic management of NEC:
- NPO for 24-48 hrs if birth asphyxiated and/or ELBW or VLBW
- Breastmilk is preferred food for po feeds, Contains IgA, macrophages, and lysozymes
- NG tube for decompression, IV antibiotics, parenteral fluids, TPN
- Bowel resection if perforation occurs

Tracheoesophageal fistula

A tracheoesophageal fistula (TEF) is a congenital or acquired communication between the trachea and esophagus. TEFs often lead to severe and fatal pulmonary complications. Most patients with TEFs are diagnosed immediately following birth or during infancy. TEFs are often associated with life-threatening complications, so they are usually diagnosed in the neonatal period. In rare cases, patients with a congenital TEF may present in adulthood.

Signs/Symptoms:
- Cyanosis
- Cough after feeding
- Salivation

Pharyngitis, tonsillitis, and influenza

Pharyngitis:
- Causes and risks- group a Beta-hemolytic strep (GABHS) increased risk for acute rheumatic fever (18 days) and acute glomerulonephritis (10 days)
- Therapeutic management- PCN is DOC

Tonsillitis:
- Pathophysiology and etiology
- Clinical manifestations- inflammation
- Nursing considerations- S/S hemorrhage (swallowing constantly)

Influenza:
- Therapeutic management- Amantadine (type A), Zanamivir and rimantadine Type B
- Prevention- IM vaccines, live nasal spray
- Nursing considerations- most contagious 24 hrs before and after onset of symptoms.

SIADH

Syndrome of Inappropriate Antidiuretic Hormone: SIADH
Produced by hypersecretion of the posterior pituitary (increased ADH)

Signs and symptoms:
- Fluid retention and hypotonicity
- Kidneys unable to reabsorb water
- Anorexia, nausea/vomiting, irritability, personality changes- mainly related to decreased sodium (do not form edema)
- Symptoms disappear when ADH is decreased

Nursing management of SIADH:
- Accurate I&O
- Daily weight
- Observe for signs of fluid overload
- Seizure precautions
- Administer ADH-antagonizing meds

Cleft Lip and/or Cleft Palate

Cleft Lip and/or Cleft Palate:
- Facial malformations that occur during embryonic development
- May appear separately or together

Surgical correction of Cleft Lip:
- Closure of lip defect precedes correction of the palate
- Z-plasty to minimize retraction of scar
- Protect suture line with Logan bow or other methods
- Typically 12-18 months of age
- Effect on speech development

Cleft Lip and Palate Feeding:
- Special feeding equipment
- Breastfeeding issues

Rh positive

The antigens of the Rhesus system are referred to as C,c, D,d, E,e. However, D has the strongest antigenic effect and for simplicity blood whose red blood cells contain the RhD antigen is termed Rh positive, those without RhD are termed Rh negative. Since the D antigen is dominant, Rh positive may mean phenotype DD or Dd.

Cerebral palsy

Cerebrum injury causing multiple nerve function deficits.

Types: Spastic CP 50%, Dyskinetic CP 20%, Mixed CP, Ataxic CP

Symptoms:
- Poor respiration status
- Intellectual disability
- Spasticity
- Speech and language deficits
- Delayed motor and sensory development
- Seizures
- Joint contractions

Tests:
- Sensory and motor skill testing
- Check for spasticity
- CT scan/MRI
- EEG

Treatment:
- PT/OT/ST
- Surgery
- Seizure medications
- Spasticity reducing medication

Phenylketonuria

Phenylketonuria is a genetic disorder related to the synthesis of phenylalanine (Phenylalanine is an essential amino acid required by the body.) As byproducts of phenylalanine accumulate in the brain the individual experiences developmental delays. Phenylketonuria is an autosomal inherited recessive trait. Symptoms of phenylketonuria include urine, and sweat with a musky odor, eczema, failure to thrive, emesis, hyperactivity, altered behavior patterns, convulsions, and developmental delay. The Guthrie test is done on all infants at birth to determine serum phenylalanine levels. Care includes a diet low in phenylalanine to decrease disease progression, and lofenalac is given to infants.

Congenital hypothyroidism

Congenital hypothyroidism occurs due to a defect in the development of the fetal thyroid gland. With congenital hypothyroidism the infant is unable to synthesize thyroxine (Free T-4). Signs and symptoms of congenital hypothyroidism include prolonged jaundice of the neonate; this means longer than the potentially expected 24 hours. Neonates with congenital hypothyroidism experience difficulty feeding, inactivity, constipation, and umbilical hernia. Infants with congenial hypothyroidism have characteristic facial expressions that include eyes that are set widely apart, broad, flat noses, constant tongue protrusion, and coarse, brittle hair with a low hair line, decreased basal metabolism that results in weight gain, delayed dentition, anemia, and developmental delays.

Cystic fibrosis

Cystic fibrosis is a generalized malfunction of the exocrine glands. Individuals with cystic fibrosis will produce excessive amounts of viscous mucous that blocks the respiratory passage ways causing respiratory distress, and failure. Cystic fibrosis is an autosomal-recessive disorder. As the infant ages disease progression causes obstruction of the alveoli and production of atelectasis. The individual will suffer multiple bouts of pneumonia, and right-sided heart failure. The pancreatic ducts may become obstructed as well with tenacious secretions that do not allow for the digestive enzymes (trypsin, lipase, and amylase) to reach the duodenum resulting in impaired fat absorption. The sweat of individuals with cystic fibrosis has increased amounts of sodium and chloride. Individuals with cystic fibrosis may also experience liver failure due to biliary duct obstruction.

Children with cystic fibrosis will require a diet that is high in calories with little protein and fat content. During the summer or hot months and with exercise the child will require increased amounts of sodium, and fluids. The child with cystic fibrosis will need to ingest artificial pancreatic enzymes with each meal as well as the artificial administration of water-soluble vitamins such as vitamin A, C, D, E, and K. The child with cystic fibrosis will require daily pulmonary hygiene. Medications will include bronchodilators and mucolytic agents to assist in the expectoration of the increased amounts of mucous produced. Antibiotics may be routinely or prophylactically prescribed. The goal of the child with cystic fibrosis is to gain weight, maintain patent airway function, and ingest a well balanced diet that accommodates the proper amount of fluids to maintain a well hydrated status.

Blunt force injuries

Blunt force injuries occur from increased amounts of mechanical injury to the body causing tears, shearing, or crushing of tissues.
- Contusion: A contusion more commonly known as a bruise is characterized by bleeding into the skin or underlying tissues as a result of ruptured blood vessels when this skin is crushed or squeezed and not broken. The progressive color changes of bruises or contusions reflect the time or duration of the bruise. Initial contusions begin as red or deep purple areas gradually fade to blue or black, then yellow, green and fading back to normal skin tone. The discoloration relates to the extent of vascular injury.
- Hematoma: A hematoma is characterized by blood that has collected or pooled into the soft tissue of an enclosed space.
- Subdural Hematoma: A subdural hematoma is a pooling or collection of blood between the dura mater and the surface of the brain. Subdural hematomas result from shearing of small veins that connect the subdural space.
- Epidermal Hematoma: An epidermal hematoma is a collection or pooling of blood between the inner surface of the skull and the dura. Epidermal hematomas are the result of arterial tears.

Clinical note: Nurses should document in detail what they see, and not diagnose contusion etc.

Abrasions

An abrasion is the removal of the superficial layers of the skin. Abrasions are caused by friction between the skin and an injuring object. An abrasion can be a fine, thin scratch or a large denuded rash area. An abrasion will initially have a pale, moist, yellow, brown appearance. As the injury dries the area will darken in color and may turn black. Abrasions characteristically ooze fluid on day one and day two of the injury, followed by a dried scab or crust covering the area. As the underlying skin begins to regenerate the scab will flake off. Abrasions may form in the pattern of the offending object.

Lacerations, avulsion, and fracture

Lacerations are tears or rips in the skin that result from ruptured tensile of the skin. Lacerations occur in soft tissue, by blunt trauma. Lacerations characteristically have jagged, and irregular edges. Laceration depth will vary depending on the amount of pressure applied at the time of the tear or rip. Types of lacerations include tears, or accidental cuts. Lacerations are categorized by location; vaginal laceration is an example. An avulsion is a large are of skin that has been torn away or pulled away causing a flap. Avulsions occur related to forced separation of the tissues. Fractures are characteristically blunt force blows or impacts that cause a bone to break or shatter. Fracture means to break.

Fractures

Types of fractures are:
- Pathological fractures: Pathological fractures are breaks at the site of an abnormality. Pathological fractures do not require an extensive amount of force related to the already weakened bone. The most common causes of pathological fractures include tumors, osteoporosis, infection, and metabolic disorders.
- Stress fractures: Stress fractures can occur in normal or abnormal bones. Stress fractures result from repeated stress placed on the bone.
- Transchondral fractures: Transchondral fractures consist of fragmented and separations at portions of a bone or joint. Transchondral fractures frequently involve the cartilage. The most typical sights of transchondral fractures include the distal femur, the ankle, kneecap, elbow and the wrist.
- Oblique fractures: Oblique fractures occur at an oblique angle across both cortices of a bone.
- Open fractures: Open fractures have broken skin and often times have soft tissue trauma.
- Occult fractures: Occult fractures are hidden fractures.
- Segmented fractures: Segmented fractures occur in 2 or more pieces or areas of the bone.

Asphyxial injuries

Asphyxial injuries occur as the result of decreased or no oxygen reaching the cells. Partial or total anoxia may occur with asphyxia. There are four categories of asphyxial injuries:
- Suffocation: Suffocation occurs when oxygen fails to reach the blood. Suffocation can occur from lack of environmental oxygen or blockage of external airways. Normal ambient oxygen is 21% room air. A level of 16% is dangerous for each individual.

- Strangulation: Strangulation is caused by compressing and causing closure of the blood vessels and air passages of the neck by external pressure. Blood flow cessation to the brain is what is occurring with strangulation. Anoxia and hypoxia are the result of strangulation.
- Chemical asphyxia: Chemical asphyxia occurs as the result of chemicals blocking oxygen from the blood or blood vessels, or blocking oxygen from the tissues. Examples of chemical asphyxiate agents include cyanide, and sewer gas.
- Drowning: Drowning results from breathing in fluid and decreasing the amount of oxygen being taken in.

Sharp force injuries

Sharp force injuries occur as the result of cuts or pierces to the skin:
- Incised wounds: Incised wounds are cuts that characteristically have more length than depth. Incised wounds are straight or jagged. Incised wounds typically have more external blood production and very little internal hemorrhage.
- Stab wounds: Stab wounds are penetrating wounds that have more depth than length. The wound characteristically is clear and distinct with very little surrounding tissue damage.
- Puncture wounds: Puncture wounds are made by sharp pointed objects that penetrate the skin. Puncture wounds are typically deep with jagged edges. Infection is a high risk for puncture wounds. The nurse will need to question the individual with a puncture wound about the last tetanus shot they had.
- Chopping wounds: Chopping wounds are made with heavy instruments such as axes, hatchets or propeller blades. Chopping wounds characteristically have sharp and blunt force attributes. Crushing of the underlying tissue often occurs with chopping wounds.

Apoptosis and necrosis

Apoptosis is cell death that occurs as the result of self-destruction of cells. Apoptosis is the natural occurrence of cell death during pregnancy with the embryo, during synaptogenesis, bone cell death during natural turnover, and lymphocyte death. Apoptosis of cells occurs as pre-programmed cell death occurs. Apoptosis is a controlled pattern of cell death. Necrosis is the pathologic death of one or more cells, a portion of tissues, or an organ. Necrosis is irreversible damage to cells, tissues and organs. Inflammatory responses often occur as the result of necrosis. When necrosis occurs there may be swelling, the cells will burst and potentially spill over into surrounding cells.

Burn injury types

The 4 types of burn injury are:
- Thermal burns-can be caused by flame, flash, scald, or contact with hot objects
- Chemical burns-are the result of tissue injury and destruction from necrotizing substances.
- Electrical burns-results from coagulation necrosis that is caused by intense heat from an electrical current
- Smoke & inhalation injury-inhaling hot air or noxious chemicals.

Thermal Burns are the most common type and result from residential fires, automobile accidents, playing with matches, improperly stored gasoline, space heaters, electrical malfunctions, or arson inhaling smoke, steam, dry heat (fire), wet heat (steam), radiation, sun, etc. Two types of chemical burns are acid and alkaline. Acids-can be neutralized and alkaline adheres to tissue, causing protein hydrolyses and liquefaction. Examples are cleaning agents, drain cleaners, and lyes, etc. With chemical burns, tissue destruction may continue for up to 72 hours afterwards.

BURNS acronym

B-*Breathing* - keep airway open. Facial burns, singed nasal hair, hoarseness, sooty sputum, bloody sputum and labored respiration indicate TROUBLE! Body Image- assist Bernie in coping by encouraging expression of thoughts and feelings.

U-*URINE OUTPUT* - in an adult, urine output should be 30-70 cc per hour, in the child 20-50 cc per hour, and in the infant, 10-20 cc per hour. Watch the K+ to keep it between 3.5-5.0 mEq/L. Keep the CVP around 12 cm water pressure!

R-*RESUSCITATION OF FLUID* - Salt & electrolyte solutions are essential over the 1st 24 hours. Maintain B/P at 90-100 systolic. ½ of the fluid for the first 24 hrs should be administered over the first 8 hour period, then the remainder is administered over the next 16 hours. First 24 hour calculation starts at the time of injury.

N-*NUTRITION* - protein & calories are components of the diet! Supplemental gastric tube feedings or hyperalimentation may be used in pts with large burned areas. Daily weights will assist in evaluating the nutritional needs!

S-*SHOCK* - Watch the B/P, CVP, and renal function. Silvadene-for infection.

Electrical burns

Injury from electrical burns results from coagulation necrosis that is caused by intense heat generated from an electric current and can cause tissue anoxia and death. The severity depends on amount of voltage, tissue resistance, current pathways, and surface area in contact with the current and length of time the current flow was sustained.

Electrical injury can cause:
- Fractures of long bones and vertebra
- Cardiac arrest or arrhythmias--can be delayed 24-48 hours after injury
- Severe metabolic acidosis--can develop in minutes
- Myoglobinuria--acute renal tubular necrosis- myoglobin released from muscle tissue whenever massive muscle damage occurs--goes to kidneys--and can mechanically block the renal tubules due to the large size.

Treatment of electrical burns:
Fluids--Ringers lactate or other fluids-flushes out kidneys--you want 75-100 cc/hr until urine sample clear an osmotic diuretic (Mannitol) may be given to maintain urine output.

Layers of skin damaged by burns

3 layers of the skin that can be damaged with burn are the:
- Epidermis-nonvascular outer layer of skin--thick as a sheet of paper.
- Dermis--30-45 x's thicker than epidermis. Consists of: connective tissue with blood vessels, hair follicles, nerve endings, sweat glands, sebaceous glands
- Subcutaneous Tissue- Contains major vesicular networks, fat, nerves, and lymphatics

The functions of the skin are as follows:
- Maintenance of body temperature
- Prevents evaporative water loss
- Produces vitamin D
- Protection from invading organisms
- Protection against the environment through the sensations of touch, pressure, and pain
- Cosmetic appearance

Burn wounds occur when there is contact between tissue and an energy source, such as heat, chemicals, electrical current, or radiation.

Smoke and inhalation injury

Smoke and inhalation injury can damage the tissues of the respiratory tract. Although damage to the respiratory mucosa can occur, it seldom happens because the vocal cords and glottis close as a protective mechanism.

Three types of smoke and inhalation injuries
- Carbon monoxide poisoning (CO poisoning and asphyxiation count for majority of deaths). Treatment- 100% humidified oxygen-draw carboxyhemoglobin level- can occur without any burn injury to the skin.
- Inhalation injury above the glottis (caused by inhaling hot air, steam, or smoke.) Mechanical obstruction can occur quickly. Watch for facial burns, signed nasal hair, hoarseness, painful swallowing, and darkened oral or nasal membranes
- 3. Inhalation injury below glottis. (above glottis-injury is thermally produced). Below glottis-it is usually chemically produced. Amount of damage related to length of exposure to smoke or toxic fumes. Can appear 12-24 hours after burn

Care of major and minor burns

Care of major burns:
- Primary excision-reduces rate of infection
- Debridement- promotes healing
- Topical antimicrobial agents
- Biologic skin coverings
- Allograft (human cadaver skin)
- Xenograft (porcine skin)
- Synthetic skin substitutes
- Split-thickness skin grafts (sheet or mesh graft)

Care of minor burns:
- Wound cleansing
- Debridement
- Controversy: removal of blisters
- Dressings

Controversy: cover wound with antimicrobial ointment or use of occlusive dressings

4 degrees of burn injury

Extent of injury described as TBSA (total body surface area)—use age-related charts

Depth of injury:
- 1st degree—superficial
- 2nd degree—partial thickness
- 3rd degree—full thickness
- 4th degree—full thickness + underlying tissue

Severity of injury- 10% of total surface area burned in school age child or younger may be fatal.

Complications of burn injuries:
- Immediate threat of airway compromise
- Profound shock
- Infection (local and systemic sepsis)
- Inhalation injuries, aspiration, pulmonary edema, pulmonary embolus.
- Tetanus if not UTD

Rule of nines

In adults, the "rule of nines" is used to determine the total percentage of area burned for each major section of the body. For children and infants, the Lund-Browder chart is used to assess the burned body surface area. Different percentages are used because the ratio of the combined surface area of the head and neck to the surface area of the limbs is typically larger in children than that of an adult.

Adults:
Anatomic Structure / Surface Area
Head and neck / 9%
Anterior torso / 18%
Posterior torso / 18%
Each leg / 18%
Each arm / 9%
Genitalia-perineum / 1%

Children:
Anatomic structure/Surface area
Head and neck / 18%

Anterior torso / 18%
Posterior torso / 18%
Each leg / 13.5%
Each arm / 9%
Genitalia-perineum / 1%

The rule of nines allows for the determination of the area of the body affected by a burn or burns to be determined. The body is categorized into percent as follows; the arms from shoulder to finger tips are 4.5 percent each, the torso (anterior and posterior) is 18 percent, the legs are each 9 percent, and the head is 4.5 percent. The posterior torso includes the buttocks in the 18 percent, while the anterior torso does not include the groin area. The anterior groin area is designated as 1 percent. A patient who has experienced a burn will require an increased number of kilocalories daily. To calculate the daily requirements of kilocalories for a burn patient add 25 kilocalories times the kg of normal body weight of the individual and 40 kilocalories times the percentage of total body surface area burned; this is referred to as the Curreri formula for adults with burns.

Phases of burn management

The three phases of burn management are emergent (resuscitative), acute, and rehabilitative.

Emergent phase
The emergent phase, (resuscitative phase) lasts from onset to 5 or more days but usually lasts 24-48 hours begins with fluid loss and edema formation and continues until fluid motorization and diuresis begins. The greatest initial threat is hypovolemic shock to a major burn patient. Arrhythmias, hypovolemic shock which may lead to irreversible shock circulation to limbs can be impaired by circumferential burns and then the edema formation. Escharotomies (incisions through eschar) done to restore circulation to compromised extremities.
Vulnerable to 2 types of injury:
- Upper airway burns that cause edema formation & obstruction of the airway
- Inhalation injury can show up 24 hrs later-watch for resp. distress such as increased agitation or change in rate or character of resp.

Pneumonia is a common complication of major burns. Most common renal complication of burns in the emergent phase is ATN. Because of hypovolemic state, blood flow decreases, causing renal ischemia. If it continues, acute renal failure may develop.

Acute phase
The acute phase begins with mobilization of extracellular fluid and subsequent diuresis. Is concluded when the burned area is completely covered or when wounds are healed. May take weeks or months., Pt is no longer grossly edematous due to fluid mobilization, full & partial thickness burns more evident, bowel sounds return, pt more aware of pain and condition.

Complications of acute phase:
- Infection due to destruction of body's 1st line of defense.
- Partial thickness wounds can convert to full-thickness wounds with infection present.

- 248 -

- Patient may get sepsis from wound infections. Signs of sepsis are: high temp., increased pulse & resp., decreased BP, and decreased urinary output, mild confusion, chills, malaise, and loss of appetite.

WBC bet. 10,000 and 20,000. Infections usually gram neg. bacteria (pseudomonas, proteus) Obtain cultures from all possible sources: IV, foley, wound, oropharynx, and sputum ROM limited, contractures can occur, Gastrointestinal-adynamic ileus results from sepsis, diarrhea or constipation (RT narcotics & decreased mobility), gastric ulcers RT stress, occult blood in stools possible, Endocrine-stress DM might occur-assess glucose prn

Predominant therapeutic interventions are:
- Fluid replacement, physical therapy, wd care, early excision and grafting, and pain management
- Fluid replacement continues from emergent phase to acute phases--given for: fluid losses, administer medications, & for transfusions.
- Physical therapy- to maintain optimal joint function
- Pain management- most critical functions as a nurse.
- Nutritional therapy-provide adequate proteins & calories
- Wound Care- the goals are cleanse and debride the area of necrotic tissue &debris, minimize further damage to viable skin, promote patient comfort, & reepithelialization or success with skin grafting.
- Care for donor site and other grafts necessary
- Excision and grafting-eschar removed to subcutaneous tissue or fascia, graft applied to tissue
- Cultured epithelial autograft (CEA) uses patient's own cells to grow skin-permanent
- Artificial skin is the latest trend. Examples: Alloderm, Life-Skin, etc.

In assessing the pain, the acronoym PQRST can help to assess/evaluate.
What **P**rovokes the pain?
What is the **Q**uality of the pain?
Does the pain **R**adiate?
What is the **S**everity of the pain?
What is the **T**iming of the pain?

Rehabilitation phase
The rehabilitation phase is defined as beginning when the patient's burn wound is covered with skin or healed and patient is capable of assuming some self-care activity. This can occur as early as 2 weeks to as long as 2-3 months after the burn injury. The goals for this time is to assist patient in resuming functional role in society & accomplish functional and cosmetic reconstruction.
Clinical Manifestations: Heals by primary intention or by grafting. Scars may form & contractures. Mature healing is reached in 6 months to 2 years. Avoid direct sunlight for 1 year on burn, new skin sensitive to trauma
Complications: Most common complications of burn injury are skin and joint contractures and hypertrophic scarring.
Because of pain, pts will assume flexed position. It predisposes wds to contracture formation. Use of physical therapy, pressure garments, splints, etc. are used.
Nursing management during rehabilitation phase: Must be directed to returning patient to society, address emotional concerns, spiritual and cultural needs, self-esteem, teaching of

wound care management, nutrition, role of exercises and physical therapy explained. A common emotional response seen is regression.

Degree of burns and nutritional goals of burns

First degree burns include only the epidermal (outer-superficial) layer of skin. No scaring is formed with first degree burns. First degree burns normally heal within 5 to 7 days. Second degree burns can take several months to heal and do form scar tissue as the healing process takes place. Second degree burns include both the epidermis and dermal layers of skin. Third degree burns involve the complete epidermis, the dermis, and often include destruction to the subcutaneous tissue, muscle or bone. Third degree burns are treated by grafting skin from other parts of the body as they do not heal. The desired nutritional outcome of burns is to maintain fluid and electrolyte balances, maintain a caloric intake to prevent a weight reduction of greater than ten percent, ensure protein intake is adequate to maintain a positive nitrogen balance for maintenance as well as replenishing visceral protein stores lost with the burn. When determining the nutritional caloric intake the size of the burn is fundamental.

Hyponatremia, hypernatremia, hyperkalemia, and hypokalemia related to wound care

Hyponatremia can occur due to silver nitrate topical ointments as a result of sodium loss through eschar, hydrotherapy, excessive GI drainage, diarrhea, or excessive water intake. Signs and symptoms of hyponatremia include weakness, dizziness, muscle cramps, fatigue, HA, tachycardia, and confusion. Hypernatremia can occur from too much hypertonic fluids, improper tube feedings, or inappropriate fluid administration. Signs and symptoms of Hypernatremia include thirst, dried furry tongue, lethargy, confusion, and possible seizures. Hyperkalemia is noted if pt is in renal failure, adrenocortical insufficiency, or massive deep muscle injury with large amounts of potassium released from damaged cells. Cardiac arrhythmias and ventricular failure can occur if K+ level greater >7mEq/L. muscle weakness & EKG changes are noted. Hypokalemia is noted with silver nitrate therapy and long hydrotherapy. Other causes include vomiting, diarrhea, prolonged GI suction, or prolonged IV therapy without K+ supplementation. Constant K+ losses occur through the burn wound.

Whirlpool treatment for wound healing

The effects of whirlpool treatment on wound healing are as follows:
- Warm water increases vasodilatation of the superficial vessels
- Increased blood flow brings oxygen and nutrients to the tissues and removes metabolites
- Increased blood flow brings antibodies, leukocytes and systemic antibiotics
- Fluid shifts into the interstitial spaces leading to edema
- Softening and loosening of necrotic tissue aides phagocytosis
- Cleansing and removal of wound exudate controls infection
- Mechanical effects of whirlpool stimulate granulation tissue formation
- Sedation and analgesia are induced by the warm water

The best types of wounds for whirlpool are those that fall into the categories of:
- Necrotic
- Moderate to heavy exudative wounds
- Wounds with debris
- Tissue which can tolerate moderate to heavy increased circulatory perfusion

The following are conditions that you would not want to use whirlpool treatment with:
- Edema of the extremity
- Lethargy
- Unresponsiveness
- Maceration
- Upper extremity infection
- Febrile conditions
- Compromised cardiovascular or pulmonary function
- Acute phlebitis
- Renal failure
- Dry gangrene - evaluate for ischemia
- Incontinence of urine or feces, if in full body whirlpool

Vacuum-assisted wound closure

Vacuum-assisted closure, also known as negative wound pressure therapy, is a technique designed to promote the formation of granulation tissue in the wound bed either as an adjunct to surgical therapy, or as an alternative to surgery in a debilitated patient. In this system, a special foam dressing with an attached evacuation tube is inserted into the wound and covered with an adhesive drape in order to create an airtight seal. Negative pressure is applied and the wound effluent is collected in a canister. Although the exact mechanism is not known, it is hypothesized that negative pressure contributes to wound healing by removing excess interstitial fluid thereby reducing edema and increasing vascularity of the wound and creating force to draw the edges of the wound closer together.

Dialysis

The two types of dialysis are hemodialysis and peritoneal dialysis. In hemodialysis, the patient's blood is passed through a tube into a machine that filters out waste products. The cleansed blood is then returned to the body. In peritoneal dialysis, a special solution is run through a tube into the peritoneal cavity, the abdominal body cavity around the intestine. The fluid is left there for a while to absorb waste products, and then removed through the tube.

There are three types of peritoneal dialysis. Continuous ambulatory peritoneal dialysis (CAPD), the most common type, needs no machine and can be done at home. Continuous cyclic peritoneal dialysis (CCPD) uses a machine and is usually performed at night when the person is sleeping. Intermittent peritoneal dialysis (IPD) uses the same type of machine as CCPD, but is usually done in the hospital because treatment takes longer. Prior to any peritoneal dialysis, a catheter is placed in the patient's abdomen, running from the peritoneum out to the surface, near the navel. This is done as a short surgery.

Peritoneal dialysis

The most common form of PD, continuous ambulatory peritoneal dialysis (CAPD), doesn't require a machine. As the word ambulatory suggests, you can walk around with the dialysis solution in your abdomen. Other forms of PD require a machine called a cycler to fill and drain your abdomen, usually while you sleep. The different types of cycler-assisted PD are sometimes called automated peritoneal dialysis, or APD.

Methods of oxygen delivery

There are two types of devices – variable performance devices and fixed performance devices. The differentiation is based on the difference between the delivered concentration of oxygen FdO_2 and the actual inspired concentration FiO_2. Variable performance devices fit into two categories, nasal cannula and facemasks. The premise behind nasal cannula is to use the dead space of the nasopharynx as a reservoir for oxygen. When the patient inspires, entrained air mixes with the reservoir air and the inspired gas is enriched. Obviously, the FiO_2 depends on the magnitude of flow of oxygen, the patient's minute ventilation and peak flow. Standard oxygen masks provide a reservoir for oxygen, but the FiO_2 is difficult to calculate unless calibrated Venturi devices are attached. With Venturis, there are slits in the oxygen delivery system which become smaller or larger depending whether a high or low FiO_2 is required. The rate of delivery of oxygen is calibrated for the size of the Venturi and amount of mixing therein.

Hyperbaric oxygen therapy

Hyperbaric oxygen therapy (HBOT) is the process whereby the patient breathes 100% oxygen in a room or chamber that is pressurized at a level greater than sea level (sea level represents one atmosphere absolute). It is a systemic therapy in which increased levels of oxygen are absorbed through the lungs. It is not a topical therapy. HBOT increases the amount of dissolved oxygen in the blood plasma which in turn delivers increased concentrations of oxygen to all areas of the body perfused by blood plasma.

The Undersea and Hyperbaric Society approved the use HBOT as a primary treatment for three conditions: air or gas embolism, decompression sickness, and carbon monoxide poisoning. It also approved it as a secondary form of treatment for the following conditions: radiation tissue damage (soft tissue and osteoradionecrosis), gas gangrene, compromised skin grafts and flaps, necrotizing soft tissue infections (subcutaneous, muscle, fascia), crush injury, compartmental syndrome, acute traumatic ischemias, chronic refractory osteomyelitis, and problem non-healing wounds.

NCLEX Test Question Strategies

Sometimes when you are testing, you may know an answer immediately on reading the choices. Other times, you may need to choose an answer without being certain. In those situations, here are some tips to help you eliminate the answer choices most likely to be incorrect. Use these strategies to dissect complex nursing questions and improve your NCLEX test taking skills.

Do NOT select an answer choice that:
- Asks "**Why**?"
- Requires you to **speculate** or read extra information into the question that isn't there.
- Is based on a scenario you may have seen at **work** or in **clinicals**; instead focus only on the information you are given.
- **Degrades** the patient, a nurse, or a colleague.
- Involves bringing up potentially **controversial** material.
- Goes against a **general rule**.
- Involves **leaving** the patient, unless absolutely necessary.
- Tries to **persuade** the patient to make a choice or agree with something; instead look for answers that are associated with **caring** about the client's feelings.
- Tells the patient not to **worry**; this minimizes the patient's concerns and feelings.
- Tries to avoid **responsibility** or passes it to someone else.
- Is **unreasonable** or under normal circumstances could/should not be done.
- Involves "**doing nothing**" or "waiting" for an unspecified period of time unless you are absolutely certain it is the best option.
- Makes **absolute** statements involving words like always, never, or must.
- Only cites a **hospital rule** for its rationale. If the hospital has a rule about something, there will be an **underlying reason**, usually patient **safety** or hospital **liability**, which you should be aware of.
- You have never heard of or are **unfamiliar** with.

Additionally, if 2 answers are exact **opposites** of each other, one of them is likely correct. If 2 or more answers are **similar**, likely none of them is correct.

If you are asked to pick which nursing action to take next, remember that every answer choice listed could be a correct action to take, but the question is asking for the **highest priority action**.

Practice Test

Practice Questions

1. A client has received 10 mg of morphine sulfate subcutaneously. When does the nurse anticipate the maximal period of respiratory depression will occur?
    a. 7 minutes
    b. 30 minutes
    c. 60 minutes
    d. 90 minutes

2. How many hours of activity per day are necessary to prevent disuse syndrome with muscle atrophy and joint contracture?
    a. 6 hours
    b. 4 hours
    c. 2 hours
    d. 1 hour

3. The nurse is one of the first on the scene of a bus accident and is triaging injured riders. **Place the following injured clients (Roman numerals) into the correct triage classification.**
    I. 40-year-old woman with arterial bleed
    II. 20-year-old male with sprained wrist, small cuts, and bruises
    III. 14-year-old female with severe crush injuries to the head and chest and dilated, non-responsive pupils
    IV. 56-year-old male with fractured femur

Minor injury (Ambulatory injured)	Immediate care	Delayed care	Unsalvageable
a.	b.	c.	d.

4. A client nearing death has an Advance Directive in his records indicating that he does not want intravenous fluids or other invasive procedures, but the client's physician has ordered IV fluids. Which of the following initial actions by the nurse is **most** appropriate?
    a. Notify the bioethics committee.
    b. Inform the physician of the Advance Directive regarding intravenous fluids.
    c. Administer intravenous fluids.
    d. Contact a supervisor to resolve the issue.

5. A client has been instructed in the application and use of anti-embolic compression stockings. Which of the following statements by the client indicates a need for more teaching? **Select all that apply.**
    a. "After I apply the stocking, I roll the top back down about 2 inches to hold the stockings in place."
    b. "I remove the stocking and reapply about every day or two."
    c. "To apply, I turn the stocking inside out while holding onto the toe."
    d. "I apply a small amount of baby powder to my legs before applying the stockings."
    e. "These stockings help prevent blood clots."

6. A client with a demand pacemaker complains that he has developed persistent chronic hiccupping and is experiencing mild discomfort in the chest. Which of the following causes does the nurse suspect?
  a. Pacemaker syndrome
  b. Dislocation of a lead
  c. Esophageal reflux
  d. Myocardial infarction

7. Which of the following are common neurological changes associated with aging? **Select all that apply.**
  a. Dementia occurs.
  b. Threshold for sensory input increases.
  c. Perspiration is reduced.
  d. Short-term memory is impaired.
  e. Muscles atrophy.

8. When examining an 80-year-old client with chronic COPD receiving home health care, the nurse notes that over the previous 48 hours the client has developed scattered painful pustular lesions on the right arm near the elbow (see photo), on the back of the neck, the face, and on both legs.

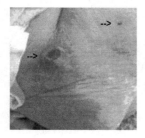

Which of the following does the nurse suspect is the **most** likely cause of the lesions?
  a. Psoriasis
  b. Herpes zoster
  c. MRSA
  d. Contact dermatitis

9. A Turkish-speaking client is scheduled for a colonoscopy, and the nurse must provide printed directions to the client, but directions are not available in Turkish. Which of the following is **most** appropriate?
  a. The nurse contacts a medical translator to translate.
  b. The client's 10-year-old daughter translates the directions.
  c. The nurse draws pictures and pantomimes directions.
  d. Client's daughter is advised to tell her parent to seek a translator.

10. While a dosage of oral morphine has approximately 25% bioavailability, what percentage is the bioavailability of an intravenous dose of morphine? **Record your answer using a whole number.**

11. The nurse is teaching the mother of a newborn to care for the umbilical cord. What should the nurse advise the mother to do if the cord becomes soiled with urine or feces?
    a. Swab with alcohol.
    b. Wipe with a dry cloth.
    c. Wash with mild soap and water, rinse and dry.
    d. Swab with povidone-iodine.

12. A client is in acute postoperative pain, and the physician orders 85 mg of meperidine (Demerol®) stat. The vial contains 100 mg in 2 mL. How many milliliters should the nurse administer? **Record your answer using a decimal number.**

13. The physician has ordered that a client recovering from back surgery be logrolled. The client has a draw sheet in place, and the nurse and an assistant are positioned with one on each side of the bed. **Place the steps to logrolling (Roman numerals) in the correct sequence from first to last.**
    I. Grasping draw sheet at shoulder and lower hips, roll patient on count of three.
    II. Place a small pillow between client's knees.
    III. Place pillows along length of client's back.
    IV. Cross client's arms across chest.
    a. (First)
    b. (Second)
    c. (Third)
    d. (Fourth)

14. The physician has ordered that a 132-pound client with increased intracranial pressure receive 0.5 g of mannitol per kg in an IV solution. How many grams should be in the total mannitol dose? **Record your answer using a whole number.**

15. When applying the leads for a 12-lead electrocardiogram, the nurse places V1 and V2 at the fourth intercostal space to the right and left of the sternum. Which of the remaining leads is placed at the fifth intercostal space on the left midclavicular line?
    a. Lead V3
    b. Lead V4
    c. Lead V5
    d. Lead V6

16. A client is recovering from a stroke and the nurse is doing range-of-motion exercises. Which movements should be included for ROM of the elbow on the weak side? **Select all that apply.**
    a. Abduction and adduction
    b. Hyperextension
    c. Supination and pronation
    d. Flexion and extension
    e. Rotation

17. The nurse is assisting a client to adjust crutches to the proper measurement. With the client in standing position, where should the tips of the crutches be placed?
    a. 2 to 3 inches directly to the side of the client's legs
    b. 4 to 6 inches to the side of the client's legs and 4 to 6 inches in front of feet
    c. 2 to 3 inches to the side of the client's legs and 4 to 6 inches in front of feet
    d. 4 to 6 inches directly to the side of the client's legs

18. A client who is very confused removed a diamond ring and threw it on the floor. Which of the following is the **most** appropriate action?
    a. Give the ring to a visiting granddaughter for safekeeping.
    b. Place the ring in the client's bedside stand in an envelope clearly marked "Valuables."
    c. Replace the ring on the client's finger.
    d. Place the ring in a secured container, according to organizational policy.

19. If the first day of a pregnant woman's last menstrual period fell on May 1, 2013, what is the expected delivery month and year? **Record your answer using the month (word) and year (whole number).**

20. Twenty micrograms (µg) are equal to how many milligrams? **Record your answer using a decimal number.**

21. A physician orders chest physiotherapy for a 4-year-old child with cystic fibrosis, but the respiratory therapists are off duty, so the physician tells the nurse to do the therapy. The nurse, however, rarely works in pediatrics, has never done chest physiotherapy, and does not know the procedure. Which of the following is the **most** appropriate response by the nurse?
    a. Ask the child's mother to explain the procedure.
    b. Check the procedure manual and attempt to do the therapy.
    c. Refuse to do the procedure.
    d. Advise the physician that the nurse will try to locate another staff person knowledgeable about chest physiotherapy.

22. A pregnant woman has experienced repeated vaginal monilial infections. When educating the client about the infection, which information should the nurse include? **Select all that apply.**
    a. Advise client to bathe daily.
    b. Explain the effects of increased estrogen production.
    c. Advise client to wear cotton panties and avoid nylon or pantyhose.
    d. Suggest client use panty liners to protect clothing.
    e. Advise the client to avoid wearing any panties.

23. When drawing up a dosage of subcutaneous heparin, how much air should be drawn into the syringe after the correct dosage is obtained?
    a. 1 mL
    b. 0.6 mL
    c. 0.2 to 0.3 mL
    d. 0.01 mL

24. Lochia serosa usually is evident on days 4 to 10 postpartum. When teaching the client about postpartum care, how should the nurse describe lochia serosa?
   a. Dark red discharge with small clots
   b. Yellowish discharge
   c. Pinkish to brownish discharge
   d. Clear watery discharge

25. The Z-track injection technique should be used with which of the following? **Select all that apply**.
   a. Iron
   b. Haloperidol
   c. Heparin
   d. Hydroxyzine (Vistaril®)
   e. Insulin

26. A Mexican-American client states that she and her family live next door to her brother and his family and that they share goods, services, and childcare. How is this type of family classified?
   a. Nuclear
   b. Dual career/dual earner
   c. Extended
   d. Extended kin network

27. The physician has ordered sublingual nitroglycerin for a client. Which of the following are contraindications for administration of sublingual or buccal medications? **Select all that apply.**
   a. Client is edentulous.
   b. Client has mild dementia.
   c. Mucous membranes are red and irritated.
   d. Client is dehydrated.
   e. Client has productive aphasia.

28. The nurse is teaching a new breastfeeding mother about breast care, but the mother has engorgement and asks if she should quit breastfeeding. Which information should the nurse include? **Select all that apply.**
   a. "Continue to nurse every 2 to 3 hours."
   b. "Gently massage the breast toward the nipple while breastfeeding."
   c. "Apply hot compresses to the breast."
   d. "Acetaminophen or ibuprofen is safe to use to relieve pain."
   e. "Engorgement usually recedes in 24 to 48 hours."

29. When administering a capsule that is individually wrapped to a client, when should the wrapping be removed?
   a. When initially obtained from the medicine cart
   b. When placed in the medicine cup
   c. Prior to entering the client's room
   d. At bedside in the client's presence

30. Which of the following are important factors in facilitating attachment between a newborn and mother?
    a. Rooming in
    b. Swaddling and holding the infant
    c. Knowledge of childcare
    d. Beginning breastfeeding within 24 hours of birth

31. Which of the following are controlled substances (Schedules I through V) regulated by the Drug Enforcement Agency (DEA)? **Select all that apply.**
    a. Codeine
    b. Ibuprofen
    c. Diphenhydramine (Benadryl®)
    d. Hydrocodone

32. Which of the following ethnic groups has the highest risk of developing diabetes mellitus type 2 and should be routinely screened for diabetes?
    a. Hispanics
    b. Asians
    c. Caucasians
    d. African-Americans

33. A hospice client is receiving high doses of opioid analgesia and is exhibiting nocturnal myoclonus with restless leg movement and involuntary jerking. Which of the following responses would the nurse expect?
    a. Discontinue opioids.
    b. Reduce dosage by half and administer a benzodiazepine.
    c. Administer naloxone.
    d. Administer flumazenil.

34. A 16-year-old female has been sexually active for two years but was recently treated for a gonorrhea infection. The nurse is teaching the adolescent about safe sex practices. Which of the following statements by the adolescent indicate a need for more information? **Select all that apply.**
    a. "I'm never going to have sex again until I'm married, so I don't need to know about safe sex!"
    b. "I should never have any kind of sex unless my partner wears a condom."
    c. "We don't need to use a condom for oral sex."
    d. "I'm confused about different birth control methods."
    e. "Birth control pills are more effective than diaphragms."

35. A client receiving high doses of hydromorphone (Dilaudid®) develops acute respiratory depression with a drop in blood pressure. Which of the following treatments is most indicated?
    a. Naloxone
    b. Naproxen
    c. Flumazenil
    d. Nortriptyline

36. A 20-year-old client has taken forty 500-mg tablets of acetaminophen with 4 ounces of alcohol in a suicide attempt. The client is **most** at risk for which of the following?
   a. Gastrointestinal hemorrhage
   b. Respiratory depression
   c. Liver failure
   d. Brain damage

37. A client with bipolar disorder is taking lithium to control symptoms. Which of the following statements indicates the need for further education?
   a. "I need to have regular tests for thyroid function."
   b. "Once I'm stabilized, I won't need further testing."
   c. "I should avoid taking ibuprofen."
   d. "It's important for me to avoid dehydration."

38. Which of the following antibiotics is contraindicated in children younger than 8 years?
   a. Tetracycline
   b. Augmentin
   c. Azithromycin
   d. Amoxicillin

39. A nurse notes that clients of one surgeon have developed at least twice as many infections as clients of other surgeons on the unit. Which of the following is the **most** appropriate action?
   a. Report the physician to the hospital administration.
   b. Ask the physician why his rate of infections is so high.
   c. Report the observations to the infection control nurse.
   d. Say nothing as infection rates vary from time to time.

40. Which type of laxative agent is usually the safest for most people?
   a. Bulk laxatives
   b. Stool softeners
   c. Stimulants
   d. Osmotics/saline

41. A client who has denied drug allergies has a telephone order for IM penicillin. Before the nurse administers the medication, the client states he thinks he may have developed a rash after "some drug." Which is the correct action?
   a. Administer the drug and document a possible previous drug reaction.
   b. Hold the drug and contact the prescribing physician.
   c. Contact the pharmacist for guidance.
   d. Contact the supervisor for guidance.

42. Which of the following blood products is indicated for a client with disseminated intravascular coagulation (DIC) to control bleeding where replacement of coagulation factors is necessary?
   a. Whole blood
   b. Irradiated red blood cells
   c. Fresh frozen plasma
   d. Platelets (multiple donors)

43. A client has requested pain medication, but after the nurse obtains the prescribed dose of codeine from the dispensing cart, the client refuses to take the medication, stating he might want it later. What should the nurse do with the medication?
    a. Return it to the dispensing cart.
    b. Leave it at the client's bedside.
    c. Dispose of the medication according to facility protocol with two appropriate witnesses.
    d. Place the medication in a tray for later use.

44. With a drop factor of 15 drops per 1 mL, what drip rate should the nurse set to deliver 1000 mL of intravenous D5W in 3 hours and 20 minutes? **Record your answer using a whole number.**

45. A client with vaginal cancer is being treated with brachytherapy, and the nurse is explaining the procedure and precautions to the client. Which of the following information should the nurse include?
    a. "Women who are pregnant and children under age 18 may not visit."
    b. "Visitors should stay at least 2 feet away from the client."
    c. "You can only leave your room for 5 to 10 minutes per day."
    d. "Visitors can stay no more than 4 hours per day."

46. When preparing to do a sterile dressing change, the nurse places sterile gauze pads on the sterile field but inadvertently touches the sterile field with an ungloved hand. Which of the following should the nurse do next?
    a. Use only gauze pads from the sterile field away from the contaminated area.
    b. Discard the gauze pads and sterile field and start over.
    c. Continue with dressing change, as the gauze pads were not contaminated.
    d. Place a new sterile field and using sterile gloves take gauze pads from the contaminated field and place on the new field.

47. If a medication is available at 100 mg per 10 mL, how many milliliters does a dose of 120 mg require? **Record your answer using a whole number.**

48. A client comes to the doctor's office with a first-degree sprained ankle. Which of the following treatments does the nurse anticipate?
    a. Cast
    b. Splint
    c. RICE (rest, ice, compression, elevation)
    d. Surgical repair

49. While observing the team leader irrigating a PICC line, a new nurse notes that the team leader has broken aseptic technique and contaminated the irrigating syringe. Which of the following actions is **most** appropriate?
    a. Report the team leader to a supervisor.
    b. Ask the team leader after the irrigation if sterile technique was required.
    c. Say nothing because the new nurse is inexperienced.
    d. Tell the team leader immediately that the irrigating syringe was contaminated.

50. A client has experienced a cardiac arrest at an office visit and the nurse is going to administer defibrillation with an automated external defibrillator (AED). Which of the following should the nurse remove prior to administering a shock?
    a. Client's watch
    b. Client's bra with metal wires
    c. Client's dentures
    d. Client's nose ring

51. A 60-kg adult is to receive a medication that is administered at 0.5 mg per kg per 24 hours. If the medication is given in 2 equal doses (every 12 hours), how many milligrams should be in each dose? **Record your answer using a whole number.**

52. A client receiving digoxin exhibits tachycardia and complains of headache and fatigue, nausea, diarrhea, and halo vision. Which of the following is probably the cause?
    a. Digoxin dosage too low
    b. Allergic response to digoxin
    c. Digoxin toxicity
    d. Disorder unrelated to digoxin

53. When teaching a client with a seizure disorder about long-term use of phenytoin, the nurse should stress the necessity for which of the following? **Select all that apply.**
    a. Dental care
    b. Hearing examinations
    c. Vitamin D therapy and evaluation for osteoporosis
    d. Drug compliance
    e. Regular exercise

54. A client is taking the loop diuretic furosemide for edema associated with heart failure. Which electrolyte imbalance resulting from the medication is of **most** concern?
    a. Hypokalemia
    b. Hyperkalemia
    c. Hypercalcemia
    d. Hypocalcemia

55. The nurse is teaching a newly diagnosed client with diabetes mellitus type 1 about self-care. Which of the following information should the nurse include? **Select all that apply.**
    a. Glucose testing
    b. Skin care
    c. Dietary compliance
    d. Bowel care
    e. Insulin administration

56. The nurse must administer eye drops to a 6-month-old infant, but the child clinches the eyes tightly to avoid the drops. Which of the following actions is the **most** appropriate?
    a. Attempt to instill the drops at a later time.
    b. Force the infant's eyes open using the thumb and index finger.
    c. Gently restrain the head and apply the drops at the inner canthus.
    d. Pull down the lower lid with the thumb and instill the drops into the conjunctival sac.

57. Which is the preferred site for intramuscular injections for both adults and children?
    a. Deltoid
    b. Ventrogluteal
    c. Dorsogluteal
    d. Vastus lateralis

58. A client is receiving a liter of normal saline intravenously but must receive 150 mL of antibiotic solution by piggyback. Which of the following is the **most** correct procedure?
    a. Clamp the primary tubing and adjust the flow rate of the piggyback unit.
    b. Hang the piggyback unit 6 inches lower than the primary unit and adjust flow rate of the piggyback unit only.
    c. Hang the piggyback unit 6 inches higher than the primary unit and adjust flow rate of the piggyback unit only.
    d. Hang the piggyback unit at the same level as the primary unit, clamp the primary tubing, and adjust flow rate of the piggyback unit.

59. Prior to administering an IV push medication, which of the following should the nurse check? **Select all that apply.**
    a. Dosage and correct dilution
    b. Recommended administration time
    c. Availability of pharmacist
    d. Client allergies
    e. Client's identification

60. How long should a woman remain in the supine position after administration of a vaginal suppository?
    a. 1 to 2 minutes
    b. 3 to 5 minutes
    c. 5 to 10 minutes
    d. 15 minutes

61. Which vitamin or mineral may alter the effect of levodopa in clients treated for Parkinson disease?
    a. Calcium
    b. Vitamin D
    c. Ascorbic acid (Vitamin C)
    d. Pyridoxine (Vitamin B6)

62. A client is admitted to a drug rehabilitation program. He appears thin with scattered lesions where he has been picking at his skin and shows evidence of severe tooth decay but is very talkative and has a rapid, irregular heartbeat. Based on these signs and symptoms, which of the following is **most** likely his drug of choice?
    a. Cocaine
    b. Methamphetamine
    c. Marijuana
    d. LSD

63. A 4-year-old child with autism spectrum disorder has verbal skills but interacts poorly. The child says "bunny" and reaches for a stuffed animal that is on a shelf. Which of the following is the **best** example of incidental teaching?
   a. The nurse asks, "What color is the bunny?" and waits for a response before giving the child the toy.
   b. The nurse states, "That's right! That is a bunny" and gives the child the toy.
   c. The nurse gives the child the toy without comment.
   d. The nurse states, "Before you get the bunny, you need to answer some questions."

64. A 7-year-old child with special needs has difficulty learning activities that require more than one step. Which of the following approaches is likely to be the **most** effective?
   a. Having the child master step one before progressing to step two
   b. Coaching and assisting the child through each step sequentially
   c. Providing posters with sequential pictures
   d. Back chaining

65. A client is scheduled to undergo a cholecystectomy. Which of the following is a required element of informed consent?
   a. Duration of operation
   b. Names of surgical staff
   c. Risks and benefits
   d. Insurance coverage

66. A woman comes to the emergency department after being badly beaten. She is shaking and appears very frightened. Which of the following is the first question the nurse should ask?
   a. "Who did this to you?"
   b. "Is the person who did this to you present here in the hospital?"
   c. "Have you called the police?"
   d. "Do you want information about women's shelters?"

67. A female client complains of sudden onset of chest and abdominal "tightness" and pressure with pain in the neck and jaw. The client feels fatigued and nauseated. She appears pale and dyspneic, and her skin is cold and clammy. Which of the following diagnostic tests does the nurse anticipate will be completed initially?
   a. Electrocardiogram
   b. Bronchoscopy
   c. Echocardiogram
   d. Complete blood count

68. A client in the mental health unit tells the nurse, "I drink too much because my job is so stressful and because I need to relax." This is an example of which type of defense mechanism?
   a. Suppression
   b. Repression
   c. Rationalization
   d. Denial

69. The nurse does an admission interview with a Native American client. The client does not make eye contact and remains silent for extended periods of time and withdraws when the nurse reaches out to touch the client's hand when reassuring her about her treatment. Which of the following is the **most** likely reason for the client's behavior?
    a. The client is frightened.
    b. The client is dishonest.
    c. The client is exhibiting cultural traits.
    d. The client speaks little English.

70. A client tells the nurse that she has always hated her mother, who left the client behind with her abusive father when the parents divorced. The mother has been trying to reestablish a relationship with the client, who is now 23 years old, but the client remains uncertain and angry. Which spiritual need is the client grappling with?
    a. Love
    b. Faith
    c. Hope
    d. Forgiveness

71. A client with Alzheimer disease has repeatedly gotten out the front door at night and run away. Which of the following suggestions may be **most** helpful to a caregiver? **Select all that apply.**
    a. Hang a curtain over the doorway.
    b. Place a latch at the top or bottom of the door.
    c. Lock the client into her bedroom.
    d. Place a motion sensor with a loud alarm on the client's bedroom door.
    e. Place bed restraints on the client.

72. Which of the following client actions **most** indicate the potential for assaultive behavior? **Select all that apply.**
    a. Passive-aggressive behavior
    b. Avoidance of eye contact
    c. Verbal threats
    d. Anger disproportionate to situation
    e. Withdrawal

73. A client recently diagnosed with colon cancer becomes furious when the nurse gives her an injection, shouting, "You hurt me, you idiot! You are so incompetent!" Which of the following is the **most** likely reason for the outburst?
    a. The nurse is incompetent.
    b. The client is in the anger stage of the grief response.
    c. The client is in the denial stage of the grief response.
    d. The client has a low pain tolerance.

74. A client with dementia says to the nurse, "I'm going to the movies now. I always go to the movies on Thanksgiving evening. I hope it doesn't snow." Which is the **most** appropriate response?
    a. "It's not Thanksgiving."
    b. "What a lovely tradition! I love movies."
    c. "Today is July 2. It's almost lunch time but after that you can watch a movie on TV."
    d. "It's snowing, so this is not a good time to go to the movies."

75. A client with terminal cancer states she is not afraid of death but is afraid of the process of dying. Which of the following is the best response?
- a. "What aspects of the dying process are you most concerned about?"
- b. "Those are normal feelings."
- c. "What can I do to help?"
- d. "I'm so sorry."

76. A client has experienced repeated panic attacks and at a visit to a clinic periodically snaps a rubber band against his wrist. Which of the following is the **most** likely reason for this action?
- a. The client has a nervous habit.
- b. The client is practicing self-injurious behavior.
- c. The client is trying to get attention.
- d. The client is practicing thought-stopping.

77. What type of initial nursing response is the **most** effective for a woman undergoing a traumatic stress crisis after being raped?
- a. Encourage the client to express feelings about the trauma.
- b. Encourage the client to talk about and describe the rape.
- c. Teach the client relaxation techniques.
- d. Tell the client about resources for rape victims.

78. Which of the following are examples of normalization for pediatric clients? **Select all that apply.**
- a. Painting children's rooms in bright colors
- b. Providing a play area
- c. Allowing siblings to visit
- d. Facilitating doll re enactment play
- e. Serving meals on trays in children's rooms

79. A client in the mental health unit has a panic-level anxiety attack and has become immobile and mute and is not processing environmental stimuli. Which of the following actions is the best nursing response?
- a. Attempt to distract the client through music or conversation.
- b. Remain with the client and speak in a calm, reassuring voice.
- c. Remind the client that the anxiety will pass.
- d. Encourage the client to use self-hypnosis techniques.

80. A schizophrenic client has frequent hallucinations and is becoming increasingly withdrawn. Which of the following are appropriate interventions for hallucinations? **Select all that apply.**
- a. Communicate frequently with the client to help present reality.
- b. Use distracting techniques.
- c. Ask client to describe the hallucinations.
- d. Encourage client to participate in reality-based activities, such as playing cards.
- e. Tell client to ignore the hallucinations.

81. Which of the following is the primary risk factor for cervical cancer?
   a. Smoking
   b. Chlamydia infection
   c. Family history of cervical cancer
   d. Human papillomavirus

82. A 36-year-old woman who smokes 2 packs of cigarettes daily seeks advice about contraception. Which of the following contraceptive methods should she avoid? **Select all that apply.**
   a. Vaginal ring
   b. Combined hormone pills
   c. Intrauterine device
   d. Progestogen-only pill
   e. All contraceptives except condoms and diaphragms

83. A client with asthma is to be discharged and must take nebulizer treatments at home. Which of the following is the best method to ensure that the client understands how to use and clean the equipment after the nurse completes a demonstration?
   a. Provide the client with written instructions.
   b. Provide the client with a telephone number to call if questions arise.
   c. Ask the client if he has any questions.
   d. Ask the client to do a return demonstration.

84. When conducting a physical examination of a 62-year-old female, the nurse notes nodules on the dorsolateral aspects of the distal interphalangeal joints (Heberden's nodes) of the right hand. Which of the following diseases does this finding suggest?
   a. Acute tenosynovitis
   b. Gout
   c. Rheumatoid arthritis
   d. Osteoarthritis

85. A mother brings her toddler to a well-baby clinic. The child is fair, and his skin is yellow-tinged, especially evident on the nose and the palms of the hands and feet; however, the sclera is white. Which of the following does the nurse anticipate should be initially assessed?
   a. Liver function tests
   b. Diet
   c. Blood count
   d. Electrolytes

86. Fetal heart tones are usually first heard with a fetoscope at what week of gestation? **Record your answer using a whole number.**

87. A new mother who is Hispanic brings her one-month-old infant for a well-baby exam and reports that she is adding yams, pureed beans, and sugar to the child's formula and has enlarged the nipple to accommodate the thickened formula. Which of the following is the **most** likely reason for this practice?
    a. The mother is following a cultural practice.
    b. The mother is uneducated about infant care.
    c. The mother cannot afford to purchase adequate amounts of formula.
    d. The mother is negligent.

88. When taking an adult client's blood pressure, the lower border of the cuff should be how far above the antecubital crease?
    a. 1 cm
    b. 5 cm
    c. 2.5 cm
    d. 7.5 cm

89. The mother of a 6-month-old child reports that she has a very good baby who is very quiet and sleeps well. The nurse notes that when the phone rings across the room, the child continues to look at the mother. Which of the following should the nurse suspect?
    a. The child has a hearing deficit.
    b. The child is anxious.
    c. The child has cognitive impairment.
    d. The child is exhibiting normal behavior for age.

90. A client complains of blurred vision, fatigue, loss of appetite, weight loss, increased thirst, and frequent urination. Which of the following laboratory assessments is **most** indicated?
    a. Blood glucose and HbA1c
    b. Serum and urine osmolality
    c. Complete blood count
    d. Urinalysis

91. Which of the following laboratory findings are consistent with hypernatremia?
    a. Increased serum sodium and decreased urine sodium
    b. Increased serum sodium and decreased urine osmolality
    c. Increased serum sodium and increased urine sodium
    d. Increased serum sodium and decreased urine specific gravity

92. The mother of a 20-month-old child reports that another toddler in daycare developed a fever 7 days previously while in contact with the other children and subsequently was diagnosed with roseola. The mother is concerned that her child will develop roseola. What information should the nurse provide to the mother? **Select all that apply.**
    a. Roseola is contagious with onset of rash.
    b. The incubation period for roseola is 9 to 10 days.
    c. Roseola is contagious with onset of fever.
    d. The incubation period for roseola is 3 to 6 days.
    e. Roseola is contagious 2 days prior to onset of fever.

93. A client has a large pressure sore on the coccygeal area. The pressure sore is draining large amounts of seropurulent discharge. Which of the following is the **most** appropriate choice for dressing material?
    a. Alginate
    b. Hydrocolloid
    c. Hydrogel
    d. Transparent film

94. A client experiences a severe generalized tonic-clonic seizure while in bed in supine position with one side rail down. Which of the following actions by the nurse are correct? **Select all that apply.**
    a. Insert a padded tongue blade between the client's teeth.
    b. Turn client to the side-lying position.
    c. Elevate and pad side rails.
    d. Leave side rail down and stand on open side to restrain client if needed.
    e. Restrain patient physically throughout the seizure.

95. A home care client has been having an Unna boot replaced every 7 days, but at a home visit the nurse finds the patient cannot ambulate because of an injury to the opposite leg. Which of the following actions is **most** correct at this time?
    a. The Unna boot should be discontinued and the leg left open.
    b. The Unna boot should be changed as scheduled.
    c. The Unna boot should be discontinued and replaced with a short stretch wrap (such as Comprilan®).
    d. The Unna boot should be discontinued and another form of compression used.

96. **Place the following metric weight measures in the correct position in the table below.**
    I. Gram
    II. Decigram
    III. Dekagram
    IV. Hectogram

Milligram	Centigram	(A)	(B)	(C)	(D)	Kilogram
a.						
b.						
c.						
d.						

97. A client has a colostomy in the following anatomic position (see diagram). When teaching the patient about colostomy care, which of the following information should the nurse include? **Select all that apply.**

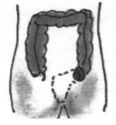

a. "You should expect to have a bowel movement every day."
b. "You may be able to regulate your bowel movements with diet or irrigations."
c. "Your stool may be soft to solid."
d. "There are different types of colostomy appliances available."
e. "Your stool will probably be semi-liquid."

98. A 68-year-old client recently had a hip replacement for which she is receiving opioid analgesia. The patient refused dinner and exhibited sudden onset of weakness and confusion. During the assessment of the client, the nurse asks the client to show her teeth.

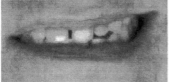

Based on the client's response (see photo), which of the following does the nurse expect is **most** likely the cause of the client's symptoms?
a. Over-medication
b. Hypoglycemia
c. Stroke
d. Delirium

99. The nurse is completing a physical examination of a client and evaluating the client for peripheral arterial and venous insufficiency. Which of the following findings are consistent with peripheral arterial insufficiency? **Select all that apply.**
a. Brownish discoloration appears about the ankles and anterior tibial area.
b. Foot exhibits rubor on dependency and pallor on elevation.
c. Ulcers are evident on end of great toe and heel.
d. Peripheral edema is marked.
e. Ulcers are superficial and irregular, often on medial or lateral malleolus.

100. A client has been recovering well from a knee replacement but has sudden onset of restlessness and anxiety and complains of chest pain, shortness of breath, and cough with frothy blood-tinged sputum. The client's pulse is 110 and temperature 101.2°F/38.4°C. The nurse notes rales in the right lung and tachypnea. Based on these findings, which of the following complications is **most** likely?
    a. Pulmonary embolism
    b. Atelectasis
    c. Pneumonia
    d. Pneumothorax

101. A client is recovering from abdominal surgery after a gunshot wound. When the nurse sees increased sanguineous drainage and changes the dressing, the nurse notes that the midline abdominal incision is dehiscing and a loop of the intestine has eviscerated through the lower third of the wound. While the client is awaiting transfer to surgery for repair, which of the following interventions should the nurse carry out? **Select all that apply.**
    a. Wearing sterile gloves, attempt to reinsert the viscera through the open wound.
    b. Cover the viscera with a dry sterile dressing.
    c. Cover the viscera with a normal saline–soaked sterile dressing.
    d. Place the client in low Fowler's position with knees slightly flexed.
    e. Place the client in Trendelenburg position.

102. A 70-year-old female states that she has difficulty falling asleep and sleeps poorly, often lying awake much of the night. The nurse should anticipate which of the following as the initial intervention?
    a. Assessment of sleep patterns
    b. Nocturnal polysomnogram
    c. Prescription for hypnotic
    d. Dietary modifications

103. The nurse is interviewing a 56-year-old male with obstructive sleep apnea (OSA) for which he has been prescribed a CPAP machine for use during sleep. The client yawns frequently during the interview. Which of the following statements by the client indicates a need for further education about OSA and CPAP?
    a. "I use only distilled water for humidification."
    b. "I try to use the CPAP most nights."
    c. "I wash the mask and tubing with soap and water and rinse with water and vinegar."
    d. "I think the nasal mask is better than the orofacial mask."

104. A 26-year-old client is going to use continuous ambulatory peritoneal dialysis (CAPD) after discharge from the hospital. Which of the following should the nurse include in teaching about CAPD? **Select all that apply.**
    a. "You will instill about 2 liters of fluid over 10 to 15 minutes."
    b. "Clamp the tubing and maintain a dwell time of about 30 minutes."
    c. "Unclamp the tubing and drain for about 20 minutes."
    d. "Immerse the dialysate bag in warm water to increase temperature."
    e. "You will instill about 2 liters of fluid over 3 to 5 hours."

105. A 5-year-old child is undergoing chemotherapy for acute lymphocytic leukemia (ALL). The child has weekly blood tests to monitor status. Which of the following abnormalities of the blood are of **most** concern during treatment for leukemia?
   a. Thrombocytopenia and neutropenia
   b. Thrombocytosis and neutropenia
   c. Thrombocytosis and neutrocytosis
   d. Thrombocytopenia and neutrocytosis

106. A 35-year-old woman is recovering from a thyroidectomy for Hashimoto's thyroiditis. The client complains that she is experiencing a tingling sensation about her mouth and fingers and muscle cramps in her legs. Which of the following complications is **most** likely the cause of these symptoms?
   a. Hypocalcemia
   b. Hypercalcemia
   c. Hypermagnesemia
   d. Hypomagnesemia

107. According to USDA dietary guidelines (see diagram), which of the following meals **most** corresponds to dietary recommendations?

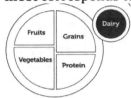

   a. One apple, 1 cup carrots, 1 cup long-grain white rice, 4 ounces poached salmon, and ½ cup sweetened yogurt
   b. One cup canned fruit cocktail, 1 cup corn, 1 cup long-grain white rice, 4 ounces fried breaded fish sticks, and 8 ounces of wine
   c. One cup steamed kale, one medium baked potato with butter and sour cream, 6 ounces rib-eye steak, and 1 cup of coffee
   d. One-half banana, 1 cup broccoli, ½ cup quinoa, 3 ounces roasted turkey, and 8 ounces of 1% milk

108. The mother of an 11-year-old boy asks the nurse what type of anticipatory guidance she should provide for her son. Which of the following are age-appropriate topics the nurse should suggest for a child of this age? **Select all that apply.**
   a. What to expect in terms of physical development and secondary sexual characteristics
   b. Responsibilities of sexual behavior, including abstinence and birth control
   c. Peer group pressures, including gangs, alcohol, and tobacco use
   d. Future goals and plans
   e. Dating and relationship issues

109. A neonate has hyperbilirubinemia and jaundice, and the physician has prescribed phototherapy, which the nurse is about to administer. **Place the actions listed below (Roman numerals) in order, beginning with the first action.**

      I. Place a protective mask over the child's eyes.
      II. Adjust light source to 15 to 20 cm above child.
      III. Turn on lights.
      IV. Remove all clothes except diaper.

    a. (First action)
    b. (Second action)
    c. (Third action)
    d. (Fourth action)

110. A client comes to a clinic with a severe cough and fever, but all of the exam rooms are full when the client arrives. Which of the following is the **best** action for the nurse to take?
    a. Tell the client to reschedule an appointment for a less busy hour.
    b. Ask the client to wait outside until an exam room becomes available.
    c. Provide the client a facemask and seat her in the waiting area with other clients.
    d. Provide the client a facemask and seat the client in a separate area as far as possible from other clients.

111. A pregnant woman at 21 weeks gestation has severe pre-eclampsia with BP of 170/120 and proteinuria of 6 g in 24 hours. What treatment does the nurse anticipate is initially indicated?
    a. Bedrest only
    b. Phenytoin
    c. Magnesium sulfate
    d. Antihypertensive, such as hydralazine

112. A full-term pregnant woman experienced premature rupture of the membranes 24 hours earlier but has not gone into labor. Which of the following does the nurse anticipate?
    a. Labor will be induced.
    b. Client is at increased risk of hemorrhage.
    c. Client will undergo Caesarean.
    d. Labor will be induced if the patient does not go into labor within 48 hours.

113. A patient had a bowel resection and has been reluctant to take deep breaths and cough because of discomfort. Which of the following interventions is most indicated initially to prevent atelectasis?
    a. Regular use of incentive spirometer
    b. Nebulizer treatments with albuterol
    c. IPPB treatments
    d. Prophylactic antibiotics

114. A client has had a pacemaker inserted recently but complains that he is experiencing heart palpitations and generalized weakness and that he has slight pain in the chest and jaw. On examination, the nurse notes that the client appears quite anxious, and the nurse observes pulsations in the neck and abdomen. Which of the following is the **most** likely cause of these findings?
    a. Pacemaker wiring has become dislodged
    b. Infection
    c. Coronary artery occlusion
    d. Pacemaker syndrome

115. A client on cardiac monitoring has dislodged his leads 6 times in a 4-hour period, setting off alarms. Each time, he makes a different excuse, but the nurse suspects the dislodgements are purposeful because the client attempts to delay the nurse's leaving after each episode. Which of the following is the **most** appropriate response?
    a. "I can see that you are doing this on purpose."
    b. "These constant alarms are disturbing to other patients."
    c. "Why are you disconnecting your leads?"
    d. "Let's talk about the reason for monitoring and what we can learn from it."

116. Which of the following should never be delegated to unlicensed assistive personnel?
    a. Monitoring and controlling blood therapy
    b. Bathing patient
    c. Ambulating patient
    d. Monitoring urinary output

117. Prior to irrigating a nasogastric (NG) tube, the nurse gently aspirates fluid and then measures the pH of the aspirate with color-coded pH paper. Which of the following pH values is consistent with gastric fluid?
    a. 6
    b. 5
    c. 4.4
    d. 3.8

118. A client has had three recent bouts of cystitis and now has urinary frequency and burning, chills, fever of 102°F/38.9°C, abdominal pain, and bilateral flank pain. Which of the following diagnostic tests does the nurse expect the physician to order initially?
    a. Complete blood count
    b. Urinalysis and urine culture and sensitivities
    c. Kidney function tests
    d. Cystoscopy

119. A client is receiving radiotherapy to the abdominal area and has developed chronic diarrhea. Which of the following should the nurse include when teaching the client ways to manage the diarrhea? **Select all that apply.**
    a. "It's important to drink 8 to 12 glasses of clear fluids each day."
    b. "It's better to eat 5 or 6 small meals than 3 large meals."
    c. "Try to increase the fiber in your diet."
    d. "You can try the BRAT diet (banana, rice, applesauce, and toast)."
    e. "Drinking milk and eating ice cream may soothe your stomach."

120. A client has been on a weight-loss program. Her waist measures 28 inches and hips 40 inches. What is her waist-to-hip ratio? **Record your answer using a decimal number.**

121. Prior to drawing blood for blood gas analysis, the nurse conducts the modified Allen test to ensure there is adequate collateral circulation. The nurse asks the client to extend the wrist over a rolled towel and make a fist. **Place the following steps (Roman numerals) in order from first to last.**
　　I. Ask the client to open and close the hand until the skin blanches.
　　II. Palpate the ulnar and radial pulses and apply pressure to both arteries.
　　III. Observe the hand for color.
　　IV. Release the ulnar artery while maintaining pressure on the radial artery.

　　a. (Step 1)
　　b. (Step 2)
　　c. (Step 3)
　　d. (Step 4)

122. What is the critical point for PO2 (the "ICU" point), the percentage point at which there is marked decrease in oxygen saturation? **Record your answer using a whole number.**

123. A client with heart failure has been prescribed the DASH diet (dietary approaches to stop hypertension) and must limit sodium intake to 2300 mg per day. Which of the following statements by the client indicates a need for further education?
　　a. "All I really have to do for this diet is stop adding salt to foods."
　　b. "I can have 2 or 3 servings of nonfat or low-fat dairy products each day."
　　c. "I should have 4 or 5 servings of both vegetables and fruits daily."
　　d. "I should limit lean meat, poultry, and fish to 6 ounces per day."

124. A client has immune thrombocytopenic purpura. The client's platelet count is 19,000. Which initial treatment does the nurse expect?
　　a. Splenectomy
　　b. Immunosuppressive therapy
　　c. Observation only
　　d. Platelet administration

125. A client is being assessed for neutropenia. The client's total white blood cell count is 5200 with 45% neutrophils and 5% bands. What is the absolute neutrophil count (ANC)? **Record your answer using a whole number.**

126. Each staff person has an individual password that allows access to electronic health records. Under which of the following circumstances should a nurse allow another staff person to use his/her password?
　　a. A physician asks to use the password to access records of a former client.
　　b. Another nurse asks to use the password because he has forgotten his own.
　　c. The nurse's supervisor asks to use the password to access client records.
　　d. The nurse should not allow anyone else to use the password, regardless of circumstances.

127. The nurse is part of an interdisciplinary team in a rehabilitation unit. Which of the following statements by a client is **most** important to be communicated to the social worker on the team?
    a. "I can't afford to hire anyone to help me when I am discharged."
    b. "I'm worried about falling when I go home."
    c. "I need to learn how to get in and out of the shower."
    d. "I'm not sure what kinds of adaptive equipment I will need."

128. An 84-year-old female with COPD in an extended-care facility is alert and responsive and has been maintained on low-flow oxygen and nebulizer treatments, but the client, who is bedridden, has removed the oxygen and refused nebulizer treatments, telling the nurse that she is ready to die and only wants comfort measures. Which of the following actions by the nurse is **most** appropriate?
    a. Insist the client take treatments as ordered by the physician.
    b. Notify the physician of the client's refusal.
    c. Ask family members to intervene.
    d. Remind the client that committing suicide is contrary to her religious beliefs.

129. If a client's LDL cholesterol is 100, HDL cholesterol is 50, and triglycerides are 150, what is the client's total cholesterol? **Record your answer using a whole number.**

130. The nurse is conducting a physical examination of a client's abdomen. **Place the examination techniques listed below (Roman numerals) in the correct sequence, from first to last.**
        I. Percussion
        II. Palpation
        III. Inspection
        IV. Auscultation
    a. (First)
    b. (Second)
    c. (Third)
    d. (Fourth)

131. The nurse is conducting an examination of the abdomen and auscultating for bruits. **Label the lettered points on the diagram with Roman numerals identifying the position of the arteries.**
        I. Femoral
        II. Aorta
        III. Iliac
        IV. Renal

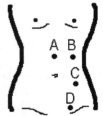

    a.
    b.
    c.
    d.

132. A female client is scheduled for a routine pelvic exam. Which of the following should the nurse ask the client to do prior to the exam?
    a. Refrain from drinking.
    b. Urinate.
    c. Wash perineal area.
    d. Perform relaxation exercises.

133. The nurse is inserting an intravenous line into the right arm and has identified a potential insertion site. **Place the steps (indicated in Roman numerals) of venipuncture in the proper sequential order.**
        I. Palpate vein.
        II. Cleanse skin.
        III. Apply tourniquet.
        IV. Perform venipuncture.
    a. (First)
    b. (Second)
    c. (Third)
    d. (Fourth)

134. A client is receiving oxygen per nasal cannula at 3L/minute. Which of the following is the approximate inspired oxygen concentration (FiO_2)?
    a. 60%
    b. 50%
    c. 40–42%
    d. 28–32%

135. A client is taking nebulizer treatments for asthma, and the nurse is instructing the client in the correct method for measuring peak expiratory flow rates (PEFR) after treatment. The nurse prepares the meter with the indicator at the base of the scale. **Place the following steps (Roman numerals) in the correct order from first to last.**
        I. Client sits upright or stands.
        II. Client places the meter in the mouth and seals lips.
        III. Client expels air through the meter as forcefully as possible.
        IV. Client takes a deep breath.
    a. (First)
    b. (Second)
    c. (Third)
    d. (Fourth)

136. Following a lumbar puncture, a client develops a severe headache that persists 24 hours and is unrelieved by bedrest or oral fluids. Which of the following interventions does the nurse anticipate?
    a. Bedrest for 3 days
    b. Opioid analgesia
    c. Epidural blood patch
    d. Intravenous fluids

137. The nurse is assisting a client who is to undergo a thoracentesis. Which of the following is the optimal position for the procedure?
    a. Lying prone with arms above head
    b. Side lying on the unaffected side
    c. Side lying on the affected side
    d. Upright position, leaning forward over an over-bed tray table

138. A client has experienced 48 hours of severe repeated bouts of vomiting. Which acid-base imbalance is of most concern?
    a. Respiratory acidosis
    b. Respiratory alkalosis
    c. Metabolic acidosis
    d. Metabolic alkalosis

139. A client is scheduled for hemodialysis twice weekly through an arteriovenous fistula in the left arm. Following each hemodialysis treatment, the nurse should evaluate the client for which of the following because of risks associated with hemodialysis? **Select all that apply.**
    a. Fluid volume deficit
    b. Fluid volume excess
    c. Bleeding
    d. Metabolic acidosis
    e. Pulmonary edema

140. A client with liver failure and ascites is having a paracentesis to relieve severe dyspnea resulting from abdominal fluid accumulation. Prior to the procedure, the nurse assists the client to urinate. Which of the following is the **most** important reason to have the patient urinate?
    a. Patient comfort
    b. Prevention of incontinence
    c. Prevention of bladder puncture
    d. Fluid displacement

141. A client is to be discharged with a tracheostomy. Which of the following should the nurse **most** stress when educating the client about home management? **Select all that apply.**
    a. Bowel care
    b. Pulmonary hygiene
    c. Dietary supplements
    d. Tracheostomy care
    e. Exercise program

142. A 72-year-old client with Parkinson disease is recovering from pneumonia and is to be discharged, but he remains weak and has poor control of his hands because of tremors. A home health aide will visit three times weekly to assist the client to bathe, and his daughter will visit every evening after work to help with laundry and housework. Which of the following referrals is **most** indicated to allow the client to remain independent in his home?
    a. Home meal delivery program (Meals on Wheels)
    b. Friendly Visitors program
    c. Hospice
    d. Occupational therapist

143. A client is receiving hospice and palliative care, including analgesia and other comfort measures. Which of the following indicates the client is undergoing life review? **Select all that apply.**
   a. The client looks through old photo albums.
   b. The client states that her analgesia is not adequate.
   c. The client reminisces about her children when they were young and her parenting skills.
   d. The client states that she is ready to die.
   e. The client states she does not want her children to have a funeral for her.

144. A mother brings her child to the clinic because of repeated bouts of head lice. Which of the following statements by the mother suggests a need for education? **Select all that apply.**
   a. "I've repeatedly used mayonnaise and olive oil treatments."
   b. "I spent hours combing nits from my child's hair."
   c. "I washed her clothing and bedding in hot water and dried in a hot dryer for 20 minutes."
   d. "I warned my child not to use anyone else's comb or brush."
   e. "I treated the dogs for lice as well."

145. A client comes to the emergency department with scalding burns covering his entire left arm, anterior and posterior surfaces. Using the rule of nines, how much total body surface area (TBSA) has been burned? **Record your answer using a whole number.**

146. A client has been on prolonged bedrest following surgery. The nurse notes that the patient has pain in the right calf on palpation with dorsiflexion of the ankle. Which of the following causes does the nurse suspect?
   a. Arthritis
   b. Muscle strain
   c. Compartment syndrome
   d. Deep vein thrombosis

147. A client had a craniotomy for a basal meningioma and is being monitored postoperatively. The client's baseline blood pressure and pulse were BP 138/72 and P 82. Temperature was 97.5°F/36.4°C. The client is awake and responding. Which of the following findings **most** indicates possible increasing intracranial pressure?
   a. Patient restless, BP 146/80 and P 90. Temperature 98.2°F/36.7°C.
   b. Patient restless and complaining of headache. BP 160/64 and P 70. Temperature 99.4°F/37.4°C.
   c. Patient sleeping. BP 142/76 and P 86. Temperature 97.8°F/36.6°C.
   d. Patient complaining of headache, BP 160/110, P 92. Temperature 98°F/36.7°C.

148. A client is being discharged with an implantable cardioverter-defibrillator (ICD), and the nurse is educating the client about home management. The client asks what he should do if the ICD fires one time but he has no other symptoms. Which of the following is the best advice?
   a. "Call 9-1-1."
   b. "Go to the emergency department when recovered from the firing."
   c. "Resume normal activities."
   d. "Lie down and rest and report the event to the physician by telephone."

149. The nurse is monitoring a client's cardiac rhythm when an abnormal rhythm occurs. Which of the following cardiac rhythms does the ECG strip (see image) indicate?

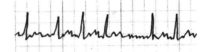

a. Ventricular fibrillation
b. Ventricular tachycardia
c. Atrial fibrillation
d. Atrial flutter

150. A client is to be discharged on warfarin (Coumadin®) therapy, and the nurse is teaching the client about the medication. Which of the following statements by the client indicates that the client's education has been effective? **Select all that apply.**

a. "I should use a soft toothbrush."
b. "My stools will routinely be black."
c. "Swimming is a good choice for exercise."
d. "I should wear a Medical Alert bracelet."
e. "I should avoid all green, leafy vegetables."

151. A client has had a central catheter inserted for administration of parenteral nutrition. An X-ray was taken to ensure correct positioning prior to commencing infusions. The X-ray report indicates that the catheter tip is in the right atrium. Which of the following actions by the nurse is correct?

a. Hold the infusion and notify the MD.
b. Gently withdraw the catheter 2 to 3 inches.
c. Begin the infusion as the catheter is placed correctly.
d. Gently insert the catheter 2 to 3 inches further.

152. A client was to receive 1 g of vancomycin intravenously in 200 mL of iso-osmotic solution over 60 minutes per infusion pump. However, the IV administration was discontinued after 45 minutes because the client developed nausea and chills. How many milligrams of vancomycin did the client receive? **Record your answer using a whole number.**

153. A client is receiving enteral feedings through a nasogastric tube, and the nurse is administering the client's medications. Which of the following can be administered through the NG tube? **Select all that apply.**

a. Hard extended-release capsules (opened, crushed, and dissolved)
b. Pills (crushed and dissolved)
c. Enteric-coated tablets (crushed and dissolved)
d. Liquid suspension
e. Soft-gel capsules (dissolved)
f. Sublingual wafer (dissolved)

154. The nurse is monitoring a client following postoperative cardiac catheterization and is checking the client's oxygen saturation (SPO2) per pulse oximetry. The nurse recognizes that the SPO2 should be maintained above what percentage in most clients to ensure adequate oxygenation? **Record your answer using a whole number.**

155. An older adult has become very confused after surgery for repair of a hip fracture. The client has repeatedly tried to climb over the bedrails and the nurse is considering placing the client in a Posey vest that is secured to the bed. Which of the following must the nurse consider when applying restraints to a client? **Select all that apply.**

    a. An alternate method should be tried prior to applying a restraint.
    b. Confused clients are almost always safer in restraints.
    c. Restraints must be removed and the client reassessed at least every 2 hours.
    d. A written policy for application of restraints must be in place.
    e. The most restrictive restraint should be applied.
    f. The nurse does not need an order for a restraint if the client is in danger.

156. The nurse is working with mothers and newborns. When educating a new mother about security measures to protect her infant, which of the following should the nurse include?

    a. "Never leave your infant unattended for more than 5 minutes."
    b. "Only allow people in hospital attire to remove the infant from the mother's room."
    c. "Notify your assigned nurse if anyone attempts to carry the child from the room in his/her arms."
    d. "Anyone with a hospital ID can be considered safe."

157. The nurse must administer 120 mg of amoxicillin oral suspension to a child. However, the only dosage available in the pharmacy is 200 mg per 5 mL. How many milliliters of suspension should the nurse administer? **Record your answer using a whole number only.**

158. Based on clinical findings, the physician suspects that a 65-year-old client has kidney disease and has ordered a blood-urea-nitrogen (BUN) test. Which of the following results is within normal limits?

    a. 5 mg/dL
    b. 15 mg/dL
    c. 40 mg/dL
    d. 100 mg/dL

159. A physician has ordered the HbA1c test for a client who complains of increased thirst and urination. Which of the following results (on two separate testings) is the lowest value considered diagnostic for diabetes mellitus?

    a. 3.5 to 4.5%
    b. 4.5 to 6%
    c. 5.7 to 6.4%
    d. ≥6.5%

160. A client with an artificial eye is too ill to remove the eye, but the lids are crusted and irritated, so the nurse must remove the prosthesis for cleaning and to inspect the eye socket. The nurse has washed hands and applied disposable gloves. **Place the remaining steps to removing the prosthesis (Roman numerals) in the correct order**.
    I. Gently retract the upper lid.
    II. Exert slight pressure below the eyelid and slip index finger under prosthesis.
    III. Break suction and slide prosthesis out of eye.
    IV. Gently retract the lower eyelid against the orbital ridge with the thumb.
    a. (First)
    b. (Second)
    c. (Third)
    d. (Fourth)

161. A client with end-stage heart failure is bedridden, and the skin in the coccygeal area is red and tender despite frequent turning because the client is occasionally incontinent of urine. The client weighs 180 pounds. Which type of pressure-relieving surface should the nurse **most** recommend at this time?
    a. Foam overlay
    b. Sheepskin
    c. Alternating pressure overlay
    d. Low air loss bed

162. A client is to receive 120 mL of normal saline per hour intravenously. The drop factor is 15 drops per mL. What drip rate should the nurse set? **Record your answer using a whole number.**

163. A client has weakness of both lower extremities, more pronounced on the right, and uses crutches to ambulate. Which of the following gaits requires the most upper body strength and balance?
    a. 4-point
    b. 3-point
    c. 2-point
    d. Swing-through

164. A client has just had a long leg cast applied to his left leg and is in bed. The cast is still damp, and the client is cold. Which of the following actions by the nurse are appropriate? **Select all that apply.**
    a. Cover the client, including the cast, with a warm blanket.
    b. Cover the client with a warm blanket, leaving the cast exposed to the air.
    c. Place a high-powered electric fan to blow directly on the cast.
    d. Turn and reposition the client every 2 to 3 hours.
    e. Place a fan in the room but directed away from the client.

165. The nurse is administering an intermittent tube feeding to a client per an NG tube. The nurse has checked placement of the tube, checked for gastric residual, and aspirated 150 mL of gastric contents. Which of the following next actions is **most** appropriate?

a. Hold feeding and notify MD of gastric residual.
b. Proceed with tube feeding.
c. Return the aspirated gastric contents to the stomach and flush the tubing with 30 mL water.
d. Return 100 mL of aspirated gastric contents to the stomach followed by the tube feeding.

166. The physician has ordered that a client with diabetes insipidus receive 50 micrograms of desmopressin acetate by oral tabs twice daily. The tablets are labeled 0.2 mg per tablet. How many tablets will the nurse administer for each dose? **Record your answer using a decimal number.**

167. Following surgical removal of an ovarian cyst, a client has not urinated in 4 hours and feels the urge to urinate but is unable to initiate urine flow. Which of the following should the nurse do initially to promote urination? **Select all that apply.**

a. Pour warm water over the client's perineum while she is on the toilet.
b. Ask the client to blow bubbles through a straw into a glass of water while trying to urinate.
c. Turn on running water while the client tries to urinate.
d. Tell the client to "just relax."
e. Catheterize the client.

168. An adult client has instilled drops into the ear to soften cerumen, and the nurse is to irrigate the ear to remove the cerumen. Which of the following statements are correct about ear irrigations? **Select all that apply.**

a. 50 mL of irrigant should be instilled at one time.
b. The tip of the syringe should be used to occlude the ear canal.
c. The pinna should be pulled up and back.
d. Allow fluid to drain out during the procedure.
e. Position client in sitting or lying position.
f. Ask client to turn the head away from the affected ear.

169. A client receiving chemotherapy for breast cancer (stage 2) tells the nurse that she is considering complementary therapy to relieve her almost constant nausea and asks the nurse for advice. Which of the following complementary therapies is **most** likely to be safe and effective?

a. Acupuncture
b. Therapeutic touch
c. Magnetic therapy
d. Herbal therapies

170. The nurse asks a Hispanic immigrant to evaluate his pain on a scale of one to ten, and the client states his pain is at level one. However, the client looks distressed and is bent over and rubbing his stomach. Which of the following approaches by the nurse is **most** indicated?
    a. Use a different type of questioning to ascertain pain level.
    b. Accept the client's word about pain.
    c. Tell the client he appears to be minimizing his discomfort.
    d. Ask the client if he is afraid to admit to pain.

171. A client is in cervical traction for a herniated cervical disc. The client complains of increasing pain in the jaw and both ears. Which of the following interventions is **most** indicated?
    a. Provide increased analgesia.
    b. Adjust weights.
    c. Correct head position.
    d. Correct body position.

172. The nurse calls a physician to report a client's sudden increase in temperature and receives a telephone order for an antibiotic. Which of the following is the correct procedure for the nurse?
    a. Write the telephone order, order from the pharmacy, and administer the medication.
    b. Write the telephone order, read it back, and ask for verbal verification before ordering the drug from the pharmacy and administering the medication.
    c. Write the order, repeating it back, and then order the drug from the pharmacy and administer the medication.
    d. Write the order and check with a supervisor before ordering the drug from the pharmacy and administering the medication.

173. The nurse believes he observes another nurse taking an opioid medication intended for a client. Which of the following initial actions is the **most** appropriate?
    a. Confront the nurse taking the client's medication.
    b. Notify a supervisor about the observation.
    c. Notify the client's physician.
    d. Carry out a personal investigation.

174. The nurse is working in the emergency department. Which of the following injuries must be reported to the police or appropriate authorities?
    a. A woman has multiple facial injuries and defensive wounds on the hands and arms but insists she fell.
    b. A 6-year-old child has severe head and face injuries and multiple broken ribs. X-rays indicate numerous old orthopedic injuries. The mother states the child fell off a swing.
    c. A client has a large open cut on his torso. He claims he was injured when a large light fixture fell on him.
    d. An 18-year-old girl who was severely intoxicated from drinking fell and broke her arm.

175. A hospitalized client calls the nurse into the room and reports that another nurse has been rude to her. Which of the following initial responses by the nurse is **most** appropriate?
    a. "I'm sure the nurse didn't mean to be rude."
    b. "The nurse was probably just very busy."
    c. "I'm sorry! There's no excuse for a nurse being rude."
    d. "I'm so sorry you felt that way. Can you tell me what happened?"

176. The nurse is documenting the interview with a client with asthma and diabetes. Which of the following documentations is correct? **Select all that apply.**
    a. "Client appears SOB and anxious."
    b. "Client took nebulizer treatment with .25 mg budesonide inhalation suspension prior to visit."
    c. "Client needs new prescription for 0.5% albuterol inhalation solution."
    d. "Client checks blood sugar Q.O.D."
    e. "Client exhibits dyspnea and tachypnea (26/min)."

177. A mother's amniotic fluid is meconium stained. Which of the following complications does the nurse anticipate the neonate may develop?
    a. Anemia
    b. Respiratory distress
    c. Growth retardation
    d. Cognitive impairment

178. Which of the following ensures minimal proper identification prior to administering medication?
    a. Nurse recognizes client.
    b. Nurse asks client's name and checks hospital ID bracelet.
    c. Nurse reads client's name on intake and output record at the foot of the client's bed.
    d. Nurse asks client's name.

179. A wheelchair-bound client is to be discharged from a rehabilitation facility to the home environment. He still needs minimal assistance for transfers because he is unable to stand and is concerned about transferring from the wheelchair to the toilet and back. Which of the following assistive devices is **most** indicated to facilitate safe transfer?
    a. Gait/transfer belt
    b. Full-body sling lift
    c. Caregiver assistance only
    d. Sliding board

180. A nurse must retrieve supplies on the top shelf of a supply room but cannot reach the shelf, which is about a foot above the nurse's reach. Which of the following is an acceptable work practice?
    a. Stand on a footstool
    b. Use a ladder
    c. Climb onto a chair
    d. Step onto the second shelf of the cabinet

181. The nurse receives a delivery of a container with this marking (see diagram). What is the meaning of this international symbol?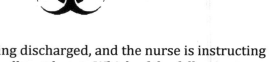
    a. Poison
    b. Medical equipment
    c. Biohazard
    d. Radioactive

182. A client with diabetes mellitus type 2 is being discharged, and the nurse is instructing the client about safe disposal of syringes and needles at home. Which of the following information should the nurse provide when educating the client? **Select all that apply.**
    a. "Place needles and syringes in a sharps disposal container immediately after use."
    b. "Keep the container in a safe place out of reach of children and pets."
    c. "Dispose of the sharps container in the regular trash can."
    d. "Dispose of the sharps container in accordance with community guidelines."
    e. "Dispose of the sharps container when it is three-quarters full."
    f. "Needles can be flushed down the toilet."

183. The hospital receives news that a train has crashed one-half mile away and that a cloud of nonlethal hazardous material has blanketed the area. Which of the following emergency responses does the nurse anticipate?
    a. Evacuation
    b. Shelter in place
    c. Relocation of staff and clients to interior of building
    d. Partial evacuation—children and critically ill only

184. The nurse is caring for a client with severe diarrhea and fecal incontinence from a *Clostridium difficile* infection. Which of the following infection control precautions should the nurse expect to implement? **Select all that apply.**
    a. Use ≥N95 respirators while caring for client.
    b. Use personal protective equipment (gown and gloves) for all contacts with the client.
    c. Maintain client in a private room or >3 feet away from other patients.
    d. Wash hands with soap and water rather than alcohol antiseptics.
    e. Wear masks for all contacts with the client.
    f. Avoid sharing electronic thermometers used by the client with other clients.

185. A 15-month-old child who weighs 10 kg is being treated with amoxicillin oral suspension at the rate of 25 mg/kg/day in two divided doses 12 hours apart. How many milligrams should the child receive at each dose? **Record your answer using a whole number only.**

186. A hospital must be evacuated because of flooding in the area. The nurse is working in the neonatal nursery and has been advised to utilize the Safe Babies® apron to transfer infants. How many infants does the nurse anticipate can be moved in one trip in the apron pockets?
    a. Two
    b. Four
    c. Six
    d. Eight

187. The nurse is about to conduct a bedside electrocardiogram of a client experiencing chest pain, but she notes that the electrical cord is frayed near the plug. Which of the following actions is **most** indicated?
a. Conduct the ECG but then label the ECG machine as "Out of Order."
b. Place tape about the frayed cord and conduct the ECG.
c. Call for repair of the ECG machine.
d. Immediately obtain a second ECG machine and conduct the ECG.

188. The nurse is working as a team leader and discussing assignments with team members. Which of the following statements to the group by a team member is a HIPAA violation of privacy?
a. "Mrs. Brown says she has no support system when she goes home."
b. "Mrs. Brown says she has been having an affair with her husband's brother!"
c. "Mrs. Brown says she dislikes her therapist, so she refuses to cooperate."
d. "Mrs. Brown seems angry all of the time and yells at her family when they visit."

189. The nurse must give a client a nebulizer treatment every 4 hours. When is the **most** appropriate time to document the treatments in the electronic health record?
a. At the beginning of the nurse's shift
b. Immediately after each treatment
c. Within 2 hours of each treatment
d. At the end of the nurse's shift

190. A homeless client has been treated in the emergency department for a small cut received in a fight with another homeless person and is about to be discharged after suturing. Which of the following information would be **most** helpful for the client in addition to information about wound care and a follow-up appointment?
a. Telephone number for Adult Protective Services
b. Telephone number of the police department
c. List of shelters and community agencies
d. List of 12-step organizations

191. A nurse is concerned that current procedures for wound care are not adequate and would like to propose changes. When pursuing process improvement, where should the nurse begin?
a. Survey literature regarding wound care.
b. Conduct interviews of physicians.
c. Dispense staff questionnaires.
d. Ask permission of the director of nursing.

192. A client is no longer responding to curative treatments. What is the best approach to initiating a discussion about the referral to palliative and hospice care?
a. "Further treatment is not going to help you."
b. "Would you like to transfer to palliative and hospice care?"
c. "Have you thought about stopping all treatments?"
d. "What do you understand about your options for care?"

193. A client has undergone gastric bypass surgery but is experiencing severe dumping syndrome after eating. Which of the following should the nurse advise the client to avoid? **Select all that apply.**
   a. Concentrated sugars
   b. Fluids with meals
   c. Whole milk and yogurt
   d. Reclining after eating
   e. Large meals

194. A client tells the nurse that he wants to designate his son to make only his healthcare decisions in the event that he is not able to do so, but he is unsure what document he needs to complete. Which of the following should the nurse advise?
   a. Living Will
   b. Advance Directive
   c. Power of Attorney
   d. Durable Power of Attorney for Healthcare

195. The nurse is preparing a mother and neonate for discharge. When educating the parents about infant car seats, which of the following information should the nurse include? **Select all that apply.**
   a. "Rear-facing car seats are safer than forward-facing car seats."
   b. "Carefully examine a car seat involved in an accident before using again."
   c. "The safest positioning of a car seat is in the middle of the back seat."
   d. "The neonate's neck should be straight, avoiding the chin-on-chest position."
   e. "The harness should be secured until only 3 or 4 fingers slide easily underneath."

196. A parent tells the nurse that her children, 5 and 10 years old, have been complaining of anal itching and have been sleeping poorly and complaining of occasional abdominal pain and nausea. What diagnostic test does the nurse anticipate?
   a. Complete blood count
   b. Tape test
   c. Abdominal x-ray
   d. Carbon urea breath test

197. A gang member who killed two children in a shooting is hospitalized under police guard and recovering from a gunshot wound. Which of the following violates the ANA Code of Ethics for Nurses?
   a. A nurse provides basic care but refuses to talk to the client.
   b. A nurse asks to be assigned to a different client.
   c. A nurse asks to take vacation time to avoid caring for the client.
   d. A nurse tells the team leader that he feels conflicted about caring for the client.

198. A patient has undergone an elective abortion, and according to hospital rules, a nurse who is morally opposed to abortions was excused from caring for the patient. However, the patient's assigned nurse is off of the floor, and as the nurse passes by the patient's room, the patient calls out, "Help, I think I'm bleeding!" Which of the following actions by the nurse is correct?

    a. Tell the patient the nurse will find another nurse to examine her.
    b. Call the nurse assigned to the patient and ask the nurse to return to examine the patient.
    c. Examine the patient for bleeding.
    d. Contact a supervisor.

199. A new mother transferring from the delivery room to her room on the unit asks the nurse if her infant will need any immunizations before they are discharged. Which of the following immunizations should the nurse advise the mother the child will require within 12 hours of birth?

    a. Polio
    b. Heptavalent pneumococcal conjugate
    c. Hepatitis B
    d. Rotavirus

200. Which of the following are examples of positive reinforcement for a client with anorexia? **Select all that apply.**

    a. The nurse tells the client, "If you don't stay with the program, you won't make progress."
    b. The client is granted an additional hour of Internet use after eating all her dinner.
    c. The nurse tells the client, "You are making good progress."
    d. The client gains one-half pound.
    e. The client loses privileges for losing one-half pound.

Answers and Explanations

1. D: The period of maximal respiratory depression after subcutaneous injection of morphine sulfate is approximately 90 minutes while it is 30 minutes for intramuscular and 7 minutes for intravenous. The respiratory center sensitivity should return to normal within 3 hours, but minute volume may remain impaired for up to 5 hours, so clients should be monitored carefully for indications of respiratory depression. IV morphine peaks at approximately 20 minutes while IM peaks at 30 to 60 minutes and SQ at 50 to 90 minutes.

2. C: Two hours of activity are necessary in each 24-hour period to prevent disuse syndrome with muscle atrophy and joint contractures, but periods of exercise should be spaced and not done all at one time. Exercises may include ambulation, active and passive range-of-motion exercises, isometric exercises, and resistive isometric exercises. Clients should be encouraged to do as much independently as possible, and children may engage in active play activities.

3.

Minor injury	Immediate care	Delayed care	Unsalvageable
A. II Sprain, cuts	B. I Arterial bleed	C. IV Fx femur	D. III Crush injuries

A-II: Minor injuries can safely be attended to later. The injured are generally alert and responsive and ambulatory ("walking wounded"). B-I: People with life-threatening injuries must be tended to immediately, so they have first priority. C-IV: People with moderate to serious injuries that are not immediately life threatening can receive delayed care and are second priority. D-III: Those who are unsalvageable, meaning their injuries are incompatible with life, have the lowest priority.

4. B: As an advocate for the client, the nurse has a responsibility to inform the physician that the client's Advance Directive specifically states he is not to receive intravenous fluids. Many times, physicians order treatments without referring to the Advance Directive, so the nurse should always be aware of client's preferences and should communicate them. If the physician insists on the treatment, then the nurse should contact a supervisor to determine if there is an organizational policy regarding the issue.

5. A and B: Anti-embolic compression stockings must be applied properly, or they can have a constrictive effect. The stocking must be without wrinkles and the top must not be turned down as this makes a constrictive band that can impair venous circulation. The stockings should be removed and reapplied at least every 8 hours so that the skin can be examined and wrinkles removed. The client correctly holds onto the toe and turns the stocking inside out before applying, and putting a small amount of baby powder or talcum powder on the skin may make application easier.

6. B: Chest discomfort and hiccupping are often indications that the atrial lead of a pacemaker has become dislodged and is stimulating the phrenic nerve, resulting in persistent hiccupping. If phrenic nerve stimulation is caused by output, then reprogramming may alleviate the problem, but if leads are displaced, then they must be replaced, and this is a medical emergency. In some cases, a lead may be too close to the diaphragm, resulting in repeated stimulation, especially if the patient is very thin.

7. B, C, D, and E: Neurological changes associated with aging include short-term memory loss, but dementia does not normally occur unless there is an underlying disorder. Peripheral nerve cells may begin to degenerate, causing muscles of the arms and legs to atrophy. The threshold for sensory input may increase and vibratory sensation may decrease. Autonomic changes cause reduced perspiration so that core temperature is higher before sweating is induced. Post-operative delirium is more likely to occur in older adults than younger.

8. C: *Staphylococcus aureus* is a common skin bacterium, and some strains, such as methicillin-resistant *Staphylococcus aureus* (MRSA), are especially virulent. Skin infections with pustular lesions may develop and spread quickly. Common manifestations of MRSA infections include impetigo, cellulitis, boils, abscesses, and rashes. Because the infection may spread systemically to internal organs, the infection must be aggressively treated with antibiotics.

9. A: While ideally printed materials should be available in a number of languages, if none are available in the language needed, then the nurse should contact a medical translator. Telephone translation services are available if speakers cannot be found locally. Children should not be asked to translate for adults as they may not completely understand and may not translate correctly. The nurse should not depend on diagrams and pantomime if medications or specific treatments are involved, and non-English speakers may not have personal access to people who can adequately translate.

10. 100%: Bioavailability refers to the amount of a drug that is absorbed unchanged into the systemic circulation. Morphine is poorly absorbed through the oral route because of the way it is metabolized in the intestines and liver, but medications that are administered intravenously immediately enter the systemic circulation and the bioavailability is 100%. Intramuscular and transdermal administration of medications also have high bioavailability, so when switching a client from oral medications to another form, the dosage may need to be adjusted.

11. C: If the umbilical cord becomes soiled with urine or feces, it should be washed with mild soap and water, rinsed, and dried. Wiping with alcohol is no longer recommended as it may increase irritation of the surrounding skin. The cord should not be covered with clothing and should be protected by folding the top of the diaper under the cord instead of covering the cord with the diaper. The baby should not be immersed in water until the cord falls off in 10 to 14 days.

12. 1.7 mL: The calculation is as follows:
Required dose X amount of solution/mg of medication.
85 X 2/100
85 X 0.02 = 1.7 mL.
Using an algebraic formula
100/2 = 85/x
100 x = 170
100x/100 = 170/100
x = 1.7 mL

13. A-II: Place a small pillow between client's knees. B-IV: Cross client's arms across chest in preparation for turn. C-I: Grasping draw sheet at shoulder and lower hips, roll patient on count of three. D-III: (Opposite nurse) Place pillows along length of client's back to provide support and maintain the person in the side-lying position. After the client is positioned, the nurse should check body alignment and client's comfort level to determine if more pillows or rolled bath blankets are needed for support.

14. 30 g: To convert pounds to kilograms, divide pounds by 2.2 (132/2.2 = 60). Then, multiply the kilograms of weight by the per-kilogram dose (60 X 0.5 = 30 g). When converting kilograms to pounds, multiply kilograms by 2.2. Mannitol is an osmotic diuretic that is used to increase excretion of sodium and water in order to reduce ICP and brain mass, especially after traumatic brain injury. Mannitol may also be used to shrink the cells of the blood-brain barrier to facilitate other medications breaching this barrier.

15. B: Lead V4. The 12-lead ECG gives a picture of electrical activity from 12 perspectives through placement of 10 body leads:
4 limb leads for both arms and both legs
Precordial leads:
V1: right sternal border at 4th intercostal space
V2: left sternal border at 4th intercostal space
V3: midway between V2 and V4
V4: left midclavicular line at 5th intercostal space
V5: horizontal to V4 at left anterior axillary line
V6: horizontal to V5 at left midaxillary line

16. B and D: The elbow range of motion should include the following:
Flexion: Bend elbow until the hand is level with the shoulder.
Extension: Straighten elbow until arm is almost vertical (150 degrees) without forcing.
Hyperextension: Bend elbow and extend lower arm as far back as possible (10 to 20 degrees) beyond vertical.
Range-of-motion exercises for the elbow can be incorporated into activities of daily living. Eating, bathing, shaving, combing the hair, and brushing the teeth all involve both flexion and extension of the elbow.

17. B: When conducting measurements for crutches with a client in standing position, the tips of the crutches should be placed approximately 4 to 6 inches to the side and 4 to 6 inches in front of the client's feet. The crutch pads should be 1.5 to 2 inches below the axilla and the client cautioned not to bear weight under the axilla but to hold the crutches against the lateral chest wall to prevent nerve damage. The client's elbows should be slightly flexed (15 to 30 degrees) when grasping the handgrip.

18. D: Because the client is confused, the nurse should place the ring in a secured container, according to organizational policy, which may vary widely. The ring should not be given to a friend or family member without consent and should not be replaced on the client's finger as the client may remove it again. The nurse should document when the ring was found, where it was found, and where it was placed for safekeeping. If witnesses are required, their names should be documented as well.

19. February 2014: Depending on the formula one uses, the exact date may vary. Starting with the first day of the last menstrual period on May 1, 2013, and using Naegele's formula, subtract 3 months and add 6 days. This would place the delivery date at February 7, 2014. Another formula adds 9 months and 7 days, placing the delivery date at February 8. Still other formulas place the date at February 5. Generally, gestation is considered to be 280 days in duration.

20. 0.02: A microgram (µg) is one-millionth of a gram (g). There are 1000 milligrams in a gram and 1000 micrograms in a milligram. In order to convert micrograms to milligrams, divide the micrograms by 1000 (20/1000 = 0.02 mg). To convert milligrams to micrograms, multiply the milligrams by 1000 (0.02mg X 1000 = 20 micrograms). Other conversions:
mg to cg = mg/10; cg to mg = cg X 10
g to cg = g X 100; cg to g = cg/100
mg to g = mg/1000; g to mg = g X 1000

21. D: The nurse should not attempt a procedure for which the nurse has not been trained and is not familiar. Chest physiotherapy may result in injury to a child if done incorrectly. The nurse should tell the physician that he has not been trained to do chest physiotherapy on children but will attempt to locate another staff person knowledgeable about the procedure. Nurses should not rely on parents or other family members to explain procedures.

22. A, B, and C: Increased estrogen production during pregnancy promotes hyperplasia of vaginal mucosa and increased production of mucus. This can create a warm, moist environment that promotes *Candida* monilial infection. The client should be advised to bathe daily and wear cotton panties but to avoid wearing nylon panties or pantyhose, panty liners, and tight clothing as these can increase the temperature and prevent airflow. The client should also be advised not to douche. Topical treatments that can be used include miconazole, butoconazole, clotrimazole, tioconazole, nystatin, or terconazole.

23. C: After withdrawing the correct dosage of heparin into a syringe, approximately 0.2 to 0.3 mL of air should be drawn into the syringe. This air helps to clear the remaining drug from the syringe and to "lock" the medication into the tissue. After the air is drawn into the syringe, the cap should be replaced carefully and the syringe pointed needle down so that the air bubble rises to the top of the syringe. Heparin injection sites should be rotated with usual sites in the upper and lower abdomen and anterior thighs.

24. C: **Lochia rubra** (days 1 to 3 or 4): Dark red discharge with small clots (smaller than nickel size). Larger clots may indicate hemorrhage or bleeding from vaginal lacerations. **Lochia serosa** (days 4 to 10): Pinkish to brownish discharge, gradually lightening as the number of red blood cells decreases. **Lochia alba** (persists an additional 2 to 85 days with average of 24 days): Yellowish discharge. Lochia alba ceases when the cervix closes. This decreases the chance of uterine infection.

25. A, B, and D: The Z-track injection technique is especially indicated for IM drugs that are irritating to the tissues, such as iron, haloperidol, hydroxyzine, and interferon. Procedure:
Fill syringe, including approximately 0.3 mL of air to provide an air lock.
Choose site (avoid deltoid). Don gloves and cleanse skin in a circular pattern.
Place 3 fingers or ulnar surface of nondominant hand on skin and pull skin laterally.
Inject at 90 degrees over 3 to 5 seconds in the spot that fingers or hand was initially placed.

Hold needle in place for 10 seconds.
Withdraw needle and release tissue.

26. D: **Extended kin network:** Two nuclear families live closely together and share goods, services, and childcare. This model is common in Hispanic families. **Nuclear:** Husband-wife-children model in which the mother usually stays home and cares for the children while the husband is the wage earner (7% of American families). **Dual career/dual earner:** Both parents work (66% of two-parent families) although one may work more than the other. **Extended:** Multigenerational or shared households with friends or family who share childcare responsibilities.

27. C and D: Sublingual and buccal medications should not be administered if the mucous membranes in the mouth are red and irritated or if the client is dehydrated, because these conditions may interfere with absorption of the medication. While severe confusion may pose a problem, as long as the client is cognizant enough to cooperate with administration, dementia alone is not a contraindication. Being edentulous is not a contraindication because sublingual wafers absorb readily and do not have to be held in place for extended periods.

28. A, B, D, and E: Production of milk sometimes outstrips demand in the first 2–3 days because the baby ingests small amounts, so the breasts often become engorged. Nursing frequently (every 2–3 hours) and gently massaging the breast toward the nipple while nursing can help reduce engorgement. If the areola is hard, some milk should be manually expressed to soften the areola before the infant latches on. Breast pumps and heat (except in a shower) may increase engorgement. Cold compresses, acetaminophen, or ibuprofen may provide relief. Engorgement usually recedes within 24 to 48 hours.

29. D: While all solid medications, such as pills, tablets, and capsules, should be delivered to the client in a disposable paper medicine cup, all individually wrapped doses should be opened in the presence of the client after verifying the client's identification with two identifiers. Prior to administration, the client should be assessed for level of consciousness, nausea and vomiting, and difficulty swallowing. Calibrated medicine cups are used for liquid preparations of 5 mL or more, but smaller amounts should be measured in a syringe for accuracy.

30. A: While knowledge of childcare is helpful to a new mother, it does not necessarily promote attachment between a newborn and mother. Important factors include frequent contact, starting as soon after birth as possible; breastfeeding, ideally starting within 60 minutes of birth; and utilizing rooming-in so that the baby stays with the mother rather than in a nursery, allowing the mother to respond readily to the infant's needs. New mothers should be reassured that bonding may take time and that it is normal if the mother does not feel an immediate attachment.

31. A and D: Schedule I drugs, such as cocaine and LSD, have high potential for abuse and no accepted medical use. Schedule II drugs pose potential for abuse and addiction and include most commonly used narcotics (codeine, hydrocodone). Schedule III drugs, such as anabolic steroids and intermediate-acting barbiturates, have lesser potential for abuse. Schedule IV drugs, including benzodiazepines, may lead to limited physical or psychological dependence. Schedule V drugs, including cough suppressants, have low potential for abuse. Schedule VI drugs include those with low potential for abuse and addiction, such as OTC drugs like ibuprofen and diphenhydramine (Benadryl®).

32. D: African-Americans have the greatest risk of developing diabetes mellitus type 2, although risks are also high for Mexican Americans, Native Americans and Hawaiians, and some Asian Americans, all of whom also have high rates of hypertension and obesity. Risk is also increased if a family member has the disease. Diabetes mellitus type 2 is the most prevalent type, accounting for 90% to 95% of cases of diabetes, and is closely associated with obesity.

33. B: Nocturnal myoclonus is a toxic effect of opioid analgesics. Toxicity may occur because they have metabolites that are neuroexcitatory. The medication dosage should be reduced by at least half and a benzodiazepine administered. The drug may also be changed to an equianalgesic, but opioids should not be discontinued as the client may experience withdrawal and inadequate pain control. Naloxone is not an effective solution for toxicity, and flumazenil is a benzodiazepine antagonist.

34. A, C, and D: Most people who are sexually active remain so, so even though the adolescent may be adamant that she is not going to have sex again until she is married, the nurse should advise her that ALL people need to know about safe sex and that she can share what she has learned with her friends. Many people believe that a condom is not necessary for oral sex, but they are mistaken. "I'm confused about different birth control methods" is a clear indication that information is needed.

35. A: Naloxone (Narcan®) is an opioid antagonist and should be administered if clients exhibit signs of acute respiratory and/or circulatory depression, although it must be used cautiously with opioid addiction as clients may experience withdrawal symptoms. For an opioid overdose in an adult client, the usual initial dose is 0.4 to 2 mg intravenously, repeated at 2- to 3-minute intervals. If the client does not have adequate response after administration of 10 mg, then other causes for the symptoms should be explored.

36. C: The maximum adult dosage of acetaminophen in 24 hours is 4 g. A single dose of 20 to 25 g can result in hepatic necrosis and liver failure with 25 g often resulting in death. The toxic reaction of acetaminophen is potentiated by alcohol. Clients often exhibit mild symptoms of nausea, vomiting, and abdominal pain in the first two days after overdose but by the second or third day, signs of liver injury become evident with elevations of transaminase, lactic hydrogenase, and bilirubin and prolonged prothrombin time. Oral N-acetylcysteine is administered to prevent or reduce liver damage.

37. B: A complete initial assessment, ongoing assessments, frequent evaluations of lithium levels, and client education are all essential. Plasma levels of lithium must be frequently monitored for lithium toxicity, which can lead to death. The normal therapeutic range of lithium is 0.6 to 1.4 mEq/L for adults. About 1 client in 25 develops goiter from lithium-induced hypothyroidism, so clients must be evaluated for thyroid disease prior to beginning therapy and on a regular basis afterward. Clients should avoid NSAIDs and dehydration.

38. A: Children younger than 8 years should not receive tetracycline because it can result in discoloration and inadequate calcification of permanent teeth if taken during the process of tooth calcification. Because this process is usually completed by the time the child is 8, the medication may be used in older children. The pediatric dose is 20 to 50 mg/kg orally in 4 equal doses over 24 hours. Discoloration and inadequate calcification of permanent teeth may also result from fetal exposure to tetracycline.

39. C: The nurse should report the observations to the infection control nurse. The nurse should avoid making assumptions about cause and effect until an investigation is concluded. While increased rates of infection may indicate surgeon negligence, they can also indicate that the physician simply has more clients on the unit than other physicians, that an operating room is contaminated, that surgical procedures are not followed by all surgical staff, or that the physician has clients who are immunocompromised or more susceptible to infection because of condition.

40. A: Bulk laxatives, such as Metamucil® and Citrucel®, are usually the safest for most people because their action most closely mimics human physiology. The polysaccharides or cellulose derivatives contained in the laxatives combine with fluids in the intestine to form gels, which stimulate peristalsis and evacuation. Clients must be advised to drink adequate liquids because bulk laxatives may induce constipation if clients are dehydrated. Clients should be encouraged to increase bulk naturally in the diet through eating bran, fruits, and vegetables.

41. B: Because penicillin may cause an anaphylactic reaction, especially in someone who has previously has a milder reaction, the correct action is to hold the drug and notify the prescribing physician that the client may have had a drug reaction so that the physician can order a skin test or an alternate antibiotic. Common adverse effects of penicillin include rash, hives, itching, and edema of face, lips, and/or tongue. Anaphylactic reactions usually occur within 60 minutes of contact with the causative agent.

42. C: **Fresh frozen plasma** replaces plasma but does not contain red blood cells or platelets. It does, however, contain most coagulation factors and complement, so it is the blood product of choice for disorders in which coagulation factors are needed. **Whole blood** is rarely used but replaces both red blood cells and plasma. **Irradiated red blood cells** are used to replace red blood cells in those who are immunocompromised. **Platelets** are used for those with thrombocytopenia.

43. C: Even though the client indicated he might want the medication at a later time, the medication must be disposed of following facility protocol with two witnesses, both of whom are licensed to dispense medications and directly observe the disposal and sign a document verifying the disposal. A medication removed from a medicine cart may not be placed back into the cart, and drugs cannot be left at a client's bedside or kept in an unsecure location, such as a tray, for later administration.

44. B: Seventy-five (75) drops per minute. In order to complete the calculation, the time needs to be converted to minutes. Three hours and 20 minutes equals 200 minutes. Then, the flow rate (mL per minute) is calculated by dividing the total volume by the minutes: 1000 mL/200 minutes equals 5 mL per minute. Since there are 15 drops per mL and 5 mL per minute, the flow rate is 15 X 5 equals 75 drops per minute.

45. A: While protocols may vary slightly, generally those receiving brachytherapy are restricted to a private room during the duration of therapy. Women who are pregnant and children under age 18 may not visit, and visitors are limited to no more than 2 hours' visit per day. Visitors must remain at least 6 feet away from the client during visits. Nurses must limit time in the room to that necessary for essential care. Housekeeping staff should be accompanied by a nurse if entering the room is necessary.

46. B: Once a sterile field is contaminated, everything within the field is also considered contaminated, so the nurse must discard the sterile field and gauze pads and start over with new supplies. When establishing a sterile field, the nurse must ensure that the area under the sterile field is clean and dry, as moisture will contaminate the field. The nurse uses clean gloves to remove the old dressing and bare hands or new clean gloves to open the sterile field and gauze packages but dons sterile gloves to apply new dressings.

47. 12 mL: The first calculation is to determine the amount of drug per milligram: 100/10 = 10 mg per mL. Then, the total dose is divided by the dose per mL: 120/10 = 12 mL. The calculation can also be done by a simple algebraic formula.
100/10 = 120/x
100x = 1200
1x = 12

48. C: The most common treatment for both strains (pulled muscles) and sprains (joint damage) is RICE therapy. **Rest** avoids further injury and lets the tissue begin to heal. **Ice/cold compresses** (15–20 minutes per hour for 24 to 48 hours) helps to reduce edema. **Compression** (such as with Ace bandages) helps to reduce edema and prevent further swelling. **Elevation** (above the heart) helps to decrease edema by increasing drainage. RICE is usually sufficient for first-degree sprains, but second- or third-degree sprains may require splinting to support the joint.

49. D: Regardless of experience or position, every nurse is responsible for the safety and welfare of clients, so the nurse should immediately tell the team leader that the irrigating syringe was contaminated and offer to retrieve new sterile supplies. Accidents happen, and one incident does not necessarily mean the team leader is negligent. This is a matter for a supervisor only if the team leader ignores the nurse and continues with the irrigation using a contaminated syringe, putting the client at increased risk of infection.

50. B: The AED kit contains cutting shears so that the nurse can quickly expose the chest. The nurse should use the shears to cut away bras with metal wires because the wires may cause arcing during defibrillation. Likewise, any metal piercings on the chest, such as nipple rings, should be removed. The defibrillator electrodes are placed on the right upper chest (negative) and below and lateral to the heart on the left side (positive). AEDs provide spoken messages and diagrams to guide people through the process.

51. 15 mg: In this case, calculation involves only multiplying the number of kilograms of weight (60) times the milligrams per kilogram (0.5). Thus, 60 X 0.5 = 30 mg per 24 hours. Since the drug is to be given in two equal doses (30/2), each dose is 15 mg.

52. C: While digoxin is used to slow the heart rate, digoxin toxicity may result in either tachycardia or bradycardia as well as almost any type of dysrhythmia. Central nervous system symptoms can include fatigue, headache, and confusion with convulsions with severe toxicity. Clients often complain of GI upsets, including lack of appetite, diarrhea, nausea, and vomiting. They may also report visual disturbances, such as halo vision, colored vision, and flickering lights. The medication should be stopped immediately and cardiac monitoring started with symptoms treated as necessary.

53. A, C, D, and E: Drug compliance is especially important for seizure disorders, and since phenytoin is usually given once or twice daily, the client should establish a routine of taking

the drug at the same times each day. Phenytoin may cause gingival hyperplasia, so careful dental care and routine dental evaluations are necessary. Long-term use of phenytoin may also cause osteoporosis, so people should take vitamin D prophylactically and exercise regularly as well as having periodic evaluations of osteoporosis to determine if other medications are necessary.

54. A: Loop diuretics, such as furosemide, block chloride and sodium resorption in the ascending limb of the loop of Henle, bringing about rapid diuresis but with major electrolyte disturbance, especially hypokalemia and hyponatremia and to a lesser degree hypocalcemia. Hypokalemia is of most importance because it can result in dysrhythmias with ECG abnormalities, hypotension, lethargy, weakness, nausea and vomiting, paresthesias, muscle cramping, and tetany. Normal values are 3.5 to 5.5 mEq/L. Potassium supplementation is often given routinely with loop diuretics.

55. A, B, C, and E: A newly diagnosed client with diabetes type 1 may feel overwhelmed with information, but the nurse must ensure the client understands basic information about glucose testing and insulin administration, skin care, and dietary compliance. The client must also be taught how to respond to signs of hypoglycemia and hyperglycemia and when to call the physician. The client also needs practical information about how to store medications, where to obtain supplies, and how often to have blood tests, such as HbA1c.

56. C: Infants are usually uncooperative with eye drops and instinctually clinch the eyes tightly to avoid them. The most appropriate method is to gently restrain the head in neutral position while the child is lying supine and place the drops at the inner canthus. When the baby opens the eyes, the fluid will flow into the eye. A caregiver, such as a parent, can assist by restraining the child's head and speaking to the child during the procedure.

57. B: The **ventrogluteal site** is the preferred site for intramuscular injections because the muscle is deep and there is no proximity to major blood vessels or nerves, making this the safest site for injections. The **deltoid site** is commonly used for immunizations in toddlers, children, and adults, but not infants. Injections to the deltoid should be limited to 1 mL. The **dorsogluteal site** is close to the sciatic nerve and should be used only if other sites are not accessible or not adequate. The **vastus lateralis** is also a safe site and is used for immunizations for infants.

58. C: Piggyback units should be hung at least 6 inches higher than the primary intravenous unit. Because of the force of gravity when the piggyback unit is infusing, the flow from the primary unit stops until the piggyback unit is empty and then it starts again, so clamping the primary unit tubing is not necessary. During infusion of the piggyback unit, a backcheck valve prevents the piggyback solution from flowing up into the primary unit.

59. A, B, D, and E: The nurse should always check client identification and allergies prior to administering any medication. With IV push medication, the manufacturer's guidelines for dosage and the correct dilution should be checked because improperly diluting a medication may result in complications. Most IV push medications are administered slowly over 1 to 5 minutes, but some medications, such as adenosine, must be injected rapidly, so the recommended administration time should be adhered to, using a watch to verify time rather than approximating.

60. C: After administration of a vaginal suppository, the woman must remain in supine position for 5 to 10 minutes to allow time for the suppository to melt and the medication to spread throughout the vagina. The suppository should be at room temperature prior to administration. If an applicator is available, it should be inserted deeply into the vagina. If inserting the suppository digitally, the finger should be inserted about 2 inches into the vagina so that the suppository rests at the cervix. The woman may want to wear a peri-pad or panty shield to contain any discharge.

61. D: Pyridoxine (Vitamin B6) can reverse the effects of levodopa in doses exceeding 10 mg. Foods high in vitamin B6 include bran, liver, fish (salmon, cod), pork tenderloin, tahini, molasses, and hazelnuts. Levodopa should be taken with meals to minimize gastrointestinal effects, but with minimal protein at the time the medication is taken. Clients should eat proteins in small frequent amounts at other times. The client should drink at least 2 liters of fluid daily.

62. B: Methamphetamine is a psychostimulant that can be snorted, ingested orally, smoked, or injected intravenously. While methamphetamine has similar effects to cocaine, the effect is much longer lasting and can persist up to 24 hours. Methamphetamine is often taken with alcohol to temper the anxiety that may occur, but the combination may increase blood pressure and risk of heart attack or stroke. Methamphetamine users often pick at their skin, leaving lesions that appear as severe acne, and may lose weight because of lack of appetite. "Meth mouth" with dental decay is a common sign.

63. A: Incidental teaching uses a child's interests as teaching opportunities and motivation to respond for those with autism spectrum disorder. This type of teaching is not classroom-based. The best example is when the nurse asks, "What color is the bunny?" and waits for a correct response before giving the child the desired toy. Questions should be appropriate for the child's age and abilities. Objective questions are easier for children with autism spectrum disorder than subjective questions.

64. D: Back chaining is an approach that teaches the last step in a process first and once that is mastered adds the next-to-the-last step, and so on until the task is mastered. For example, if teaching a child to make a peanut butter and jelly sandwich, the last step would be to place the sandwich on a plate, so the nurse would do everything except that and then ask the child to put the completed sandwich on the plate, waiting until the child masters this successfully before adding the next-to-the-last step.

65. C: According to the American Medical Association, informed consent must include the following:
Explanation of diagnosis
Nature and reason for treatment or procedure
Risks and benefits
Alternative options (regardless of cost or insurance coverage)
Risks and benefits of alternative options
Risks and benefits of not having a treatment or procedure
Providing informed consent is a requirement of all states. The client should be given full and clear information prior to signing the consent form and should be encouraged to ask questions to clarify any information that is not clear.

66. B: Because abusers often accompany victims of domestic abuse to the hospital, the first question should be "Is the person who did this to you present here in the hospital?" If the client answers affirmatively, then security should be called immediately for the client's and nurse's protection. Even if the client answers negatively, the nurse should observe carefully any interactions the client has with someone accompanying her, as she may be too frightened or too ashamed to answer truthfully.

67. A: The initial diagnostic test should be the electrocardiogram because these symptoms are consistent with myocardial infarctions in females, who may not experience the "classic" symptoms of crushing chest pain more associated with males. Females often complain of chest or abdominal tightness and pressure and pain in the neck, jaw, shoulders, or arms rather than the chest. Some clients may complain of "indigestion" and most feel severe fatigue. Nausea, dyspnea, and cold, clammy skin are common findings.

68. C: This is an example of **rationalization** because the client is attempting to make excuses for drinking excessively. Clients often try to find logical reasons for their actions and often blame their situations, family members, or friends for their problems. With **repression**, the client involuntarily blocks the awareness of negative feelings and experiences. **Suppression** is similar to repression, but the blocking of awareness is voluntary. **Denial** is a refusal to acknowledge that a problem exists at all.

69. C: While all of these are possibilities, the most likely reason is simply that the client is exhibiting cultural traits common to Native Americans. Native Americans often avoid direct eye contact as a way to show respect and politeness, and they tend to be more comfortable with silence during a conversation than is typical in American culture. Native Americans also value personal space and may be uncomfortable with touch. They may feel more comfortable with folk approaches to healing rather than Western medicine and may want to combine both during treatment.

70. D: The client is grappling with the spiritual need to forgive. Forgiveness can be very difficult—both forgiving the self and others—and clients may obsess over mistakes they or others have made. Clients may believe that forgiving someone means accepting or condoning the behavior; however, forgiving can be freeing for the client and relieve the stress associated with anger towards someone. Even if clients are unable to forgive, they may be able to make peace with what has occurred and move forward more positively.

71. A and B: Disguising the doorway by hanging a curtain across it or placing a painting on the door is enough to prevent some clients with dementia from opening the door. A good way to keep clients inside is to place a latch at the top or bottom of the door as Alzheimer clients rarely look beyond the doorknob when trying to open a door. Clients should never be locked into a room, and motion sensors with alarms are often terrifying to clients, increasing their stress and need to get away.

72. C and D: While clients who are angry may exhibit passive-aggressive behavior and may avoid eye contact or stare at others, those who have the potential for assaultive behavior are usually more threatening and may make verbal threats ("I'll kill you!") or physical threats (pushing, shoving) with anger disproportionate to situation. They are often very tense and agitated, pacing and exhibiting restlessness. They often use a loud intimidating voice with shouting and obscenities. They may respond excessively to environmental stimuli and have disturbed thought processes and suspicions of others.

73. B: The client is probably in the anger stage of the grief process (Kübler-Ross). Upon receiving bad news, many clients initially experience **denial**, although this period usually only lasts one to two weeks. Within a few hours of receiving bad news, many also begin to experience **anger**, and this anger is often directed at family members and caregivers because clients feel helpless and terrified. Many also go through a **bargaining** stage where they may begin attending religious services or seek other opinions. **Depression** may be prolonged as the client comes to grips with loss and finally reaches **acceptance**.

74. C: As much as possible, clients with dementia should be oriented to what is true but without directly challenging them or telling them they are wrong, and the nurse should avoid humoring clients by playing along with their confused statements. In this case, telling the date (July 2) and the time (lunch time) helps to orient the client, and offering to allow the client to watch a movie responds to the client's stated desire to go a movie. If the client becomes extremely agitated at being contradicted, then the best response may be to refocus the client's attention.

75. A: "What aspects of the dying process are you most concerned about?" is the best response because it encourages the client to express her concerns and allows the nurse to assess what can be done to alleviate those concerns. For example, many people facing death are afraid of dying in pain, and the nurse can assure that client that adequate control of pain is almost always possible. This provides a good opportunity also to discuss hospice care. Some clients may express concern about family or financial obligations. These clients may benefit from the assistance of a social worker.

76. D: The client is probably practicing thought-stopping. This is a technique that people sometimes use to stop the intrusion of negative thoughts or anxiety. Initially, clients learn the technique by imagining something that causes them to have negative thoughts, such as the fear of being in public, and then they shout, "STOP," and attempt to redirect thoughts. Over time, they speak the word "stop" and then may substitute a silent thought. Some people use the snap of a rubber band against the skin to stop thoughts.

77. A: While all of these things have value, clients who have been raped often find it difficult to talk about the rape itself initially but may more easily discuss their feelings—fear, anger, shame—so that is a good place to begin. Providing too much information too early, such as about relaxation techniques and resources, often serves little purpose because the client is too traumatized to process the information. Clients undergoing a traumatic stress crisis are victims of stressors over which they have no control, and this can leave them feeling overwhelmed and depressed.

78. A, B, and C: Normalization is the process of providing a child with as normal an environment as possible in a facility, such as a hospital. Rooms may be painted in bright colors and play areas provided. Visiting hours are usually unrestricted, and siblings (and sometimes therapy animals) are allowed to visit. Children may eat in communal areas and be allowed more choices related to foods and sleeping hours. Planned play activities and group activities may be available for children as well. Doll reenactment is a therapeutic play technique.

79. B: Panic attacks usually subside within 5 to 30 minutes, and the best nursing response is to stay with the client while the panic attack occurs, speaking in a calm reassuring voice even though the client in the acute stage may not be processing verbal input. Maintaining

the client's safety is a primary concern because during panic attacks clients may bolt and run, even sometimes injuring themselves in the process. Quieting the environment and reducing stimuli may help reduce the client's anxiety.

80. A, C, and D: The nurse should ask the client to describe hallucinations because this information is necessary to help the nurse calm the client and to determine if the client or others are at risk because of the hallucinations. The nurse should communicate frequently with the client, helping to keep the client oriented and presenting a model of reality. The nurse should also encourage the client to participate in reality-based activities, such as playing cards or badminton. Using distracting techniques is helpful when intervening for delusions but less successful with hallucinations.

81. D: The primary risk factor for cervical cancer is a history of human papillomavirus infection. HPV comprises >100 viruses. About 40 are sexually transmitted and invade mucosal tissue, causing genital warts (condylomata). HPV infection causes changes in the mucosa, which can lead to cervical cancer. Over 99% of cervical cancers are caused by HPV, and 70% are related to HPVs 16 and 18. The HPV vaccine, Gardasil®, protects against HPVs 6 and 11 (which cause genital warts), 16 and 18 (which cause cancer). Protection is only conveyed if the female has not yet been infected with these strains.

82. A and B: While most contraceptives are relatively safe for women who smoke, smokers over age 35 are usually advised to avoid combined hormone pills and vaginal rings, such as NuvaRing® (which releases both estrogen and progestogen). The women may more safely take progestogen-only pills or use an intrauterine device, intrauterine system, or diaphragm as well as implanted contraceptives and the contraceptive injection.

83. D: While there is value in all of these approaches—written instructions, help number, questions—the best method is to ask the client to do a return demonstration. This allows the nurse to directly observe and evaluate the client's ability to carry out the needed actions. The client should be able to refer to written directions during the demonstration, but if the client requires the nurse's assistance or becomes confused, this indicates the need for further education.

84. D: Heberden's nodes are characteristic of osteoarthritis. Other findings may include radial deviation of the distal phalanx (finger tip tilted toward the thumb) and Bouchard's nodes, nodules on the proximal interphalangeal joints. Osteoarthritis is usually caused by previous injury to joints, so it may occur on one side only, and is associated with cartilage deterioration. It is slowly progressive with symptoms usually occurring after age 60.

85. B: Carotemia causes a yellowing of the skin but does not affect the sclera, so the nurse should first ask about the child's diet. Carotemia results from increased levels of beta-carotene in the blood, usually related to high dietary intake of yellow-orange foods, such as sweet potatoes and carrots. Carotemia is common in children if caregivers give the child large amounts of carrots but can also occur in adult vegetarians or people who take excessive carotene nutritional supplements.

86. 20 weeks: While the fetal heartbeat may be observed on ultrasound at about 6½ weeks gestation, it cannot usually be detected by fetoscope until 20 weeks. In early pregnancy, fetal heart tones are often more easily heard above the symphysis pubis, but this position shifts later according to fetal growth and position. Fetal heart tones are more easily

detected through the fetus's back, so at later weeks of gestation, the nurse should palpate the fetal position before auscultating.

87. B: In the traditional Hispanic culture, people often believe that children should be started on regular foods early as it will promote increased growth and development, because a common belief is that a large baby is healthier and stronger even though this practice may, in fact, limit growth and increase risk of choking. Some people also believe that the infant must be exposed to cultural foods early to acquire a taste for them. It can be challenging to change cultural ideas, but the nurse should provide as much education about infant nutritional needs as possible.

88. C: The lower border of the blood pressure cuff should be placed at about 2.5 cm above the antecubital crease. The arm should be flexed slightly at the elbow and positioned so that the antecubital crease is at heart level. The inflatable bladder of the cuff should be over the brachial artery. The nurse should palpate the radial pulse while increasing pressure on the cuff, and when the pulse is no longer palpable, raise cuff pressure another 30 mm Hg.

89. A: Careful observation can detect hearing deficits at an early age. By 3 months, an infant should exhibit a positive Moro reflex (startle) to sound and may awaken with noise and react to sound by opening or blinking the eyes. Between 3 and 6 months, and infant should begin to coo and try to emulate sounds and should look in the direction of sounds, such as a ringing telephone, and should begin to respond to his or her name. Babies usually begin to say first words by 12 to 15 months, imitate sounds, and follow vocal directions.

90. A: The symptoms are consistent with diabetes mellitus type 1, so the laboratory assessment that is most indicated is blood glucose and HbA1c. The blood glucose level indicates the current level of glucose in the blood (normal value ≤100 mg/dL), but the level may fluctuate throughout the day and vary according to dietary intake. HbA1c provides a more accurate assessment because it shows the average glucose level over a 3-month period. The normal value for HbA1c is <6%.

91. A: Hypernatremia results from water deprivation, such as can occur with dehydration, watery diarrhea, burns, diabetes insipidus, heatstroke, and excess sodium chloride administration. Indications include increased serum sodium level (>145 mEq/L) but decreased urine sodium as sodium is reabsorbed by the body rather than excreted through the urine. Urine specific gravity and osmolality are increased because sodium retention results in fluid retention (as the body attempts to compensate) and concentrated urine. Normal value: 135–145 mEq/L; Hyponatremia: <135 mEq/L; Hypernatremia: >145 mEq/L.

92. B and C: Roseola is a contagious disease for which there is no vaccine. It occurs primarily in children between 6 and 24 months of age after the decline of maternal antibodies makes them more susceptible to infection. Roseola is contagious with onset of fever, so the child has been exposed to the virus and may still develop the infection, as the incubation period is 9 to 10 days. Roseola is characterized by high fever for 3 to 8 days followed by a pale pink maculopapular rash that lasts 1 to 2 days.

93. A: Alginate dressings are appropriate for wounds with a large amount of exudate as they absorb the discharge and form a hydrophilic gel that conforms to the shape of the wound. Because the dressing material (wafers, ropes, fibers) swells in contact with discharge, the wound should be packed loosely. The alginate is covered with a secondary dressing.

Hydrocolloid dressings are effective for clean wounds or those with small to moderate exudate. Hydrogel is for dry wounds or those with a small amount of exudate. Transparent film is used with dry wounds.

94. B and C: During a severe generalized tonic-clonic seizure, the client should be turned to side-lying position to prevent aspiration. Padded tongue blades are no longer utilized with seizures and may cause damage to the mouth and teeth. The side rails should be elevated during the seizure and padded, using pillows or blankets, to prevent a fall from the bed and other injuries. The nurse should not physically restrain a client during a seizure as this may cause injury.

95. D: The Unna boot provides support to the calf muscle pump when the client ambulates, so it cannot be used for clients who are not ambulatory. In this case, it should be discontinued until the client is able to resume ambulation but should be replaced with an alternate form of compression, such as compression stockings, to decrease the danger of deep vein thrombosis. Short stretch wrap, such as Comprilan®, is also used only with ambulatory clients.

96. **Metric weight measures**

Milligram	Centigram	A-II Decigram	B-I Gram	C-III Dekagram	D-IV Hectogram	Kilogram

97. B, C, and D: This is a sigmoid colostomy, so much of the reabsorptive properties of the colon remain. Because of this, the stool may range from soft to solid. Many clients only expel stool every 2 to 3 days, so the client needs to find what is normal for him. Clients with sigmoid colostomies can often use irrigations to control bowel movements, and some are even able to trigger movements with certain foods or to expel stool on a predictable schedule. Clients should be advised of all of the options for appliances and stoma covers.

98. C: While over-medication, delirium, and hypoglycemia may all result in weakness and confusion, when the client was asked to show her teeth, the lips clearly lifted more on the left side than on the right side and more teeth can be observed on the left side. This suggests a weakness or paralysis, consistent with a stroke. Since the weakness is on the right side, the stroke is on the left side. When assessing a stroke patient for facial palsy, the nurse can ask the patient to show her teeth or pantomime the action.

99. B and C: With peripheral arterial insufficiency, the foot exhibits rubor on dependency and pallor on elevation. The skin often feels cool and appears pale and shiny with loss of hair on the leg, foot, and toes. Because of impaired circulation, the toenails may appear thick and ridged. Pedal pulses are weak or absent. Ulcers tend to occur on the tips of toes or between toes and on heels or other pressure areas. Ulcers are usually deep, circular, and painful and may be necrotic. Because the venous system may be intact, peripheral edema is usually minimal.

100. A: Because the onset of symptoms is rapid, these findings are consistent with pulmonary embolism. Acute pulmonary embolism occurs when a thrombus from the venous system or the right side of the heart travels to the lungs and blocks a pulmonary artery or arteriole, resulting in increased alveolar dead space in which ventilation occurs but gas exchange is impaired because of ventilation/perfusion mismatching or

intrapulmonary shunting. Common originating sites for thrombus formation are the deep veins in the legs, the pelvic veins, and the right atrium.

101. C and D: The nurse should never attempt to push protruding viscera back through an incision but should examine the viscera for indications of ischemia or other tissue damage and cover it with normal saline–soaked dressings to protect the tissue. The client should be placed in low Fowler's position with head of bed elevated 15 to 45 degrees and knees slightly flexed to reduce tension on the abdominal wound. The client's vital signs must be monitored carefully at least every 15 minutes and the client reassured.

102. A: The initial intervention when a client reports disturbed sleeping is to complete an assessment of sleep patterns. This should involve questions regarding hours of sleep, quality of sleep, arousals, as well as the number and duration of naps during the day. The client may be asked to keep a sleep diary around the clock, recording sleeping and awakening times, for a few days. Some other initial conservative interventions may include limiting naps and increasing daytime activity, limiting caffeine, maintaining room heat at 70° to 75°F, and playing soft soothing music at bedtime.

103. B: The client needs to understand the critical importance of using the CPAP machine every time he sleeps. The client's frequent yawning probably indicates that he is not using the machine routinely. Obstructive sleep apnea is characterized by passive collapse of the pharynx during sleep because of upper airway narrowing, often associated with obesity. Patients usually snore loudly with cycles of breath cessation caused by apneic periods lasting up to 60 seconds. These may occur 30 or more times a night despite continued chest wall and abdominal movements, indicating an automatic attempt to breathe.

104. A and C: With continuous ambulatory peritoneal dialysis (CAPD) the client instills about 2 liters of fluid over 10 to 15 minutes and then clamps the tubing and folds the tubing and bag over the abdomen and secures it with clothing, maintaining a dwell time of 3 to 5 hours. After this, the tubing is unclamped and dialysate and waste products drained for about 20 minutes. This drainage is discarded and new dialysate instilled to begin the cycle again.

105. A: The blood abnormalities of most concern during treatment of leukemia and most other cancers as well are thrombocytopenia and neutropenia. About 10% of clients with ALL initially present with disseminated intravascular coagulation (DIC) because of thrombocytopenia. As the platelet level falls, the ability of the blood to clot is impaired and the client is at risk for hemorrhage. The absolute neutrophil count is monitored closely because, as the ANC falls, the risk for exogenous and endogenous infections increases markedly.

106. A: Hypoparathyroidism with hypocalcemia is a complication of thyroidectomy. Hypocalcemia may occur because of inadvertent removal of all or some of the parathyroid glands but may also occur temporarily after surgery because of edema or manipulation of the parathyroid glands during the thyroidectomy. Typical symptoms include a tingling sensation about the mouth and in the fingers and toes. Some may develop severe muscle cramps and tetany. Transient mild hypoparathyroidism may require no treatment, but IV calcium gluconate is indicated for calcium levels below 7 mg/dL.

107. D: The meal that most corresponds to the dietary guidelines is one-half banana, 1 cup broccoli, ½ cup quinoa, 3 ounces roasted turkey, and 8 ounces of 1% milk. The dietary guidelines advise that half of a plate should be filled with fruits and vegetables and that grains should be whole grains (such as quinoa and brown rice). Milk products should be low- or nonfat, and protein should be lean and include limited red meat as well as nonmeat sources of protein, such as beans, eggs, and soy products.

108. A and C: The pre-adolescent child needs to be aware of bodily changes to expect as he develops secondary sexual characteristics, including normal variations among children and changes in height, weight, and body structure. The mother should allow the child to express changes in the way he thinks and awareness and should stress the importance of education. She should also ask the child about issues related to peer pressure, such as bullying, gangs, drugs, tobacco, and alcohol use.

109. A-IV, B-I, C-II, D-III: The nurse should prepare the child for the treatment by removing all clothes except the diaper so that as much skin as possible is exposed to the light. The nurse should apply a protective mask over the child's eyes and adjust the light source to 15 to 20 cm above the child prior to turning on the lights and administering the treatment. Indications include:

Weight	Serum bilirubin level
500 to 750 g	5 to 8 mg/dL
751 to 1000 g	6 to 10 mg/dL
1001 to 1250 g	8 to 10 mg/dL
1251 to 1500 g	10 to 12 mg/dL

110. D: A client with a severe cough and fever requires both standard precautions and droplet precautions. The best action is to provide the client with a facemask and seat the client in a separate area as far away from other clients as possible to reduce the chance of the infection spreading. A client who is ill should not be sent away or asked to wait outside. The nurse should thoroughly wash his/her hands after contact with the client.

111. C: While bedrest alone with much time in the lateral decubitus position to maximize uterine blood flow is often indicated for clients with mild pre-eclampsia, those with severe pre-eclampsia (BP >160–180/>110 and proteinuria >5 g/24 hours) are usually treated initially with magnesium sulfate (IM or IV) as a prophylaxis to prevent seizures. An antihypertensive, such as hydralazine, is given if the diastolic pressure remains above 110. If seizures (eclampsia) occur, magnesium sulfate or other anticonvulsants, such as diazepam and phenytoin, may be used to prevent recurrence.

112. A: Women who experience premature rupture of the membranes at term and do not go into labor within 12 to 24 hours are induced because the risk of infection increases with time. About 9 out of 10 women with premature rupture of the membranes go into labor within 24 hours. In some cases, such as a woman with a history of current or recent vaginal infection or multiple digital vaginal exams, labor may be induced at any time after the membranes rupture.

113. A: Pulmonary hygiene is especially important after surgery because inactivity and failure to breathe deeply and cough, aggravated by pain, can result in atelectasis. Patients should be instructed in the use of the incentive spirometer both before surgery and after

surgery and use should be monitored to ensure compliance. Patients with atelectasis typically initially become short of breath and may develop a cough and low-grade fever as secretions pool and the lung collapses. Untreated, the patient may develop hypoxemia, pneumonia, or respiratory failure.

114. D: These symptoms are consistent with mild pacemaker syndrome and occur when the atrial and ventricular contractions are not synchronized properly. This causes decreased cardiac output because the atria do not adequately fill the ventricles. Peripheral vascular resistance increases to compensate initially. Moderate pacemaker syndrome is characterized by increasing dyspnea and orthopnea, dizziness, vertigo, confusion, and sensation of choking. Severe pacemaker syndrome includes pulmonary edema with rales and marked dyspnea, syncope, and heart failure.

115. D: Clients are often quite nervous about cardiac monitoring, especially if they are fearful about their condition, and they may dislodge leads so that they can get attention from nurses because they are afraid to be alone or need reassurance. Challenging a client or attempting to make the person feel guilty does not solve the underlying problem. A better approach is for the nurse to take time to talk with the client, explaining how telemetry works, what the numbers and tracings on the monitor mean, and what the staff is learning from the monitoring.

116. A: The nurse should always remember the five rights of delegation: right task, right circumstances, right person, right direction or communication, and right supervision. The nurse should never delegate tasks for which assistive personnel have not been trained, and this includes administration of medications and blood therapy. Assistive personnel can monitor vital signs during blood therapy and should be taught to recognize and report signs of adverse effects, but the responsibility for primary monitoring lies with the nurse.

117. D: Gastric fluid is acidic, usually with a pH value of 4 or less. Intestinal aspirate is usually greater than 4 and respiratory secretions greater than 5.5. However, the nurse should not rely on pH alone, but should carefully observe the color and consistency of aspirate. Gastric fluids may vary in color from green and cloudy (most common) to white, tan, red-tinged (from blood), or brown. If the tube is placed in the duodenum, aspirate may be yellow or bile-stained. If the end of the NG tube is in the esophagus, the aspirate may be clear and look like saliva.

118. B: Because the client has systemic symptoms (fever, chills) and flank pain, these symptoms suggest a kidney infection rather than cystitis. The initial diagnostic tests include a urinalysis and urine culture and sensitivities to determine the causative organism. Clients are usually started on a broad-spectrum antibiotic while awaiting the culture and sensitivity report. In most cases, symptoms recede rapidly once antibiotics are started, so if the infection is severe or the client's condition deteriorates, the client may need hospitalization for intravenous antibiotic therapy.

119. A, B, and D: Radiotherapy to the abdominal area and pelvis often damages cells in the intestines, resulting in diarrhea. Clients should be advised to drink 8 to 12 glasses of clear liquids, eat 5 to 6 small meals daily, and limit fiber, fat, and lactose (milk products) as they may increase diarrhea. Some people benefit from the BRAT diet, especially when diarrhea is acute—banana, rice, applesauce, and toast. Clients should also avoid fried and spicy foods, cruciferous vegetables and beans, and soy products.

120. 0.7: The formula for calculating the waist-to-hip ratio is: waist (inches) divided by hips (inches).

In this case 28/40 = 0.7. The waist must be measured at its smallest circumference and the hips at the widest. This measurement determines whether a person's body type is classified as "pear" or "apple." People with "apple" shapes have increased abdominal fat, which is a higher health risk than fat in the hips.

Gender	Ideal	Increased risk	High risk
Male	0.9 to 0.95	0.96 to 1.0	>1.0
Female	0.7 to 0.8	0.81 to 0.85	>0.85

121. A-II, B-I, C-IV, D-III: The modified Allen test is conducted to ensure that the ulnar artery provides adequate circulation, including collateral circulation, so that the radial artery can be used to obtain an arterial blood sample. The patient extends the wrist over a rolled towel and makes a fist. Steps:
A. (Step 1) II. Palpate the ulnar and radial pulses and apply pressure to both arteries.
B. (Step 2) I. Ask the client to open and close the hand until the skin blanches.
C. (Step 3) IV. Release the ulnar artery while maintaining pressure on the radial artery.
D. (Step 4) III. Observe the hand for color. The hand should regain natural color within 5 seconds if circulation is adequate.

122. 60 percent: Each hemoglobin molecule has four iron-containing heme sites to which oxygen can bind. As oxygen binds to the heme, the hemoglobin becomes saturated. The SO_2 level is the percentage of total heme sites in the blood saturated with oxygen. At 80 to 90 PO_2, hemoglobin is fully saturated so increased PO_2 can't increase saturation. The critical point for PO_2 is 60% because below this point there is a marked decrease in saturation. PO_2 of 60 usually corresponds to SO_2 of 91%, which is referred to as the "ICU" point.

123. A: Simply not adding extra salt to food is insufficient because many foods, especially processed foods, are very high in sodium. Clients need to follow dietary guidelines and learn to read labels. DASH nutrient goals (based on a 2100 calorie diet) limit Na to 1500 to 2300 mg, total fat 27%, protein 18%, and carbohydrates 55%.
Grains (whole grains preferred): 6 to 8 daily
Vegetables and fruits: 4 to 5 each daily
Milk products (non- or low-fat): 2 to 3 daily
Lean meat, poultry, fish: ≤6 ounces daily
Nuts, seeds, legumes: 4 to 5 weekly
Fats and oils: 2 to 3 daily
Sweet/added sugar: ≤5 weekly

124. D: Once the platelet count drops below 50,000, the blood's ability to clot is impaired. If a client is scheduled for an invasive procedure, the risk of bleeding increases at this level; otherwise, risk is not generally significant until the platelet count drops to below 20,000. At this level, clients usually begin to develop signs of bleeding, such as petechial, nosebleeds, bleeding gums, and increased menstrual flow and require administration of platelets. For milder thrombocytopenia, observation and steroids are indicated with immunosuppressive therapy and splenectomy used for more severe disease.

125. 2600: The absolute neutrophil count (ANC) is calculated indirectly based on the total white blood cell count and percentages of neutrophils and bands:
ANC = Total WBC X (% neutrophils + % bands/100)
ANC = 5200 X (45 + 5/100) = 5200 X 0.50 = 2600 mm³
A normal ANC for adults is 1800 to 7700, so this is within normal range. The risk of infection increases markedly when the ANC falls to 1000, and risk is severe at 500.

126. D: Passwords are used to protect client's records from unauthorized access, so anyone who is authorized should be able to access the records with his/her own password. Therefore, the nurse should not allow anyone else to use his/her password. Passwords can also be used to track an individual nurse's activity in the electronic health record, so the nurse may be putting his/her own career in jeopardy by allowing someone else to use the password.

127. A: The nurse should communicate the client's financial concerns to the social worker: "I can't afford to hire anyone to help me when I am discharged." The social worker will have knowledge about resources and qualifications for applying for assistance, such as Medicaid. The social worker can assess the client's income and support system to help determine the best plan for the client. Concerns about necessary equipment and managing self-care, such as showering safely, should be communicated to physical and occupational therapists.

128. B: Clients who are alert and responsive have the right to refuse any treatment, so the most appropriate action is for the nurse to notify the physician and ensure that orders are in place for comfort measures, such as adequate analgesia. The nurse should not insist that the client accept treatments against her wishes, as this may be construed as coercion, and should not ask family members to intervene. Most religions view refusing life-prolonging treatments as different from active suicide, but it is inappropriate to use religious beliefs to make clients feel guilty.

129. 180: The formula for calculating total cholesterol is LDL + HDL + (triglycerides/5).
100 + 50 + (150/5) = 100 + 50 +30 = 180
An alternate formula is LDL + HDL + (Triglycerides X 0.20).
100 + 50 + (150 X 0.20) = 100 + 50 +30 = 180
The optimal total cholesterol level is below 200. Optimal LDL is below 100. Optimal HDL is ≥60. Normal triglyceride level is below 150.

130. A: (First) III Inspection, B (Second) IV Auscultation, C (Third) I Percussion, D (Fourth) II Palpation. While the usual order of examination techniques is to begin with examination and then progress to palpation, percussion, and finally auscultation, because stimulating the abdomen may increase bowel sounds and contractions, the nurse should examine the abdomen differently from least invasive to most, beginning with inspection. This is followed by auscultation to assess normal bowel sounds, then percussion to assess for gas, fluid, and consolidated masses, and finally to palpation.

131. A-II Aorta, B-IV Renal, C-III Iliac, D-I Femoral:

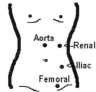

Auscultation should be done gently to avoid stimulating bowel contractions over the sites indicated on the diagram. For hypertensive patients, the renal arteries should be assessed bilaterally as bruits may be heard, suggesting arterial occlusion. Systolic bruits are fairly common and often benign, but bruits that have both systolic and diastolic components indicate turbulent blood flow. Aortic, iliac, and femoral bruits may be heard with peripheral arterial insufficiency.

132. B: The client should always urinate prior to a pelvic exam. When positioning the client for the exam, the client's head should be elevated slightly as this helps relax abdominal muscles. The client should be advised to keep her arms at her side or folded across her chest and not over her head as this position may cause the abdominal muscles to tense. The nurse should explain the steps to the procedure and ensure that the speculum is warmed prior to the examination.

133. A-III Apply tourniquet, B-I Palpate vein, C-II Cleanse skin, and D-IV Perform venipuncture: The nurse should carefully examine the veins for potential puncture sites prior to performing the venipuncture. The nurse may apply a tourniquet or heat and hold the arm in dependent position. Once a vein has been selected, the tourniquet can be released while the nurse prepares materials. Then the tourniquet is applied, the vein palpated, and the skin cleansed, with venipuncture last. The nurse should avoid palpating the vein after the skin is cleansed unless wearing sterile gloves.

134 D: A nasal cannula at 3L/min delivers an FiO_2 of approximately 28–32%. The flow rate for nasal cannulas ranges from 0.5 L/min (21–24% FiO_2) to 6 L/min (40–44% FiO_2), but should not be administered at a higher flow rate because the FiO_2 will not increase, and it can result in drying of the mucous membranes. Face masks, non-rebreathing masks, partial re-breathing masks, and Venturi masks can be used if a higher FiO_2 is needed.

135. A-I Client sits upright or stands. B-IV Client takes a deep breath. C-II Client places the meter in the mouth and seals lips. D-III Client expels air through the meter as forcefully as possible. The client should repeat this procedure 2 to 5 times, noting the highest number achieved. Following treatment, the client's PEFR should be within 20% of personal best, and if results are <80% of personal best, treatment may be inadequate for client's condition.

136. C: Headaches occur in about one-fifth of clients following lumbar puncture, but the headaches are usually relieved by the client's lying flat and drinking ample fluids. If headaches are severe and persistent, then this usually indicates a hole in the dura mater, and an epidural blood patch may be applied with an autologous blood specimen. The blood is injected in a small amount at the site of the lumbar puncture to create a blood clot that serves as a "patch."

137. D: The optimal position for a thoracentesis is an upright position with the client sitting and leaning over an over-bed tray table with the shoulders and upper arms supported by a pillow as this position expands the intercostal space, making insertion easier. If the client is unable to tolerate a sitting position, then the client should be positioned in the side-lying position on the unaffected side so that the thoracentesis insertion site is easily accessed.

138. D: Severe vomiting can result in metabolic alkalosis because of loss of chloride in the emesis. In a compensating measure for chloride loss, bicarbonate increases. Metabolic alkalosis may also result from gastric suctioning, diuresis, hypokalemia, and excessive mineralocorticoid or sodium bicarbonate intake. Other laboratory findings include increased pH, normal PCO2 if compensated but increased if noncompensated. Symptoms include dizziness, confusion, anxiety, muscle cramping, tingling, seizures, tetany, tachycardia, arrhythmias, nausea, vomiting, anorexia, and compensatory hypoventilation.

139. A and C: Excess fluid is removed quickly from the body during hemodialysis. This can sometimes result in fluid deficit, especially if the client has run a fever or had inadequate fluid intake. Because heparin is administered during the treatment to prevent clots from forming, the client is at increased risk of bleeding. The presence of fluid volume excess, metabolic acidosis, and pulmonary edema should be evaluated prior to hemodialysis since clients are unable to excrete adequate fluids or waste products because of impaired kidney function.

140. C: The large accumulation of fluid that can occur with ascites makes palpating the bladder difficult, so the bladder must be emptied prior to a paracentesis in order to prevent inadvertent puncture of the bladder when the needle or trocar is inserted. Clients should be positioned in upright or high Fowler's position because this helps to keep the intestines toward the back of the peritoneal cavity, preventing intestinal laceration. Usually only 4 to 5 L of fluid are removed at one time. If larger volumes are removed, the client is at risk of hypotension.

141. A, B, and D: Clients with a tracheostomy are at increased risk of fecal impaction because they cannot perform the Valsalva maneuver to bear down, so they need to be educated about bowel care and advised to use stool softeners routinely and laxatives and suppositories as needed. Additionally, they need to understand the importance of pulmonary hygiene to prevent atelectasis and infection and should be confident in all aspects of tracheostomy care, including information about what to do if the tracheostomy tube falls out.

142. A: Because of his weakness and tremors, the client will probably have difficulty preparing meals, so referral to a home meal delivery program (such as Meals on Wheels) is probably the best referral since arrangements have already been made for personal care and housekeeping. Home meal delivery programs usually provide meals 5 to 7 days a week at low cost ($2 to $4 is common). The meals are often delivered midday with a hot entrée, and many programs also provide a sandwich or other light meal for evening as well as breakfast foods (such as cereal) for the next day.

143. A and C: During a life review, clients reflect on their lives, their successes and failures, and their relationships. Some clients may begin to organize old photographs or look through photo albums. Others may want to reminisce and talk about their lives and families. Some talk about their children and parenting skills. They may talk about things they regret or choices they have made. People often try to validate that their lives had purpose through their life reviews.

144. A and E: The mother is using nonstandard treatments with mayonnaise and olive oil. While some anecdotal reports suggest this is helpful, according to the CDC there is no evidence to support these treatments. The mother should use OTC or prescription shampoos intended to treat lice. While linens and clothes used by the child should be washed and dried in a hot air cycle for at least 5 minutes to prevent spread, treating pets, such as cats and dogs, does no good as they do not spread head lice.

145. 9%: According to the rule of nines, body surface area (BSA) is sectioned into areas that are primarily multiples of 9:
Head: 9%

Anterior trunk: 18% (9% chest and 9% abdomen)
Posterior trunk: 18% (9% upper back and 9% lower back and buttocks)
Legs: 18% each (9% anterior and 9% posterior)
Arms: 9% each (4.5% anterior and 4.5% posterior)
Genitals: 1%
The percentage of BSA that is burned is important when calculating potential fluid loss and the need for fluid and electrolyte replacement.

146. D: A positive Homan's sign—pain on palpation of the calf with dorsiflexion of the ankle—is indicative of deep vein thrombosis (DVT) although this sign occurs in only about 10%, so the absence does not preclude DVT. DVT is associated with inactivity, such as prolonged bedrest or sitting for long periods while flying, and is a complication of surgery. Clients may have pain and tenderness, erythema, elevated temperature, and unilateral edema although some exhibit no overt symptoms.

147. B: Increasing intracranial pressure is indicated by increasing BP with widening pulse pressure, decreasing pulse, and increasing temperature. The client's initial BP was 138/72 with a pulse pressure of 66 but is now 160/64 with a pulse pressure of 96. The initial pulse was 83 and has decreased to 70. Baseline temperature was 97.5°F/36.4°C and is now increased to 99.4°F/37.4°C. Restlessness and headache are early indications of increasing intracranial pressure. Clients may also have an alteration in consciousness, change in pupillary reactions, and increasing dyspnea.

148. D: If an implantable cardioverter-defibrillator fires one time and is not associated with other cardiac symptoms, this is not a medical emergency, and the patient should be advised to lie down to rest until he feels recovered from the stress of the firing and to telephone the physician to report the event. Multiple firings are a medical emergency, and the client or family member should call 9-1-1 as the firings may indicate recurrent ventricular fibrillation/ventricular tachycardia or a fractured lead. A single firing associated with symptoms (chest pain, dizziness, syncope, and shortness of breath) is also a medical emergency.

149. C: The irregular rhythm is an atrial fibrillation, which is characterized by a rapid, very irregular pulse with an atrial rate of 300 to 600 and ventricular rate of 120 to 200. Because the beats are rapid and ineffectual, the atria do not empty adequately, so blood begins to pool, increasing risk of thrombus formation and emboli. Because stroke volume decreases, cardiac output decreases, leading to myocardial ischemia and palpitations.

150. A, C, and D: Because clients are at risk for bleeding, they should use soft toothbrushes. Swimming is a good choice for exercise because the water exerts even pressure. Clients should always wear a Medical Alert bracelet or necklace indicating they are taking the anticoagulant. Stools should not be black as this is a sign of bleeding. While green leafy vegetables are high in vitamin K, they can be eaten in normal amounts and do not need to be restricted.

151. A: The nurse should hold the infusion and notify the MD that the catheter tip is incorrectly placed, as it should be in the superior vena cava rather than the right atrium. Infusing the solutions directly into the right atrium may result in tissue damage. While the catheter needs to be withdrawn a few inches and another X-ray taken to ensure correct placement, this procedure should only be done by a physician or a specially trained nurse.

152. 750 mg: The simplest solution to the problem is to convert 1 g to 1000 mg and then, since the infusion was set for 60 minutes and three-fourths of the time elapsed, simply multiply 1000 X 0.75 = 750 mg. If using an algebraic formula:

1000/60 = x/45
60x = 45,000
6 x = 4500
6x/6 = 4500/6
x = 750 mg

153. B, D, and E: Pills may be crushed and diluted in 10 to 15 mL of water to be added to the NG tube feeding. Liquid forms of medications are easiest to add. Soft-gel capsules can be opened at one end and drained, but some dosage is usually lost, so dissolving the capsule in warm water first (and removing the remains of the gel capsule) is a better solution. Extended-release capsules should be opened but NOT crushed before adding to the tube. Enteric-coated tablets should not be crushed or administered per NG tube, and sublingual wafers are not absorbed through the GI tract.

154. 95%: The oximeter uses light waves to determine oxygen saturation (SPO2) and utilizes an external oximeter attached to a finger or earlobe. If a client has marked vasoconstriction, the earlobe may provide more accurate readings than the finger. Oxygen saturation should be maintained >95% although some patients with chronic respiratory disorders, such as COPD, may have lower SPO2. Oximetry is often used postoperatively to assess peripheral circulation and when patients are on mechanical ventilation.

155. A, C, and D: Restraints are used to restrict movement, activity, and access. Guidelines for restraints not part of routine care (surgical restraints, arm boards) include:
A written policy must be in place.
An assessment must be completed prior to application of restraints.
An alternative method should be tried before applying a restraint.
Restraints cannot be applied without a written order.
The least restrictive effective restraint should be used.
The nurse must remove the restraint, assess, and document findings at least every 2 hours.

156. C: While security measures may vary somewhat, generally infants should only be removed from the mother's room in a crib and never carried in someone's arms. Mothers should be informed to never leave their infants unattended, even for a few minutes to use the bathroom. If no family member is present, the mother should call her nurse. The mother should not assume hospital attire or ID alone are sufficient identification and should remain wary of any strangers asking questions about the infant.

157. 3 mL: A simple algebraic formula provides the answer:
Mg in suspension/mL = Desired dose/x (mL needed)
200/5 = 120/x
200x = 600
200x/200 = 600/200
x = 3 mL dose

158. B: Fifteen mg/dL is within normal limits (range is 8–21 for ages 14 to adult; 5–17 for newborns; 7–17 for children to 13 years; 10–31 for adults >90 years. Urea (nonprotein

nitrogen compound) is an end product of protein metabolism. BUN is usually evaluated with creatinine. The normal ratio of BUN/creatinine is 15:1 to 24:1. A BUN >100 mg/dL is a critical value. Signs of an elevated BUN include restlessness, confusion, acidemia, nausea and vomiting, and coma.

159. D: While there is not total agreement about the results of HbA1c tests, generally levels of ≥6.5% are considered diagnostic of diabetes mellitus. Values of 5.7 to 6.4% are considered pre-diabetic by most authorities. Lower values are within normal limits. Because hemoglobin retains excess blood glucose and red blood cells live about 120 days, the HbA1c test shows the average blood glucose levels over a 3-month period. HbA1c is used to diagnose diabetes and monitor long-term diabetic therapy.

160. A-IV Gently retract the lower eyelid against the orbital ridge with the thumb. B-I Gently retract the upper lid. C-II Exert slight pressure below the eyelid and slip the index finger under the prosthesis. D-III Break suction and slide the prosthesis out of the eye. Once the prosthesis is removed, clean the prosthesis with soap and water and rinse well with running water to remove all soap and residue. Dry and polish the prosthesis. Retract eyelids, wash socket with clean washcloth or gauze pad moistened with warm water or NS. Wash eyelid margins with mild soap and water and dry.

161. C: Both foam overlays and sheepskin are inappropriate for incontinent clients. The alternating pressure overlay is the best choice because it is liquid-resistant and has cells or cylinders that alternately inflate and deflate at intervals, controlled by a pump. They should only be used with clients <250 pounds, so the client fits this criterion. While the low air loss bed provides a superior support surface, it is much more expensive and must be monitored carefully and maintained properly, and it can result in hypothermia because of the constant flow of air.

162. 30: The problem can be calculated using dimensional analysis:
Desired: drops per minute
120 mL/1 hour X 15 drops/1 mL X 1 hour/60 minutes
Eliminate like terms (mL and hour) and reduce 120 and 60 by removing zeroes
12/1 X 15 drops/1 X 1/6 minutes
12 X 15 X 1 = 180/6 = 30 drops per minute

163. B: The 3-point gait requires the client to have the most upper body strength and balance because the client must support the entire weight of the body with the arms. The sequence for ambulation is to start with both feet together and the crutch tips slightly to the front and side of the feet. Then, the client advances the weaker leg and both crutches at the same time with the toe even with the crutches, followed by the stronger leg with the toe advancing slightly past the crutches. Note: the crutches are advanced only with the weaker leg.

164. B, D, and E: The nurse should cover the client with a warm blanket, leaving the cast exposed to the air so that it can dry properly. The client should be turned and repositioned every 2 to 3 hours so that all sides of the cast can dry evenly. While some facilities use heat cradles or commercial cast dryers at low temperatures, high-powered electric fans should not blow directly on the cast as this may result in the outside drying and the inside remaining damp. Fans may be used away from the cast to increase air circulation in the room.

165. A: While protocols regarding tube feedings may vary somewhat, generally if gastric residual is less than 100 mL, it is returned to the stomach and the tubing flushed with 30 mL of water, but if it is more than 100mL (in this case 150 mL) it may indicate that an obstruction has occurred, and the nurse should hold the feeding and notify the MD before proceeding. The amount of residual gastric contents should be aspirated and measured at least every 8 hours.

166. 0.25: To complete the calculation, first convert micrograms to milligrams: 50 mcg = 0.05 mg.
The formula:
Desired dose/Available dose = Number of tablets needed for correct dosage
0.05/0.2 = 0.25 tablets

167. A, B, and C: Difficulty urinating is a common problem after surgery, and conservative methods should be tried before catheterization. Methods to promote urination include pouring warm water over the client's perineum, asking the client to blow bubbles through a straw into a glass of water, and turning on running water while the client attempts to urinate. Telling a client to "just relax" may increase stress. It's more helpful to lead the client through relaxation exercises.

168. C, D, and E: The irrigating syringe should be filled with about 50 mL of irrigant but it should be instilled slowly, using care not to occlude the ear canal with the syringe tip as this may result in increased pressure and rupture of the eardrum. The client should be positioned lying flat or sitting with the head turned toward the affected ear to facilitate drainage and help secure the drainage basin. On those over 3 years old, the pinna is pulled up and back. The solution should drain out freely during the irrigation.

169. A: Acupuncture has been demonstrated to relieve chemotherapy-induced nausea and vomiting in a number of studies. Some studies also seem to indicate that ginger (usually in tea form) can reduce the intensity of nausea but not vomiting. The nurse may recommend both of these therapies. However, there is no evidence to suggest that therapeutic touch or magnetic therapy are effective in relieving nausea, and herbal therapies must be evaluated individually as some may interact negatively with the client's medications.

170. A: While pain is usually considered to be that which the client states it is, the one-to-ten scale that is commonly used in the United States is not always used in other countries. People from Hispanic countries often describe pain in terms of small amount, normal, or strong. The nurse should use a different type of questioning to ascertain pain and might state, "I see that you are rubbing your stomach and seem to be in pain" to encourage dialogue.

171. C: If a client in cervical traction complains of increasing pain in the jaw and ears, the chinstrap may be exerting excess pull on the chin, resulting in increased pressure on the temporomandibular joint. The nurse should gently correct the client's head position by tilting the head slightly forward to relieve the pull on the chin. If the pain occurs on only one side, then the traction may be uneven, and the client's body may need to be positioned correctly.

172. B: When taking a verbal order of any kind, including a telephone order, the nurse should write the order and then read it back, asking for verbal verification that the order is correct, before notifying the pharmacy of the order or administering the medication. In an emergency situation only, such as may occur with a cardiac arrest, the nurse may repeat back an order for verification. Verbal orders should not be accepted if the physician is present on the unit.

173. B: Unless the client is in danger, the nurse should not confront the nurse he suspects of taking an opioid medication intended for a client, because a confrontation may end badly. The other nurse may deny the accusation and place blame on the first nurse or may even react violently. Instead, the observing nurse should immediately notify a supervisor of his concerns so that the administration can carry out an investigation according to facility protocol, which also determines whether an incident report needs to be completed.

174. B: While state laws vary regarding how to report and what to report, all states require mandatory reporting of suspected child abuse. Because the type and extent of injuries to the child are not consistent with a fall off of a swing and the child has evidence of multiple previous injuries, the incident must be reported to the proper authorities. In most states, the report is made to Child Protective Services, who in turn may notify the police.

175. D: The most appropriate response to a client's complaint is to express empathy and gather information without placing blame or making excuses: "I'm so sorry you felt that way. Can you tell me what happened?" Allowing a client to ventilate feelings is often sufficient, but if the issue is serious, the nurse should describe the client's response to the nurse involved and then follow the same procedures in listening to the nurse in order to try to reach a resolution.

176. C and E: Decimal numbers should contain a leading zero, such as with "0.5% albuterol inhalation solution." If the zero is missing, such as with ".25 mg budesonide inhalation solution," the initial period may be overlooked or read as a number one and the statement misread as "25 mg" or "125 mg." Similarly, trailing zeroes should be avoided after whole numbers, "10 mg" instead of "10.0 mg." Abbreviations such as "SOB," which may be misinterpreted as a pejorative or as "short of breath" or "side of bed" should also be avoided and the words written out.

177. B: If the neonate swallowed amniotic fluid, the child may be born in acute respiratory distress, but symptoms may be delayed for a few hours, so the child must be monitored carefully. If the neonate cries at delivery and shows no signs of distress, then the mouth and throat are suctioned, but if respiratory distress is evident, the child should be intubated and tracheobronchial suctioning done to remove meconium plugs. The gastric contents may be suctioned as well to prevent the infant from regurgitating and aspirating meconium.

178. B: Two forms of identifiers should always be used prior to administering medication to any client, even if the nurse recognizes the client and is relatively sure of the client's identity. Asking the client's name and checking the hospital ID bracelet meet minimal requirements. In some cases, clients may be identified by asking their names and birthdates. The nurse should always double check the name on the medication as well. An ID bracelet that is not on the client but elsewhere, such as on a bedside stand, should not be used for identification.

179. D: While a gait/transfer belt may be used by a caregiver until the client is independent, a sliding board is most indicated because the client cannot stand and requires sitting transfer. Use is quite simple and sliding boards are relatively inexpensive. They are usually made of rigid plastic material with low friction so that the client can easily slide from the chair onto the toilet or another surface. Any caregiver who will be assisting should be instructed in methods to use to assist the client without causing injury to the caregiver or the client.

180. B: According to OSHA guidelines, if items are out of reach, the acceptable work practice is to get a properly maintained ladder and use that to climb up to reach the objects. The nurse should never use stools, chairs, or boxes in place of a ladder or try to "climb" up a cabinet by standing on a lower shelf. It's important to climb high enough on the ladder that the nurse is not lifting items over the head because this can result in injuries and falls.

181. C:

 This is the international symbol for biohazards. Biohazards are biological materials (plants, animals, organisms), such as bacteria, viruses, and parasites, which are dangerous to people's health or pose the risk of infection. In medical facilities, items that must be labeled as biohazards include used hypodermic needles and contaminated dressings because they may contain infectious biological material. Each facility should establish protocols for handling and disposing of biohazardous materials. Biohazardous waste products are generally disposed of in red plastic bags with the biohazard symbol on the bag.

182. A, B, D, and E: The client should dispose of syringes and needles in a sharps disposal container (or glass jar) immediately after use, being sure to maintain the container out of reach of children and pets. The container should be disposed of when it is about three-quarters full because if the container is too full, the risk of accidental puncture increases. While the container may be disposed of in the regular trash in some areas, other areas are more restrictive, so the client must check with the local community garbage disposal company for guidelines. Needles should never be flushed down the toilet.

183. B: Because attempting to evacuate clients from the facility is likely to increase exposure to the hazardous material, the most likely emergency response is to shelter in place. This applies to both staff and clients. Guidelines may vary according to the type of waste but can include locking doors, sealing doors and windows, and shutting off air-conditioning and forced-air systems. Many facilities have windows that do not open, but if not, windows should be closed immediately. Staff should monitor news reports because emergency personnel may not be readily available to provide information.

184. B, C, D, and F: Clients with gastrointestinal disorders and diarrhea should be maintained on both standard precautions and contact precautions. The nurse should use personal protective equipment (gown and gloves) for all contact with the client but does not need to wear a mask or N95 respirator. The client should be in a private room or ≥3 feet away from other clients. Because *C. difficile* spreads readily, special care must be taken with environmental cleaning. Nurses should wash hands with soap and water rather than alcohol antiseptic and should avoid sharing electronic thermometers used by the client with others.

185. 125 mg: Because the child is to receive 25 mg for each kilogram of weight, the calculation is to simply multiply 25 X 10 = 250 mg. Since the total dosage is to be given in two divided doses, the nurse will administer 125 mg (250/2) at each dose.

186. B: The Safe Babies® apron is a one-piece apron that fits over the head and attaches on the side with Velcro closures. The apron contains two large pockets in the front and two in the back, so the nurse can carry 4 infants at one time. Infants should be wrapped in blankets for warmth prior to being placed in the pockets. The apron is designed so the person's arms are free. This allows the nurse to carry supplies or even additional infants if necessary.

187. D: Because this is an emergency situation, the nurse should immediately obtain a second ECG machine and conduct the ECG. This may involve sending another staff member to a different unit, but the nurse should remain with the client. Once finished, the nurse should label the first machine as "Out of Order" and follow facility procedures for initiating repairs. Under no circumstances should the nurse use equipment that is damaged and may cause a spark because of the danger this poses to the clients and staff.

188. B: Because nurses work closely with clients, a client often divulges confidential information, such as the fact that she has been having an affair with her husband's brother. However, the nurse must evaluate communications to determine if they are health related and can and should be reported or if they are private communications. In this case, no purpose is served by reporting the client's statement except to spread gossip, so this is a HIPAA violation of privacy.

189. B: If at all possible, each treatment should be documented immediately after completion. Treatments should never be documented in advance, even if they are routine and the nurse is relatively sure they will be completed. The longer the period of time following completion of a treatment, the greater the chance that an error in documenting (such as forgetting to chart) will occur. If the nurse cannot document immediately, then the nurse should make a note of the time and essential information. Documenting should not be left until the end of shift.

190. C: The most helpful information for the homeless client is probably a list of shelters and community agencies, especially those with programs to assist the homeless. Adult Protective Services investigates abuse, but cuts resulting from a fight are not usually considered abusive situations. Many homeless people are very reluctant to deal with the police in any way. Providing a list of 12-step organizations is not indicated unless the client is inebriated or there is other evidence of a drinking problem.

191. A: If a nurse believes that current procedures should be changed, then the best place to begin is with a survey of the literature regarding wound care to determine what best practices are recommended. Armed with this information, the nurse can approach the director of nursing or other appropriate person and discuss other methods, such as interviews and questionnaires, which might help to determine the need for change, those interested in assisting, and the best way to proceed.

192. D: The best approach is "What do you understand about your options for care?" The nurse should never suggest that treatment won't help because even those in hospice and palliative care receive treatment. However, the focus of treatment is different, so the nurse should stress that the goal of hospice and palliative care is to keep the client as comfortable

as possible. Clients may feel they are being abandoned if the nurse suggests stopping all treatments.

193. A, B, C, and E: Clients who have undergone gastric bypass surgery should avoid concentrated sugars as they accelerate emptying of the stomach. Clients should drink liquids at least 30 minutes before meals rather than with foods and should eat 5 or 6 small meals a day rather than 3 large meals. Dairy products should be restricted to low-fat products, but many people find dairy products cause diarrhea, so they should be introduced cautiously. Those with dumping syndrome may find that reclining after eating slows emptying of the stomach and reduces symptoms.

194. D: A Durable Power of Attorney for Healthcare remains in effect (durable) if the client is unable to make decisions, so this is the best option. While state laws vary somewhat, a Durable Power of Attorney for Healthcare is generally limited to healthcare decisions only. In some states, a healthcare proxy can be established as part of an Advance Directive, but in other states two different documents are required, so the nurse should always be familiar with state regulations.

195. A, C, and D: Rear-facing car seats are safest, and neonates should always be placed in rear-facing seats. Car seats should be secured in the middle of the back seat, away from airbags, or airbags should be disconnected. Neonates are at risk for hypoxia in car seats, so the parents should ensure the child's neck is straight, avoiding the chin-to-chest position, and should limit time in the car seat to short trips of ≤60 minutes. Harnesses should be secure so that only one finger can easily slide underneath. No car seat involved in an accident should be used again even if no damage is evident.

196. B: While some children with pinworms (*Enterobius vermicularis*) may be essentially asymptomatic, common findings include intense anal itching and vulvovaginitis in girls. Those infected often are restless at night and sleep poorly and may complain of intermittent abdominal pain and nausea. The tape test (tape across the anus at bedtime) is the most common diagnostic procedure because the mature worms crawl through the anus to lay eggs in the perineal folds and become attached to the tape.

197. A: Providing basic care but refusing to talk to the client is a violation of provision 1 of the ANA Code of Ethics for Nurses. This provision requires that the nurse practice with compassion and show respect for each individual, regardless of social/economic status, personal attributes, or type of health problems. It's the nurse's responsibility to provide care to the highest standard to all patients. Attempting to avoid caring for a particular client does not violate the Code of Ethics but it may be construed as unprofessional.

198. C: Even if hospital policy allows nurses to avoid caring for clients undergoing abortions, this does not excuse the nurse from the ethical responsibility of attending to emergency situations, such as the possibility that the client is hemorrhaging. The nurse should immediately evaluate the client to determine whether emergency intervention is needed. If so, the nurse should follow protocol; if not, the nurse should reassure the client and notify the client's nurse when he or she returns.

199. C: While most immunizations of infants begin at 6 to 8 weeks, the hepatitis B vaccine should be administered within 12 hours of birth to all infants because hepatitis B is transmitted through body fluids and can be contracted during birth. A series of three

injections of monovalent HepB are required, with the second injection between one and two months and the third at or after 24 weeks. If the mother tests positive for hepatitis B, then the infant should be given both the monovalent HepB vaccination as well as HepB immune globulin within 12 hours of birth.

200. B, C, and D: Positive reinforcement provides something in return for a change in behavior. This can include tangible rewards, such as an additional hour of Internet use or some type of privilege, or supportive statements, such as "You are making good progress." Sometimes positive reinforcement occurs naturally as a result of behavioral change, such as when the client gains one-half pound. When possible, positive reinforcement should occur immediately after a behavioral change so that the client makes a positive association with the behavior.

Secret Key #1 - Time is Your Greatest Enemy

Pace Yourself

Wear a watch. At the beginning of the test, check the time (or start a chronometer on your watch to count the minutes), and check the time after every few questions to make sure you are "on schedule."

If you are forced to speed up, do it efficiently. Usually one or more answer choices can be eliminated without too much difficulty. Above all, don't panic. Don't speed up and just begin guessing at random choices. By pacing yourself, and continually monitoring your progress against your watch, you will always know exactly how far ahead or behind you are with your available time. If you find that you are one minute behind on the test, don't skip one question without spending any time on it, just to catch back up. Take 15 fewer seconds on the next four questions, and after four questions you'll have caught back up. Once you catch back up, you can continue working each problem at your normal pace.

Furthermore, don't dwell on the problems that you were rushed on. If a problem was taking up too much time and you made a hurried guess, it must be difficult. The difficult questions are the ones you are most likely to miss anyway, so it isn't a big loss. It is better to end with more time than you need than to run out of time.

Lastly, sometimes it is beneficial to slow down if you are constantly getting ahead of time. You are always more likely to catch a careless mistake by working more slowly than quickly, and among very high-scoring test takers (those who are likely to have lots of time left over), careless errors affect the score more than mastery of material.

Secret Key #2 - Guessing is not Guesswork

You probably know that guessing is a good idea. Unlike other standardized tests, there is no penalty for getting a wrong answer. Even if you have no idea about a question, you still have a 20-25% chance of getting it right.

Most test takers do not understand the impact that proper guessing can have on their score. Unless you score extremely high, guessing will significantly contribute to your final score.

Monkeys Take the Test

What most test takers don't realize is that to insure that 20-25% chance, you have to guess randomly. If you put 20 monkeys in a room to take this test, assuming they answered once per question and behaved themselves, on average they would get 20-25% of the questions correct. Put 20 test takers in the room, and the average will be much lower among guessed questions. Why?

1. The test writers intentionally write deceptive answer choices that "look" right. A test taker has no idea about a question, so he picks the "best looking" answer, which is often wrong. The monkey has no idea what looks good and what doesn't, so it will consistently be right about 20-25% of the time.
2. Test takers will eliminate answer choices from the guessing pool based on a hunch or intuition. Simple but correct answers often get excluded, leaving a 0% chance of being correct. The monkey has no clue, and often gets lucky with the best choice.

This is why the process of elimination endorsed by most test courses is flawed and detrimental to your performance. Test takers don't guess; they make an ignorant stab in the dark that is usually worse than random.

$5 Challenge

Let me introduce one of the most valuable ideas of this course—the $5 challenge:

You only mark your "best guess" if you are willing to bet $5 on it.
You only eliminate choices from guessing if you are willing to bet $5 on it.

Why $5? Five dollars is an amount of money that is small yet not insignificant, and can really add up fast (20 questions could cost you $100). Likewise, each answer choice on one question of the test will have a small impact on your overall score, but it can really add up to a lot of points in the end.

The process of elimination IS valuable. The following shows your chance of guessing it right:

If you eliminate wrong answer choices until only this many remain:	Chance of getting it correct:
1	100%
2	50%
3	33%

However, if you accidentally eliminate the right answer or go on a hunch for an incorrect answer, your chances drop dramatically—to 0%. By guessing among all the answer choices, you are GUARANTEED to have a shot at the right answer.

That's why the $5 test is so valuable. If you give up the advantage and safety of a pure guess, it had better be worth the risk.

What we still haven't covered is how to be sure that whatever guess you make is truly random. Here's the easiest way:

Always pick the first answer choice among those remaining.

Such a technique means that you have decided, **before you see a single test question**, exactly how you are going to guess, and since the order of choices tells you nothing about which one is correct, this guessing technique is perfectly random.

This section is not meant to scare you away from making educated guesses or eliminating choices; you just need to define when a choice is worth eliminating. The $5 test, along with a pre-defined random guessing strategy, is the best way to make sure you reap all of the benefits of guessing.

Secret Key #3 - Practice Smarter, Not Harder

Many test takers delay the test preparation process because they dread the awful amounts of practice time they think necessary to succeed on the test. We have refined an effective method that will take you only a fraction of the time.

There are a number of "obstacles" in the path to success. Among these are answering questions, finishing in time, and mastering test-taking strategies. All must be executed on the day of the test at peak performance, or your score will suffer. The test is a mental marathon that has a large impact on your future.

Just like a marathon runner, it is important to work your way up to the full challenge. So first you just worry about questions, and then time, and finally strategy:

Success Strategy

1. Find a good source for practice tests.
2. If you are willing to make a larger time investment, consider using more than one study guide. Often the different approaches of multiple authors will help you "get" difficult concepts.
3. Take a practice test with no time constraints, with all study helps, "open book." Take your time with questions and focus on applying strategies.
4. Take a practice test with time constraints, with all guides, "open book."
5. Take a final practice test without open material and with time limits.

If you have time to take more practice tests, just repeat step 5. By gradually exposing yourself to the full rigors of the test environment, you will condition your mind to the stress of test day and maximize your success.

Secret Key #4 - Prepare, Don't Procrastinate

Let me state an obvious fact: if you take the test three times, you will probably get three different scores. This is due to the way you feel on test day, the level of preparedness you have, and the version of the test you see. Despite the test writers' claims to the contrary, some versions of the test WILL be easier for you than others.

Since your future depends so much on your score, you should maximize your chances of success. In order to maximize the likelihood of success, you've got to prepare in advance. This means taking practice tests and spending time learning the information and test taking strategies you will need to succeed.

Never go take the actual test as a "practice" test, expecting that you can just take it again if you need to. Take all the practice tests you can on your own, but when you go to take the official test, be prepared, be focused, and do your best the first time!

Secret Key #5 - Test Yourself

Everyone knows that time is money. There is no need to spend too much of your time or too little of your time preparing for the test. You should only spend as much of your precious time preparing as is necessary for you to get the score you need.

Once you have taken a practice test under real conditions of time constraints, then you will know if you are ready for the test or not.

If you have scored extremely high the first time that you take the practice test, then there is not much point in spending countless hours studying. You are already there.

Benchmark your abilities by retaking practice tests and seeing how much you have improved. Once you consistently score high enough to guarantee success, then you are ready.

If you have scored well below where you need, then knuckle down and begin studying in earnest. Check your improvement regularly through the use of practice tests under real conditions. Above all, don't worry, panic, or give up. The key is perseverance!

Then, when you go to take the test, remain confident and remember how well you did on the practice tests. If you can score high enough on a practice test, then you can do the same on the real thing.

General Strategies

The most important thing you can do is to ignore your fears and jump into the test immediately. Do not be overwhelmed by any strange-sounding terms. You have to jump into the test like jumping into a pool—all at once is the easiest way.

Make Predictions

As you read and understand the question, try to guess what the answer will be. Remember that several of the answer choices are wrong, and once you begin reading them, your mind will immediately become cluttered with answer choices designed to throw you off. Your mind is typically the most focused immediately after you have read the question and digested its contents. If you can, try to predict what the correct answer will be. You may be surprised at what you can predict.

Quickly scan the choices and see if your prediction is in the listed answer choices. If it is, then you can be quite confident that you have the right answer. It still won't hurt to check the other answer choices, but most of the time, you've got it!

Answer the Question

It may seem obvious to only pick answer choices that answer the question, but the test writers can create some excellent answer choices that are wrong. Don't pick an answer just because it sounds right, or you believe it to be true. It MUST answer the question. Once you've made your selection, always go back and check it against the question and make sure that you didn't misread the question and that the answer choice does answer the question posed.

Benchmark

After you read the first answer choice, decide if you think it sounds correct or not. If it doesn't, move on to the next answer choice. If it does, mentally mark that answer choice. This doesn't mean that you've definitely selected it as your answer choice, it just means that it's the best you've seen thus far. Go ahead and read the next choice. If the next choice is worse than the one you've already selected, keep going to the next answer choice. If the next choice is better than the choice you've already selected, mentally mark the new answer choice as your best guess.

The first answer choice that you select becomes your standard. Every other answer choice must be benchmarked against that standard. That choice is correct until proven otherwise by another answer choice beating it out. Once you've decided that no other answer choice seems as good, do one final check to ensure that your answer choice answers the question posed.

Valid Information

Don't discount any of the information provided in the question. Every piece of information may be necessary to determine the correct answer. None of the information in the question is there to throw you off (while the answer choices will certainly have information to throw you off). If two seemingly unrelated topics are discussed, don't ignore either. You can be confident there is a relationship, or it wouldn't be included in the question, and you are probably going to have to determine what is that relationship to find the answer.

Avoid "Fact Traps"

Don't get distracted by a choice that is factually true. Your search is for the answer that answers the question. Stay focused and don't fall for an answer that is true but irrelevant. Always go back to the question and make sure you're choosing an answer that actually answers the question and is not just a true statement. An answer can be factually correct, but it MUST answer the question asked. Additionally, two answers can both be seemingly correct, so be sure to read all of the answer choices, and make sure that you get the one that BEST answers the question.

Milk the Question

Some of the questions may throw you completely off. They might deal with a subject you have not been exposed to, or one that you haven't reviewed in years. While your lack of knowledge about the subject will be a hindrance, the question itself can give you many clues that will help you find the correct answer. Read the question carefully and look for clues. Watch particularly for adjectives and nouns describing difficult terms or words that you don't recognize. Regardless of whether you completely understand a word or not, replacing it with a synonym, either provided or one you more familiar with, may help you to understand what the questions are asking. Rather than wracking your mind about specific detailed information concerning a difficult term or word, try to use mental substitutes that are easier to understand.

The Trap of Familiarity

Don't just choose a word because you recognize it. On difficult questions, you may not recognize a number of words in the answer choices. The test writers don't put "make-believe" words on the test, so don't think that just because you only recognize all the words in one answer choice that that answer choice must be correct. If you only recognize words in one answer choice, then focus on that one. Is it correct? Try your best to determine if it is correct. If it is, that's great. If not, eliminate it. Each word and answer choice you eliminate increases your chances of getting the question correct, even if you then have to guess among the unfamiliar choices.

Eliminate Answers

Eliminate choices as soon as you realize they are wrong. But be careful! Make sure you consider all of the possible answer choices. Just because one appears right, doesn't mean that the next one won't be even better! The test writers will usually put more than one good answer choice for every question, so read all of them. Don't worry if you are stuck between two that seem right. By getting down to just two remaining possible choices, your odds are now 50/50. Rather than wasting too much time, play the odds. You are guessing, but guessing wisely because you've been able to knock out some of the answer choices that you know are wrong. If you are eliminating choices and realize that the last answer choice you are left with is also obviously wrong, don't panic. Start over and consider each choice again. There may easily be something that you missed the first time and will realize on the second pass.

Tough Questions

If you are stumped on a problem or it appears too hard or too difficult, don't waste time. Move on! Remember though, if you can quickly check for obviously incorrect answer choices, your chances of guessing correctly are greatly improved. Before you completely give up, at least try to knock out a couple of possible answers. Eliminate what you can and then guess at the remaining answer choices before moving on.

Brainstorm

If you get stuck on a difficult question, spend a few seconds quickly brainstorming. Run through the complete list of possible answer choices. Look at each choice and ask yourself, "Could this answer the question satisfactorily?" Go through each answer choice and consider it independently of the others. By systematically going through all possibilities, you may find something that you would otherwise overlook. Remember though that when you get stuck, it's important to try to keep moving.

Read Carefully

Understand the problem. Read the question and answer choices carefully. Don't miss the question because you misread the terms. You have plenty of time to read each question thoroughly and make sure you understand what is being asked. Yet a happy medium must be attained, so don't waste too much time. You must read carefully, but efficiently.

Face Value

When in doubt, use common sense. Always accept the situation in the problem at face value. Don't read too much into it. These problems will not require you to make huge leaps of logic. The test writers aren't trying to throw you off with a cheap trick. If you have to go beyond creativity and make a leap of logic in order to have an answer choice answer the question, then you should look at the other answer choices. Don't overcomplicate the problem by creating theoretical relationships or explanations that will warp time or space. These are normal problems rooted in reality. It's just that the applicable relationship or explanation may not be readily apparent and you have to figure things out. Use your common sense to interpret anything that isn't clear.

Prefixes

If you're having trouble with a word in the question or answer choices, try dissecting it. Take advantage of every clue that the word might include. Prefixes and suffixes can be a huge help. Usually they allow you to determine a basic meaning. Pre- means before, post- means after, pro - is positive, de- is negative. From these prefixes and suffixes, you can get an idea of the general meaning of the word and try to put it into context. Beware though of any traps. Just because con- is the opposite of pro-, doesn't necessarily mean congress is the opposite of progress!

Hedge Phrases

Watch out for critical hedge phrases, led off with words such as "likely," "may," "can," "sometimes," "often," "almost," "mostly," "usually," "generally," "rarely," and "sometimes." Question writers insert these hedge phrases to cover every possibility. Often an answer choice will be wrong simply because it leaves no room for exception. Unless the situation calls for them, avoid answer choices that have definitive words like "exactly," and "always."

Switchback Words

Stay alert for "switchbacks." These are the words and phrases frequently used to alert you to shifts in thought. The most common switchback word is "but." Others include "although," "however," "nevertheless," "on the other hand," "even though," "while," "in spite of," "despite," and "regardless of."

New Information

Correct answer choices will rarely have completely new information included. Answer choices typically are straightforward reflections of the material asked about and will directly relate to the question. If a new piece of information is included in an answer choice that doesn't even seem to relate to the topic being asked about, then that answer choice is likely incorrect. All of the information needed to answer the question is usually provided for you in the question. You should not have to make guesses that are unsupported or choose answer choices that require unknown information that cannot be reasoned from what is given.

Time Management

On technical questions, don't get lost on the technical terms. Don't spend too much time on any one question. If you don't know what a term means, then odds are you aren't going to get much further since you don't have a dictionary. You should be able to immediately recognize whether or not you know a term. If you don't, work with the other clues that you have—the other answer choices and terms provided—but don't waste too much time trying to figure out a difficult term that you don't know.

Contextual Clues

Look for contextual clues. An answer can be right but not the correct answer. The contextual clues will help you find the answer that is most right and is correct. Understand the context in which a phrase or statement is made. This will help you make important distinctions.

Don't Panic

Panicking will not answer any questions for you; therefore, it isn't helpful. When you first see the question, if your mind goes blank, take a deep breath. Force yourself to mechanically go through the steps of solving the problem using the strategies you've learned.

Pace Yourself

Don't get clock fever. It's easy to be overwhelmed when you're looking at a page full of questions, your mind is full of random thoughts and feeling confused, and the clock is ticking down faster than you would like. Calm down and maintain the pace that you have set for yourself. As long as you are on track by monitoring your pace, you are guaranteed to have enough time for yourself. When you get to the last few minutes of the test, it may seem like you won't have enough time left, but if you only have as many questions as you should have left at that point, then you're right on track!

Answer Selection

The best way to pick an answer choice is to eliminate all of those that are wrong, until only one is left and confirm that is the correct answer. Sometimes though, an answer choice may immediately look right. Be careful! Take a second to make sure that the other choices are not equally obvious. Don't make a hasty mistake. There are only two times that you should stop before checking other answers. First is when you are positive that the answer choice you have selected is correct. Second is when time is almost out and you have to make a quick guess!

Check Your Work

Since you will probably not know every term listed and the answer to every question, it is important that you get credit for the ones that you do know. Don't miss any questions through careless mistakes. If at all possible, try to take a second to look back over your answer selection and make sure you've selected the correct answer choice and haven't made a costly careless mistake (such as marking an answer choice that you didn't mean to mark). The time it takes for this quick double check should more than pay for itself in caught mistakes.

Beware of Directly Quoted Answers

Sometimes an answer choice will repeat word for word a portion of the question or reference section. However, beware of such exact duplication. It may be a trap! More than likely, the correct choice will paraphrase or summarize a point, rather than being exactly the same wording.

Slang

Scientific sounding answers are better than slang ones. An answer choice that begins "To compare the outcomes..." is much more likely to be correct than one that begins "Because some people insisted..."

Extreme Statements

Avoid wild answers that throw out highly controversial ideas that are proclaimed as established fact. An answer choice that states the "process should used in certain situations, if..." is much more likely to be correct than one that states the "process should be discontinued completely." The first is a calm rational statement and doesn't even make a definitive, uncompromising stance, using a hedge word "if" to provide wiggle room, whereas the second choice is a radical idea and far more extreme.

Answer Choice Families

When you have two or more answer choices that are direct opposites or parallels, one of them is usually the correct answer. For instance, if one answer choice states "x increases" and another answer choice states "x decreases" or "y increases," then those two or three answer choices are very similar in construction and fall into the same family of answer choices. A family of answer choices consists of two or three answer choices, very similar in construction, but often with directly opposite meanings. Usually the correct answer choice will be in that family of answer choices. The "odd man out" or answer choice that doesn't seem to fit the parallel construction of the other answer choices is more likely to be incorrect.

Special Report: How to Overcome Test Anxiety

The very nature of tests caters to some level of anxiety, nervousness, or tension, just as we feel for any important event that occurs in our lives. A little bit of anxiety or nervousness can be a good thing. It helps us with motivation, and makes achievement just that much sweeter. However, too much anxiety can be a problem, especially if it hinders our ability to function and perform.

"Test anxiety," is the term that refers to the emotional reactions that some test-takers experience when faced with a test or exam. Having a fear of testing and exams is based upon a rational fear, since the test-taker's performance can shape the course of an academic career. Nevertheless, experiencing excessive fear of examinations will only interfere with the test-taker's ability to perform and chance to be successful.

There are a large variety of causes that can contribute to the development and sensation of test anxiety. These include, but are not limited to, lack of preparation and worrying about issues surrounding the test.

Lack of Preparation

Lack of preparation can be identified by the following behaviors or situations:

Not scheduling enough time to study, and therefore cramming the night before the test or exam
Managing time poorly, to create the sensation that there is not enough time to do everything
Failing to organize the text information in advance, so that the study material consists of the entire text and not simply the pertinent information
Poor overall studying habits

Worrying, on the other hand, can be related to both the test taker, or many other factors around him/her that will be affected by the results of the test. These include worrying about:

Previous performances on similar exams, or exams in general
How friends and other students are achieving
The negative consequences that will result from a poor grade or failure

There are three primary elements to test anxiety. Physical components, which involve the same typical bodily reactions as those to acute anxiety (to be discussed below). Emotional factors have to do with fear or panic. Mental or cognitive issues concerning attention spans and memory abilities.

Physical Signals

There are many different symptoms of test anxiety, and these are not limited to mental and emotional strain. Frequently there are a range of physical signals that will let a test taker know that he/she is suffering from test anxiety. These bodily changes can include the following:

Perspiring
Sweaty palms
Wet, trembling hands
Nausea
Dry mouth
A knot in the stomach
Headache
Faintness
Muscle tension
Aching shoulders, back and neck
Rapid heart beat
Feeling too hot/cold

To recognize the sensation of test anxiety, a test-taker should monitor him/herself for the following sensations:

The physical distress symptoms as listed above
Emotional sensitivity, expressing emotional feelings such as the need to cry or laugh too much, or a sensation of anger or helplessness
A decreased ability to think, causing the test-taker to blank out or have racing thoughts that are hard to organize or control.

Though most students will feel some level of anxiety when faced with a test or exam, the majority can cope with that anxiety and maintain it at a manageable level. However, those who cannot are faced with a very real and very serious condition, which can and should be controlled for the immeasurable benefit of this sufferer.

Naturally, these sensations lead to negative results for the testing experience. The most common effects of test anxiety have to do with nervousness and mental blocking.

Nervousness

Nervousness can appear in several different levels:

The test-taker's difficulty, or even inability to read and understand the questions on the test
The difficulty or inability to organize thoughts to a coherent form
The difficulty or inability to recall key words and concepts relating to the testing questions (especially essays)
The receipt of poor grades on a test, though the test material was well known by the test taker

Conversely, a person may also experience mental blocking, which involves:

Blanking out on test questions
Only remembering the correct answers to the questions when the test has already finished.

Fortunately for test anxiety sufferers, beating these feelings, to a large degree, has to do with proper preparation. When a test taker has a feeling of preparedness, then anxiety will be dramatically lessened.

The first step to resolving anxiety issues is to distinguish which of the two types of anxiety are being suffered. If the anxiety is a direct result of a lack of preparation, this should be considered a normal reaction, and the anxiety level (as opposed to the test results) shouldn't be anything to worry about. However, if, when adequately prepared, the test-taker still panics, blanks out, or seems to overreact, this is not a fully rational reaction. While this can be considered normal too, there are many ways to combat and overcome these effects.

Remember that anxiety cannot be entirely eliminated, however, there are ways to minimize it, to make the anxiety easier to manage. Preparation is one of the best ways to minimize test anxiety. Therefore the following techniques are wise in order to best fight off any anxiety that may want to build.

To begin with, try to avoid cramming before a test, whenever it is possible. By trying to memorize an entire term's worth of information in one day, you'll be shocking your system, and not giving yourself a very good chance to absorb the information. This is an easy path to anxiety, so for those who suffer from test anxiety, cramming should not even be considered an option.

Instead of cramming, work throughout the semester to combine all of the material which is presented throughout the semester, and work on it gradually as the course goes by, making sure to master the main concepts first, leaving minor details for a week or so before the test.

To study for the upcoming exam, be sure to pose questions that may be on the examination, to gauge the ability to answer them by integrating the ideas from your texts, notes and lectures, as well as any supplementary readings.

If it is truly impossible to cover all of the information that was covered in that particular term, concentrate on the most important portions, that can be covered very well. Learn these concepts as best as possible, so that when the test comes, a goal can be made to use these concepts as presentations of your knowledge.

In addition to study habits, changes in attitude are critical to beating a struggle with test anxiety. In fact, an improvement of the perspective over the entire test-taking experience can actually help a test taker to enjoy studying and therefore improve the overall experience. Be certain not to overemphasize the significance of the grade - know that the result of the test is neither a reflection of self worth, nor is it a measure of intelligence; one grade will not predict a person's future success.

To improve an overall testing outlook, the following steps should be tried:

Keeping in mind that the most reasonable expectation for taking a test is to expect to try to demonstrate as much of what you know as you possibly can.
Reminding ourselves that a test is only one test; this is not the only one, and there will be others.
The thought of thinking of oneself in an irrational, all-or-nothing term should be avoided at all costs.
A reward should be designated for after the test, so there's something to look forward to. Whether it be going to a movie, going out to eat, or simply visiting friends, schedule it in advance, and do it no matter what result is expected on the exam.

Test-takers should also keep in mind that the basics are some of the most important things, even beyond anti-anxiety techniques and studying. Never neglect the basic social, emotional and biological needs, in order to try to absorb information. In order to best achieve, these three factors must be held as just as important as the studying itself.

Study Steps

Remember the following important steps for studying:

Maintain healthy nutrition and exercise habits. Continue both your recreational activities and social pass times. These both contribute to your physical and emotional well being.
Be certain to get a good amount of sleep, especially the night before the test, because when you're overtired you are not able to perform to the best of your best ability.
Keep the studying pace to a moderate level by taking breaks when they are needed, and varying the work whenever possible, to keep the mind fresh instead of getting bored.
When enough studying has been done that all the material that can be learned has been learned, and the test taker is prepared for the test, stop studying and do something relaxing such as listening to music, watching a movie, or taking a warm bubble bath.

There are also many other techniques to minimize the uneasiness or apprehension that is experienced along with test anxiety before, during, or even after the examination. In fact, there are a great deal of things that can be done to stop anxiety from interfering with lifestyle and performance. Again, remember that anxiety will not be eliminated entirely, and it shouldn't be. Otherwise that "up" feeling for exams would not exist, and most of us depend on that sensation to perform better than usual. However, this anxiety has to be at a level that is manageable.

Of course, as we have just discussed, being prepared for the exam is half the battle right away. Attending all classes, finding out what knowledge will be expected on the exam, and knowing the exam schedules are easy steps to lowering anxiety. Keeping up with work will remove the need to cram, and efficient study habits will eliminate wasted time. Studying should be done in an ideal location for concentration, so that it is simple to become interested in the material and give it complete attention. A method such as SQ3R (Survey, Question, Read, Recite, Review) is a wonderful key to follow to make sure that the study habits are as effective as possible, especially in the case of learning from a textbook. Flashcards are great techniques for memorization. Learning to take good notes will mean that notes will be full of useful information, so that less sifting will need to be done to seek out what is pertinent for studying. Reviewing notes after class and then again on occasion will keep the information fresh in the mind. From notes that have been taken summary sheets and outlines can be made for simpler reviewing.

A study group can also be a very motivational and helpful place to study, as there will be a sharing of ideas, all of the minds can work together, to make sure that everyone understands, and the studying will be made more interesting because it will be a social occasion.

Basically, though, as long as the test-taker remains organized and self confident, with efficient study habits, less time will need to be spent studying, and higher grades will be achieved.

To become self confident, there are many useful steps. The first of these is "self talk." It has been shown through extensive research, that self-talk for students who suffer from test anxiety, should be well monitored, in order to make sure that it contributes to self confidence as opposed to sinking the student. Frequently the self talk of test-anxious students is negative or self-defeating, thinking that everyone else is smarter and faster, that they always mess up, and that if they don't do well, they'll fail the entire course. It is important to decreasing anxiety that awareness is made of self talk. Try writing any negative self thoughts and then disputing them with a positive statement instead. Begin self-encouragement as though it was a friend speaking. Repeat positive statements to help reprogram the mind to believing in successes instead of failures.

Helpful Techniques

Other extremely helpful techniques include:

Self-visualization of doing well and reaching goals
While aiming for an "A" level of understanding, don't try to "overprotect" by setting your expectations lower. This will only convince the mind to stop studying in order to meet the lower expectations.
Don't make comparisons with the results or habits of other students. These are individual factors, and different things work for different people, causing different results.
Strive to become an expert in learning what works well, and what can be done in order to improve. Consider collecting this data in a journal.
Create rewards for after studying instead of doing things before studying that will only turn into avoidance behaviors.
Make a practice of relaxing - by using methods such as progressive relaxation, self-hypnosis, guided imagery, etc - in order to make relaxation an automatic sensation.
Work on creating a state of relaxed concentration so that concentrating will take on the focus of the mind, so that none will be wasted on worrying.
Take good care of the physical self by eating well and getting enough sleep.
Plan in time for exercise and stick to this plan.

Beyond these techniques, there are other methods to be used before, during and after the test that will help the test-taker perform well in addition to overcoming anxiety.

Before the exam comes the academic preparation. This involves establishing a study schedule and beginning at least one week before the actual date of the test. By doing this, the anxiety of not having enough time to study for the test will be automatically eliminated. Moreover, this will make the studying a much more effective experience, ensuring that the learning will be an easier process. This relieves much undue pressure on the test-taker.

Summary sheets, note cards, and flash cards with the main concepts and examples of these main concepts should be prepared in advance of the actual studying time. A topic should never be eliminated from this process. By omitting a topic because it isn't expected to be on the test is only setting up the test-taker for anxiety should it actually appear on the exam. Utilize the course syllabus for laying out the topics that should be studied. Carefully go over the notes that were made in class, paying special attention to any of the issues that the professor took special care to emphasize while lecturing in class. In the textbooks, use the chapter review, or if possible, the chapter tests, to begin your review.

It may even be possible to ask the instructor what information will be covered on the exam, or what the format of the exam will be (for example, multiple choice, essay, free form, true-false). Additionally, see if it is possible to find out how many questions will be on the test. If a review sheet or sample test has been offered by the professor, make good use of it, above anything else, for the preparation for the test. Another great resource for getting to know the examination is reviewing tests from previous semesters. Use these tests to review, and aim to achieve a 100% score on each of the possible topics. With a few exceptions, the goal that you set for yourself is the highest one that you will reach.

Take all of the questions that were assigned as homework, and rework them to any other possible course material. The more problems reworked, the more skill and confidence will form as a result. When forming the solution to a problem, write out each of the steps. Don't simply do head work. By doing as many steps on paper as possible, much clarification and therefore confidence will be formed. Do this with as many homework problems as possible, before checking the answers. By checking the answer after each problem, a reinforcement will exist, that will not be on the exam. Study situations should be as exam-like as possible, to prime the test-taker's system for the experience. By waiting to check the answers at the end, a psychological advantage will be formed, to decrease the stress factor.

Another fantastic reason for not cramming is the avoidance of confusion in concepts, especially when it comes to mathematics. 8-10 hours of study will become one hundred percent more effective if it is spread out over a week or at least several days, instead of doing it all in one sitting. Recognize that the human brain requires time in order to assimilate new material, so frequent breaks and a span of study time over several days will be much more beneficial.

Additionally, don't study right up until the point of the exam. Studying should stop a minimum of one hour before the exam begins. This allows the brain to rest and put things in their proper order. This will also provide the time to become as relaxed as possible when going into the examination room. The test-taker will also have time to eat well and eat sensibly. Know that the brain needs food as much as the rest of the body. With enough food and enough sleep, as well as a relaxed attitude, the body and the mind are primed for success.

Avoid any anxious classmates who are talking about the exam. These students only spread anxiety, and are not worth sharing the anxious sentimentalities.

Before the test also involves creating a positive attitude, so mental preparation should also be a point of concentration. There are many keys to creating a positive attitude. Should fears become rushing in, make a visualization of taking the exam, doing well, and seeing an A written on the paper. Write out a list of affirmations that will bring a feeling of confidence, such as "I am doing well in my English class," "I studied well and know my material," "I enjoy this class." Even if the affirmations aren't believed at first, it sends a positive message to the subconscious which will result in an alteration of the overall belief system, which is the system that creates reality.

If a sensation of panic begins, work with the fear and imagine the very worst! Work through the entire scenario of not passing the test, failing the entire course, and dropping out of school, followed by not getting a job, and pushing a shopping cart through the dark alley where you'll live. This will place things into perspective! Then, practice deep breathing and create a visualization of the opposite situation - achieving an "A" on the exam, passing the entire course, receiving the degree at a graduation ceremony.

On the day of the test, there are many things to be done to ensure the best results, as well as the most calm outlook. The following stages are suggested in order to maximize test-taking potential:

Begin the examination day with a moderate breakfast, and avoid any coffee or beverages with caffeine if the test taker is prone to jitters. Even people who are used to managing caffeine can feel jittery or light-headed when it is taken on a test day.
Attempt to do something that is relaxing before the examination begins. As last minute cramming clouds the mastering of overall concepts, it is better to use this time to create a calming outlook.
Be certain to arrive at the test location well in advance, in order to provide time to select a location that is away from doors, windows and other distractions, as well as giving enough time to relax before the test begins.
Keep away from anxiety generating classmates who will upset the sensation of stability and relaxation that is being attempted before the exam.
Should the waiting period before the exam begins cause anxiety, create a self-distraction by reading a light magazine or something else that is relaxing and simple.

During the exam itself, read the entire exam from beginning to end, and find out how much time should be allotted to each individual problem. Once writing the exam, should more time be taken for a problem, it should be abandoned, in order to begin another problem. If there is time at the end, the unfinished problem can always be returned to and completed.

Read the instructions very carefully - twice - so that unpleasant surprises won't follow during or after the exam has ended.

When writing the exam, pretend that the situation is actually simply the completion of homework within a library, or at home. This will assist in forming a relaxed atmosphere, and will allow the brain extra focus for the complex thinking function.

Begin the exam with all of the questions with which the most confidence is felt. This will build the confidence level regarding the entire exam and will begin a quality momentum. This will also create encouragement for trying the problems where uncertainty resides.

Going with the "gut instinct" is always the way to go when solving a problem. Second guessing should be avoided at all costs. Have confidence in the ability to do well.

For essay questions, create an outline in advance that will keep the mind organized and make certain that all of the points are remembered. For multiple choice, read every answer, even if the correct one has been spotted - a better one may exist.

Continue at a pace that is reasonable and not rushed, in order to be able to work carefully. Provide enough time to go over the answers at the end, to check for small errors that can be corrected.

Should a feeling of panic begin, breathe deeply, and think of the feeling of the body releasing sand through its pores. Visualize a calm, peaceful place, and include all of the sights, sounds and sensations of this image. Continue the deep breathing, and take a few minutes to continue this with closed eyes. When all is well again, return to the test.

If a "blanking" occurs for a certain question, skip it and move on to the next question. There will be time to return to the other question later. Get everything done that can be done, first, to guarantee all the grades that can be compiled, and to build all of the confidence possible. Then return to the weaker questions to build the marks from there.

Remember, one's own reality can be created, so as long as the belief is there, success will follow. And remember: anxiety can happen later, right now, there's an exam to be written!

After the examination is complete, whether there is a feeling for a good grade or a bad grade, don't dwell on the exam, and be certain to follow through on the reward that was promised...and enjoy it! Don't dwell on any mistakes that have been made, as there is nothing that can be done at this point anyway.

Additionally, don't begin to study for the next test right away. Do something relaxing for a while, and let the mind relax and prepare itself to begin absorbing information again.

From the results of the exam - both the grade and the entire experience, be certain to learn from what has gone on. Perfect studying habits and work some more on confidence in order to make the next examination experience even better than the last one.

Learn to avoid places where openings occurred for laziness, procrastination and day dreaming.

Use the time between this exam and the next one to better learn to relax, even learning to relax on cue, so that any anxiety can be controlled during the next exam. Learn how to relax the body. Slouch in your chair if that helps. Tighten and then relax all of the different muscle groups, one group at a time, beginning with the feet and then working all the way up to the neck and face. This will ultimately relax the muscles more than they were to begin with. Learn how to breathe deeply and comfortably, and focus on this breathing going in and out as a relaxing thought. With every exhale, repeat the word "relax."

As common as test anxiety is, it is very possible to overcome it. Make yourself one of the test-takers who overcome this frustrating hindrance.

Special Report: Additional Bonus Material

Due to our efforts to try to keep this book to a manageable length, we've created a link that will give you access to all of your additional bonus material.

Please visit http://www.mometrix.com/bonus948/nclexrn to access the information.